MYELODYSPLASTIC SYNDROMES

Edited by **Ota Fuchs**

Myelodysplastic Syndromes
http://dx.doi.org/10.5772/61879
Edited by Ota Fuchs

Contributors

Albert Breier, Khalid Al-Anazi, Andreas Himmelmann, Argiris Symeonidis, Alexandra Kouraklis-Symeonidis, Lale Olcay, Ota Fuchs

Published by InTech

Janeza Trdine 9, 51000 Rijeka, Croatia

Publishing Process Manager Andrea Koric

Technical Editor SPi Global

Cover InTech Design team

First published August, 2016

Printed in Croatia

Additional hard copies can be obtained from orders@intechopen.com

Myelodysplastic Syndromes, Edited by Ota Fuchs

p. cm.

Print ISBN 978-953-51-2586-0
Online ISBN 978-953-51-2587-7

INTECH

open science | open minds

Contents

Preface

Despite efforts in studies of the biology of myelodysplastic syndromes (MDS), a diagnosis of MDS in individual patient relies mainly on morphological and cytogenetic examinations of the bone marrow and blood. Genomic instability, gene mutations, deregulated gene expression, and epigenetic changes play the key role in the pathogenesis of MDS. High-throughput genetic technologies such as single nucleotide polymorphism and comparative genomic hybridization and next-generation sequencing helped in performing mutation profiling but are preferentially used in clinical trials and not in routine laboratories. These laboratories are limited by the cost-effective care and interpretation barriers, and they do not currently use mutational profiling for diagnosis of MDS. Many mutations are not specific for MDS, and they also occur in other myeloid malignancies. Besides somatic mutations, cytokine aberrations, immune dysregulation, alterations in the bone marrow microenvironment (niche), abnormal RNA splicing, and changes in telomers and signal pathways are involved in the MDS pathogenesis.

This book provides a concise review of advances in myelodysplastic syndromes and will be useful not only to the researchers and clinicians involved in this topic but also to medical students. Introduction chapter is a brief review of current knowledge of MDS prognostication, pathogenesis, and therapy. Chapter 2 discusses disorders mimicking MDS and difficulties in MDS diagnosis. Chapter 3 analyzes the role of inflammation and immune suppression in the pathogenesis of MDS. The application of immunosuppressive treatment may relieve the autoimmune manifestations but also improves hematopoiesis. Chapter 4 focuses on the 5q- syndrome first described by Van den Berghe et al. in 1974. Patients with 5q- syndrome have refractory anemia with del(5q) as the sole karyotypic abnormality and medullary blast count of less than 5 %. The del(5q) occurs in approximately 10–20 % of patients with de novo MDS. Pathogenesis of the 5q- syndrome has been intensively studied in last years, and immunomodulatory or cereblon-binding drug lenalidomide is used for the treatment of transfusion-dependent anemia in these lower-risk del(5q) MDS patients. MDS cases with del(5q) and additional karyotypic abnormalities and secondary MDS cases with del(5q) have a poor prognosis in contrast to the good prognosis of the 5q- syndrome. Chapters 5 and 6 review higher-risk MDS, monosomy 7, and chronic myelomonocytic leukemia, treated by hypomethylating agents (azacitidine and decitabine). Allogeneic stem cell transplantation is the only treatment option with curative potential for higher-risk MDS patients but is limited by age of patients. Resistance to chemotherapy is a serious obstacle to the successful treatment. This important topic is discussed in an overview in Chapter 7.

Each chapter is written by scientists and clinicians with specific expertise in the field.

Ota Fuchs, PhD
Institute of Hematology and Blood Transfusion
Department of Genomics
Prague, Czech Republic

Chapter 1

Introductory Chapter: Myelodysplastic Syndromes

Ota Fuchs

Additional information is available at the end of the chapter

http://dx.doi.org/10.5772/64729

Myelodysplastic syndromes (MDS) are a heterogeneous group of clonal hematopoietic stem cell disorders characterized by ineffective hematopoiesis, peripheral cytopenias, frequent karyotypic abnormalities, and risk of transformation to acute myeloid leukemia (AML) [1–5]. MDS are rare in young people, and median age of patients with MDS is approximately 70 years [6, 7]. Current management in MDS includes supportive care, drug therapy, and allogeneic stem cell transplantation. MDS patients older than age 70 years are not good candidates for allogeneic stem cell transplantation [8, 9]. The major complication of MDS patients after allogeneic stem cell transplantation with reduced intensity conditioning is relapse of malignant disease. Relapse can be predicted by monitoring of Wilms' tumor 1 (WT1) gene expression by real-time PCR and $CD34^+$ donor chimerism analysis [10].

Single-nucleotide polymorphism array (SNP-A) analysis, standard metaphase cytogenetics, and rapid progress in flow cytometric analysis, genes mutation analysis, and gene expression profiling have identified key deregulated genes and signaling pathways important for accurate prognostication and risk stratification for individual patients with MDS [11–18]. The initial French–British–American (FAB) classification system of MDS was published in 1982 [19] and was later refined to the International Prognostic Scoring System (IPSS) [20] and to World Health Organization (WHO) Prognostic Scoring System (WPSS) [21, 22]. The new revised IPSS (IPSS-R) integrated marrow cytogenetic subset, marrow blast percentage, and depth of cytopenias (hemoglobin, platelet, and absolute neutrophil count) and was published in 2012 [23]. Validation of WPSS for MDS and comparison with IPSS-R has been recently described [24]. Two other prognostic systems for MDS subgroups (M.D. Anderson lower risk MDS prognostic scoring system; chronic myelomonocytic leukemia /CMML/ prognostic scoring system) exist [18, 25].

In lower risk MDS, treatment focuses on amelioration of consequences of cytopenias and transfusions and improving of quality of life. The first line of therapy of lower risk MDS with normal chromosome 5 is treatment with erythropoiesis-stimulating agents (erythropoietin) with or without of granulocyte colony-stimulating factor [26]. Transfusion-dependent lower risk MDS patients with del(5q) are treated with immunomodulatory or cereblon-binding drug lenalidomide [27]. Thrombocytopenia occurring sometimes in combination with anemia or without anemia can be treated with romiplostin (thrombopoietin agonist) [27]. Neutropenia is treated with growth factors (G-CSF and GM-CSF) [27]. Higher-risk MDS if untreated have median survival only about 12 months. Two hypomethylating agents (azacitidine and decitabine) inhibit DNA methyltransferases 3A and 3B and reverse the aberrant methylation involved in MDS progression to AML. The development of novel therapeutic strategies in MDS is dependent on recent advances in the molecular pathogenesis of MDS [6, 16, 28–39]. Various combination therapies in MDS are also intensively studied [27, 40, 41].

Author details

Ota Fuchs*

Address all correspondence to: Ota.Fuchs@uhkt.cz

Institute of Hematology and Blood Transfusion, Prague, Czech Republic

References

[1] Nimer SD. Myelodysplastic syndromes. Blood. 2008; 111: 4841–4851. doi:10.1182/blood-2007-08-078139.

[2] Tefferi A, Vardiman JW. Myelodysplastic syndromes. N Engl J Med. 2009; 361: 1872–1885. doi:10.1056/NEJMra0902908.

[3] Adès L, Itzkson R, Fenaux P. Myelodysplastic syndromes. Lancet. 2014; 383: 2239–2252. doi:10.1016/S0140-6736(13)61901-7.

[4] Bejar R, Steensma DP. Recent developments in myelodysplastic syndromes. Blood. 2014; 124: 2793–2803. doi:10.1182/blood-2014-04-522136.

[5] Pellagatti A, Boultwood J. The molecular pathogenesis of the myelodysplastic syndromes. Eur J Haematol. 2015; 95: 3–15. doi:10.1111/ejh.12515.

[6] Zahr AA, Ramirez CB, Wozney J, Prebet T, Zeidan AM. New insights into the pathogenesis of MDS and the rational therapeutic opportunities. Expert Rev Hematol 2016; 9: 377–388. doi:10.1586/17474086.2016.1135047.

[7] Rollison DE, Howlader N, Smith MT, Strom SS, Merritt WD, Ries LA, Edwards BK, List AF Epidemiology of myelodysplastic syndromes and chronic myeloproliferative disorders in the United States, 2001–2004, using data from the NAACCR and SEER-programs. Blood. 2008; 112: 45–52. doi:10.1182/blood-2008-01-134858.

[8] Tamari R, Castro-Malaspina H. Transplant for MDS: challenges and emerging strategies. Best Pract Res Clin Haematol. 2015; 28: 43–54. doi:10.1016/j.beha.2014.11.006

[9] Brierley CK, Steensma DP. Allogeneic stem cell transplantation in myelodysplastic syndromes: does pretransplant clonal burden matter? Curr Opin Hematol. 2016; 23: 167–174. doi:10.1097/MOH.0000000000000217.

[10] Lange T, Hubmann M, Burkhardt R, Franke GN, Cross M, Scholz M, Leiblein S, Al-Ali HK, Edelmann J, Thiery J, Niederwieser D. Monitoring of WT1 expression in PB and CD34(+) donor chimerism of BM predicts early relapse in AML and MDS patients after hematopoietic cell transplantation with reduced-intensity conditioning. Leukemia. 2011; 25: 498–505. doi:10.1038/leu.2010.283.

[11] Tiu RV, Visconte V, Traina F, Schwandt A, Maciejewski JP. Updates in cytogenetics and molecular markers in MDS. Curr Hematol Malig Rep. 2011; 6: 126–135. doi:10.1007/s11899-011-0081-2.

[12] Otrock ZK, Tiu RV, Maciejewski JP, Sekeres MA. The need for additional genetic markers for myelodysplastic syndrome stratification: what does the future hold for prognostication? Expert Rev Hematol. 2013; 6: 59–68. doi:10.1586/ehm.12.67.

[13] Bejar R. Clinical and genetic predictors of prognosis in myelodysplastic syndromes. Haematologica. 2014; 99: 956–964. doi:10.3324/haematol.2013. 085217.

[14] Pellagatti A, Boultwood J. The molecular pathogenesis of the myelodysplastic syndromes. Eur J Haematol. 2015; 95: 3–15. doi:10.1111/ ejh.12515.

[15] Gerstung M, Pellagatti A, Malcovati L, Giagounidis A, Porta MG, Jädersten M, Dolatshad H, Verma A, Cross NC, Vyas P, Killick S, Hellström-Lindberg E, Cazzola M, Papaemmanuil E, Campbell PJ, Boultwood J. Combining gene mutation with gene expression data improves outcome prediction in myelodysplastic syndromes. Nat Commun. 2015; 6: 5901. doi:10.1038/ ncomms6901.

[16] Zahid MF, Patnaik MS, Gangat N, Hashmi SK, Rizzieri DA. Insight into the molecular pathophysiology of myelodysplastic syndromes: targets for novel therapy. Eur J Haematol. 2016; doi:10.1111/ejh.12771. [Epub ahead of print].

[17] Alhan C, Westers TM, Cremers EM, Cali C, Witte BI, Ossenkoppele GJ, van de Loosdrecht AA. The myelodysplastic syndromes flow cytometric score: a three-parameter prognostic flow cytometric scoring system. Leukemia. 2016; 30: 658–665. doi:10.1038/leu.2015.295.

[18] Jonas BA, Greenberg PL. MDS prognostic scoring systems – past, present, and future. Best Pract Res Clin Haematol. 2015; 28: 3–13. doi:10.1016/ j.beha.2014.11.001.

[19] Bennett JM, Catovsky D, Daniel MT, Flandrin G, Galton DA, Gralnick HR, Sultan C. Proposals for the classification of the myelodysplastic syndromes. Br J Haematol. 1982; 51:189–199.

[20] Greenberg P, Cox C, LeBeau MM, Fenaux P, Morel P, Sanz G, Sanz M, Vallespi T, Hamblin T, Oscier D, Ohyashiki K, Toyama K, Aul C, Mufti G, Bennett J. International scoring system for evaluating prognosis in myelodysplastic syndromes. Blood. 1997; 89: 2079–2088.

[21] Malcovati L, Porta MG, Pascutto C, Invernizzi R, Boni M, Travaglino E, Passamonti F, Arcaini L, Maffioli M, Bernasconi P, Lazzarino M, Cazzola M. Prognostic factors and life expectancy in myelodysplastic syndromes classified according to WHO criteria: a basis for clinical decision making. J Clin Oncol. 2005; 23: 7594–7603. doi:10.1200/JCO. 2005.01.7038.

[22] Malcovati L, Germing U, Kuendgen A, Della Porta MG, Pascutto C, Invernizzi R, Giagounidis A, Hildebrandt B, Bernasconi P, Knipp S, Strupp C, Lazzarino M, Aul C, Cazzola M. Time-dependent prognostic scoring system for predicting survival and leukemic evolution in myelodysplastic syndromes. J Clin Oncol. 2007; 25: 3503–3510. doi:10.1200/JCO. 2006.08. 5696.

[23] Greenberg PL, Tuechler H, Schanz J, Sanz G, Garcia-Manero G, Solé F, Bennett JM, Bowen D, Fenaux P, Dreyfus F, Kantarjian H, Kuendgen A, Levis A, Malcovati L, Cazzola M, Cermak J, Fonatsch C, Le Beau MM, Slovak ML, Krieger O, Luebbert M, Maciejewski J, Magalhaes SM, Miyazaki Y, Pfeilstöcker M, Sekeres M, Sperr WR, Stauder R, Tauro S, Valent P, Vallespi T, van de Loosdrecht AA, Germing U, Haase D. Revised international prognostic scoring system for myelodysplastic syndromes. Blood. 2012; 120: 2454–2465. doi:10.1182/blood-2012-03-420489.

[24] Della Porta MG, Tuechler H, Malcovati L, Schanz J, Sanz G, Garcia-Manero G, Solé F, Bennett JM, Bowen D, Fenaux P, Dreyfus F, Kantarjian H, Kuendgen A, Levis A, Cermak J, Fonatsch C, Le Beau MM, Slovak ML, Krieger O, Luebbert M, Maciejewski J, Magalhaes SM, Miyazaki Y, Pfeilstöcker M, Sekeres MA, Sperr WR, Stauder R, Tauro S, Valent P, Vallespi T, van de Loosdrecht AA, Germing U, Haase D, Greenberg PL, Cazzola M. Validation of WHO classification-based Prognostic Scoring System (WPSS) for myelodysplastic syndromes and comparison with the revised International Prognostic Scoring System (IPSS-R). A study of the International Working Group for Prognosis in Myelodysplasia (IWG-PM). Leukemia. 2015; 29: 1502–1513. doi:10.1038/leu.2015.55.

[25] Zeidan AM, Sekeres MA, Wang XF, Al Ali N, Garcia-Manero G, Steensma DP, Roboz G, Barnard J, Padron E, DeZern A, Maciejewski JP, List AF, Komrokji RS. MDS Clinical research consortium. Comparing the prognostic value of risk stratifying models for patients with lower-risk myelodysplastic syndromes: Is one model better? Am J Hematol. 2015; 90: 1036–1040. doi:10.1002/ajh.24173.

[26] Greenberg PL, Sun Z, Miller KB, Bennett JM, Tallman MS, Dewald G, Paietta E, van der Jagt R, Houston J, Thomas ML, Cella D, Rowe JM. Treatment of myelodysplastic syndrome patients with erythropoietin with or without granulocyte colony-stimulating factor: results of a prospective randomized phase 3 trial by the Eastern Cooperative

Oncology Group (E1996). Blood. 2009; 114: 2393–2400. doi:10.1182/blood-2009-03-211797.

[27] Ornstein MC, Mukherjee S, Sekeres MA. More is better: combination therapies for myelodysplastic syndromes. Best Pract Res Clin Haematol. 2015; 28: 22–31. doi:10.1016/j.beha.2014.11.002.

[28] Bejar R, Steensma DP. Recent developments in myelodysplastic syndromes. Blood. 2014; 124: 2793–2803. doi:10.1182/blood-2014-04-522136.

[29] Loiseau C, Ali A, Itzykson R. New therapeutic approaches in myelodysplastic syndromes: hypomethylating agents and lenalidomide. Exp Hematol. 2015; 43: 661–672. doi:10.1016/j.exphem.2015.05.014.

[30] List A. New therapeutics for myelodysplastic syndromes. Leuk Res. 2012; 36: 1470–1474. doi: 10.1016/j.leukres.2012.08.010.

[31] Carrancio S, Markovics J, Wong P, Leisten J, Castiglioni P, Groza MC, Raymon HK, Heise C, Daniel T, Chopra R, Sung V. An activin receptor IIA ligand trap promotes erythropoiesis resulting in a rapid induction of red blood cells and haemoglobin. Br J Haematol. 2014; 165: 870–882. doi:10.1111/ bjh.12838.

[32] Thepot S, Boehrer S, Seegers V, Prebet T, Beyne-Rauzy O, Wattel E, Delaunay J, Raffoux E, Hunault M, Jourdan E, Chermat F, Sebert M, Kroemer G, Fenaux P, Adès L; Groupe Francophone des Myelodysplasies (GFM). A phase I/II trial of Erlotinib in higher risk myelodysplastic syndromes and acute myeloid leukemia after azacitidine failure. Leuk Res. 2014; 38: 1430–1434. doi:10.1016/ j.leukres. 2014.09.014.

[33] Platzbecker U, Wong RS, Verma A, Abboud C, Araujo S, Chiou TJ, Feigert J, Yeh SP, Götze K, Gorin NC, Greenberg P, Kambhampati S, Kim YJ, Lee JH, Lyons R, Ruggeri M, Santini V, Cheng G, Jang JH, Chen CY, Johnson B, Bennett J, Mannino F, Kamel YM, Stone N, Dougherty S, Chan G, Giagounidis A. Safety and tolerability of eltrombopag versus placebo for treatment of thrombocytopenia in patients with advanced myelodysplastic syndromes or acute myeloid leukaemia: a multicentre, randomised, placebo-controlled, double-blind, phase 1/2 trial. Lancet Haematol. 2015; 2: e417–e426. doi: 10.1016/S2352-3026(15)00149-0.

[34] Santini V. Life after hypomethylating agents in myelodysplastic syndrome: new strategies. Curr Opin Hematol. 2015; 22: 155–162. doi:10.1097/MOH.0000000000000117.

[35] Santini V, Fenaux P. Treatment of myelodysplastic syndrome with thrombomimetic drugs. Semin Hematol. 2015; 52: 38–45. doi:10.1053/j.seminhematol. 2014.10. 005.

[36] Borthakur G, Popplewell L, Boyiadzis M, Foran J, Platzbecker U, Vey N, Walter RB, Olin R, Raza A, Giagounidis A, Al-Kali A, Jabbour E, Kadia T, Garcia-Manero G, Bauman JW, Wu Y, Liu Y, Schramek D, Cox DS, Wissel P, Kantarjian H. Activity of the oral mitogen-activated protein kinase kinase inhibitor trametinib in RAS-mutant

relapsed or refractory myeloid malignancies. Cancer. 2016; 122: 1871–1879. doi:10.1002/cncr.29986.

[37] Garcia-Manero G, Fenaux P, Al-Kali A, Baer MR, Sekeres MA, Roboz GJ, Gaidano G, Scott BL, Greenberg P, Platzbecker U, Steensma DP, Kambhampati S, Kreuzer KA, Godley LA, Atallah E, Collins R Jr, Kantarjian H, Jabbour E, Wilhelm FE, Azarnia N, Silverman LR. ONTIME study investigators. Rigosertib versus best supportive care for patients with high-risk myelodysplastic syndromes after failure of hypomethylating drugs (ONTIME): a randomised, controlled, phase 3 trial. Lancet Oncol. 2016; 17: 496–508. doi:10.1016/S1470-2045(16)00009-7.

[38] Komrokji RS. Searching for a light at the end of the tunnel? Beyond hypomethylating agents in myelodysplastic syndromes. Am Soc Clin Oncol Educ Book. 2016; 35: e345–e352. doi:10.14694/EDBK_161221.

[39] Mies A, Bulycheva E, Rogulj IM, Hofbauer LC, Platzbecker U. Alterations within the Osteo-Hematopoietic Niche in MDS and their Therapeutic Implications. Curr Pharm Des. 2016; 22: 2323–2332.

[40] Issa JP, Garcia-Manero G, Huang X, Cortes J, Ravandi F, Jabbour E, Borthakur G, Brandt M, Pierce S, Kantarjian HM. Results of phase 2 randomized study of low-dose decitabine with or without valproic acid in patients with myelodysplastic syndrome and acute myelogenous leukemia. Cancer. 2015; 121: 556–561. doi:10.1002/cncr.29085.

[41] DiNardo CD, Daver N, Jabbour E, Kadia T, Borthakur G, Konopleva M, Pemmaraju N, Yang H, Pierce S, Wierda W, Bueso-Ramos C, Patel KP, Cortes JE, Ravandi F, Kantarjian HM, Garcia-Manero G. Sequential azacitidine and lenalidomide in patients with high-risk myelodysplastic syndromes and acute myeloid leukemia: a single arm, phase 1/2 study. Lancet Haematol. 2015; 2: e12–e20. doi:10.1016/ S2352-3026(14)00026-X.

Chapter 2

Immune Dysregulation in Myelodysplastic Syndromes: Pathogenetic-Pathophysiologic Aspects and Clinical Consequences

Argiris Symeonidis and
Alexandra Kouraklis-Symeonidis

Additional information is available at the end of the chapter

http://dx.doi.org/10.5772/64618

Abstract

Myelodysplastic syndromes are clonal hematopoietic stem cell disorders, in which the immune system plays a substantial pathogenetic role. Patients manifest frequent infections, mainly attributed to neutropenia, but sometimes opportunistic pathogens are isolated in non-neutropenic patients. They also exhibit autoimmune diseases or syndromes with a background of immune activation and various "abnormalities" of T-lymphocytes, B-lymphocytes, and NK cells. The most typical profile includes reduced total T lymphocytes (mainly CD4+ helper T-cells, resulting in decrease or inversion of the CD4/CD8 cell ratio) and impaired NK cell function. Many TH1 direction cytokines, and particularly sIL-2R, IL-6, and TNF-α are usually found increased in the serum and bone marrow, which have been strongly associated with advanced disease, anemia, and other disease-related features. Clonal origin of lymphocytes has been confirmed only in few cases. Mixed lymphocyte cultures and genomic assays have shown severely impaired immunoregulatory abnormalities, probably induced by the hematopoietic cells. In a minority of patients, immune activation is capable to prevent or delay clonal expansion, but these patients have more profound hematopoietic impairment. Immunosuppressive treatment may not only relieve the autoimmune manifestations but also improve hematopoiesis. However, this kind of treatment is not well tolerated, is associated with severe infections, and in some cases may enhance AML evolution.

Keywords: myelodysplastic syndromes, pathogenesis, immune abnormalities, autoimmune diseases, immunosuppressive treatment

1. Introduction

Myelodysplastic syndromes (MDS) are diseases emerging from somatic mutations of a pluripotent hematopoietic stem cell, affecting its functional capacity for maturation and differentiation, but preserving it alive and capable to escape from apoptotic signals. The affected cell creates a clone, gradually suppressing nonclonal cells, and finally dominating in the bone marrow. Clonal cells are prone to additional genetic events, promoting survival advantage and further impairing differentiation and maturation, thus generating a neoplastic phenotype, with the evolution to acute myelogenous leukemia (AML). Since such genetic events occur serially, but with a variable evolutionary potential, MDS represent probably the best *in vivo* model of "step-by-step" progression from a premalignant state to a high-potential neoplasm, such as AML. The multiparametric study of MDS can draw messages and conclusions, potentially applicable for the pathogenesis and pathophysiology of all types of neoplasia.

One rather unexpected aspect of MDS pathophysiology is the strong involvement of the immune system. Soon after the initial description of MDS, many "immune abnormalities" were reported in the literature. The "easy" initial interpretation of the participation of the immune system to the dysplastic clone was quickly changed, in favor of other explanations. But even now, a clear interpretation and a definite treatment strategy for these "abnormalities" have not been established. In this chapter, we describe the spectrum of "*immune abnormalities*" of MDS and briefly discuss treatment approaches, targeting the immune system. Besides a thorough literature review, we have used our personal experience, based on the study of more than 1500 patients. Thus, this chapter includes also original data, presented at various meetings, but not yet published as full papers, emerged from personal/institutional research activities at the Department of Hematology of the University Hospital of Patras.

2. Infections unrelated to the severity of neutropenia among patients with MDS

Infections of various etiologies are common among MDS patients and represent one of the major presenting features, but also a leading cause of morbidity and mortality. Beside the usually advanced patient age and comorbidity, the major predisposing factor in many retrospective studies analyzing the frequency and severity of infections is the depth of neutropenia. Functional neutrophil abnormalities have also been reported, such as impaired locomotion and chemotaxis, reduced complement receptor-1 and -3 expressions, and reduced enzymatic armamentarium, resulting in impaired respiratory burst and reduced bactericidal and fungicidal capacity. These defects have been observed in all types of MDS but are more frequent in the higher risk groups [1]. However, severe common and opportunistic infections may be manifested in nonneutropenic patients. In these cases, besides the functional neutrophil impairment, various acquired defects of the adaptive immunity, affecting immunocompetent cell populations have been proposed as predisposing factors. Finally, transfusions, transfusion-induced iron overload, and the newer treatment modalities, such as lenalidomide and hypomethylating agents, may hamper immune functions and contribute to the development of infections.

There are several published cases or small series of patients manifesting pyogenic collections/abscesses, not only at common sites (perianal, splenic, liver), but also at rare and uncommon (pararenal, intramuscular, paracolic, etc.), without the development of strong inflammatory reaction [2, 3]. It has been suggested that mature granulocytes of MDS patients may not produce effective inflammatory reaction to eliminate pathogens, and induce the formation of granulomas or abscesses [1, 2]. MDS patients, even when nonneutropenic, may exhibit delayed healing of infections and have increased intracellular neutrophil collagenase activity, irrespective of WHO or IPSS subgroup [3].

Other patients manifest bacterial, viral, and fungal infections, from rare/opportunistic pathogens, before any immunosuppressive or cytotoxic treatment, similar to those encountered among patients with underlying congenital or acquired immunodeficiency. Among such rare bacterial pathogens, coagulase-negative *Staphylococci*, rare Enterococci, *Myc. avium-intracellulare, Myc. Kansasii, Myc. Malmoense, Bacillus cereus, Corynebacterium* and *Phenylobacterium* spp., *Aeromonas hydrophila, Brevundimonas diminuta, Rhodococcus corynebacterioides,* and *Bordetella hinzii* are included. Among viral, fungal, and other pathogens, CMV and EBV reactivation, HHV-6 infection, JCV-induced progressive multifocal leukoencephalopathy (PML), *Pneumocystis iirovecii,* and *Legionella pneumophila* are included. Invasive fungal infections are rather uncommon and may emerge during the myelosuppression, which follows cytotoxic chemotherapy and/or allogeneic stem cell transplantation, in patients receiving prophylactically or therapeutically strong combinations of antibacterial antibiotics. However, many cases have been reported in the absence of these recognized predisposing factors. Involved pathogens are both, yeasts, including *C. albicans, Candida* non-*albicans* spp., and *Cryptococcus neoformans* and molds, such as *Aspergillus* and zygomycetes, and the usually affected organs are the lungs, liver, spleen, and central nervous system (CNS), and more rarely the skin, soft tissues, and other organs.

3. Association of autoimmune and immune-mediated diseases, with the manifestation of MDS

3.1. Clinical syndromes of immune overactivity associated with myelodysplastic syndromes

3.1.1. Clearly autoimmune diseases

Only few years after the recognition of MDS as separate entities and the proposal of their first classification system (FAB classification), it was obvious that they were associated with increased frequency of various immune abnormalities, either abnormal laboratory findings, such as organ- and non-organ-specific autoantibodies, or true clinical syndromes or diseases, reflecting severely impaired adaptive immunity.

Among the autoimmune or immune-mediated clinical syndromes, described in association with MDS, Coombs-positive immunohemolytic anemia (AIHA) [4], immune thrombocytopenia (ITP) [5], Evans' syndrome, autoimmune neutropenia, and pure red cell aplasia (usually drug-related) are included. AIHA is somewhat more common, and is usually of warm type, associated with mild to moderate chronic hemolysis [4]. It can be automatically presented or triggered by red blood cell transfusions. Treatment is mainly based on corticosteroids, but response rate is lower than in the idiopathic cases, and even when a "complete" response is achieved, this cannot be objectively evaluated due to coexistence of the basic disease, which has as a major manifestation anemia, although not clearly hemolytic. When corticosteroids are ineffective or associated with unacceptable toxicity, cyclosporine-A, mofetil mycophenolate, or pulses of vinca alkaloids may be used. In some instances immunosuppressive treatment may be accompanied by trilineage response, improving also neutrophil and platelet counts.

Immune thrombocytopenia particularly of chronic type, when manifested in elderly patients may mimic true MDS, particularly when there is additional underlying comorbidity and patients also have anemia of chronic disease. In such instances, the differential diagnosis is difficult and this is clearly an overlapping area of hematological disorders [6]. More complicating is the fact that these two different entities may share some common pathogenetic features, concerning premature megakaryocyte cell death [7]. However, true immune thrombocytopenia with high titers of antiplatelet autoantibodies may be the presenting feature [6, 8] or may complicate the course of a previously diagnosed MDS [9]. In some instances, ITP may precede and MDS may follow some months or years, even after the achievement of complete response of the ITP. Thrombocytopenia has been related to higher amount of glycocalicin and platelet-associated IgG, higher MPV, more advanced disease, and worse prognosis in patients with MDS. The occurrence of ITP has been more frequently reported in chronic myelomonocytic leukemia (CMML) and the del-5q syndrome, whereas relatively severe thrombocytopenia, with mild-moderate or absence of anemia and neutropenia has been reported among patients with isolated del-20q [10]. Retrospective evaluation of 123 patients with CMML revealed the presence of auto-/hyperimmune disorders in 19.5% of them, compared to 3–4% incidence in the general population [11]. CMML has been considered the MDS, most frequently associated with "paraneoplastic" manifestations. Finally, high frequency of hypocomplementemia, often associated with severe cytopenia, particularly in patients with lower risk MDS has been reported, suggesting the possible contribution of autoimmune mechanisms in its pathogenesis [12].

3.1.2. Common clinical syndromes with a dominantly immune pathogenesis

Dominant position among the immune hyperactivity/autoimmunity syndromes possess the various systemic vasculitides, such as febrile neutrophilic dermatosis (Sweet's syndrome) [13], other leucocytoclastic vasculitides, and necrotizing panniculitis, most commonly localized in the skin and accompanied by rashes or resulting in extended skin ulcerations. Large vessel arteritis (Takayasu's disease), aortitis, and other organ-specific vasculitides, such as Wegener's granulomatosis, have been reported. Additional cutaneous manifestations associated with the occult or prominent presence of an MDS include granulomatous eruptions, pyoderma gangrenosum, erythema nodosum, erythema elevatum diutinum, bullous pemphigoid, cutaneous lupus, Behçet's disease, dermatomyositis, and Raynaud's syndrome.

http://dx.doi.org/10.5772/64618

Hematological	(Other) Cutaneous syndromes
Immunohemolytic anemia	Erythema nodosum
Immune thrombocytopenia	Pyoderma gangrenosum
Evans' syndrome	Erythema elevatum diutinum
Chronic cold agglutinin disease	Bullous pemphigoid
Autoimmune neutropenia	Cutaneous lupus
Pure red cell aplasia	Granulomatous eruptions
	Raynaud phenomenon
Connective tissue type	
Systemic lupus erythematosus	**Other syndromes**
Classical seropositive rheumatoid arthritis	Fever of unknown origin (disease related)
Seronegative rheumatoid arthritis	Sarcoidosis – sarcoidotic-type granulomata
Sjögren's syndrome	Iridocyclitis – uveitis
Mixed connective tissue disease	Sterile osteomyelitis
Polymyalgia rheumatica	Hashimoto's thyroiditis
Seronegative migratory synovitis	Addison disease
Remitting symmetrical synovitis with pitting edema	Behcet disease
Eosinophilic fasciitis	Pericarditis
Relapsing polychondritis	Pleural effusions
Polymyosistis	Chronic autoimmune hepatitis
Dematomyosistis	Inflammatory bowel disease
	Ulcerative colitis
Vasculitic type	Autoimmune pancreatitis
Sweet's syndrome	Pulmonary alveolar proteinosis
Leucocytoclastic vasculitis	Bronchiolitis obliterans organizing pneumonia
Periarteritis nodosa	Nephrotic syndrome
Wegener granulomatosis	Segmental glomerulosclerosis
Large vessel arteritis (Takayasu disease)	Peripheral demyelinating polyneuropathy
Aortitis	Expressive aphasia
Necrotizing panniculitis	

Table 1. Clinical syndromes of auto-/hyperimmune basis associated with myelodysplasia.

Fever of unknown origin in the absence of any known underlying condition has been described in association with MDS and may be accompanied by mild lymphadenopathy and sarcoidic-type noncaseating granulomata, high serum ferritin, and polyclonal hyper-γ-globulinemia.

Various rheumatic manifestations may also be associated with an MDS and some patients are diagnosed following an initial presentation of a typical rheumatic disease. Remitting seronegative symmetrical synovitis with pitting edema has been reported as an initial presentation of MDS, with subsequent manifestation of relapsing polychondritis. Besides the more frequent than expected classical rheumatoid arthritis and systemic lupus erythematosus, seronegative migratory synovitis, various seropositive and seronegative polyarthritic syndromes, polymyositis, polymyalgia rheumatica, eosinophilic fasciitis, Sjögren's syndrome, and mixed connective tissue disease have also been reported.

Less common syndromes are noninfectious serosal effusions, usually pleural, but sometimes also pericarditis, chronic autoimmune hepatitis, Hashimoto's thyroiditis, Addison's disease, inflammatory bowel disease, glomerulonephritis and nephrotic syndrome, focal and segmental glomerulosclerosis, chronic autoimmune pancreatitis, ulcerative colitis, and various syndromes reflecting immune-based inflammatory processes of the CNS, such as seizures, expressive aphasia and paresis, and peripheral demyelinating polyneuropathy [14]. Finally, noninfectious pulmonary infiltrates, sometimes typical for alveolar proteinosis and bronchiolitis obliterans organizing pneumonia (BOOP), in the absence of previous allogeneic transplantation have also been reported. **Table 1** summarizes the various auto-/hyperimmune syndromes, sometimes called "paraneoplastic," associated with MDS.

3.1.3. Relapsing polychondritis

Of particular interest is the syndrome of relapsing polychondritis, which, besides the presentation as an idiopathic autoimmune syndrome, has almost exclusively been reported in association with MDS and very rarely with other diseases. Thus, among newly diagnosed polychondritis, without any evidence for a hematological disorder, BM examination may reveal the presence of an as yet undiagnosed MDS [15]. Polychondritis is manifested as painful inflammation of the cartilaginous areas of the body, such as the external ear, the basal area of the nose and the nasal septum, the synovial cartilage, and the tracheal and bronchial cartilaginous rings. Symptomatic period may persist for many days or some weeks, followed by resolution, but symptoms reappear after weeks or months. The cartilage is finally destroyed, resulting in anatomical malformation and functional disturbances. The syndrome may be associated with fever, renal, cardiovascular, or ocular manifestations, as well as by symptoms, related to organ-specific dysfunction, not clearly containing cartilaginous tissue [16]. Pathogenesis is clearly immune-based and may reflect immunological reaction against some marrow stromal elements, which also exist in the cartilaginous tissue. Prompt intervention with corticosteroids accelerates resolution of the inflammatory reaction and may reduce tissue destruction and malformations.

3.1.4. Overview of patient series and epidemiological data on autoimmune manifestations

Autoimmune diseases have been reported on average in 10–30% of MDS patients, in all age groups and disease subtypes sometimes more frequently among females and in patients with higher risk MDS or CMML [9, 17]. In some early studies, the frequency of true autoimmune diseases among series of MDS patients was not found increased compared to non-MDS subjects of similar age. Moreover, the detection of various autoantibodies, directed against erythrocytic, neutrophilic, and platelet components, in the serum of MDS patients has been disputed, whether it really represents an immune abnormality, and has been attributed to the advanced patient age to thorough searching processes or to alloimmunization from the frequent transfusions. It has been suggested, although not proved, that similar results could be obtained from multiply transfused non-MDS patients of advanced age [18]. In another study, patients exhibiting immune abnormalities were younger and had mainly therapy-related MDS with complex chromosomal aberrations [9]. Among the reported cases with available cytogenetics, trisomy 8 cases are rather overrepresented, but in the majority of described series of patients no clear preponderance of any demographic, cytogenetic, or histological feature was found [19]. In some studies, the frequency of autoimmune diseases is higher, but there is the possibility of misinterpretation of dysplastic bone marrow changes attributed to the advanced patient age or to the underlying autoimmune disease as indicative of primary MDS [17]. In a large French multicenter retrospective analysis of 123 MDS patients, exhibiting systemic inflammatory and autoimmune diseases (SIADs), vasculitic syndromes were more frequently encountered among CMML, and a comparison of this group with 665 patients without such manifestations revealed that patients exhibiting SIADs were younger, male, without RARS, with higher risk disease, and a poor karyotype, but without survival difference [20].

Autoimmune manifestations may not be a single clinical syndrome, but a clustering of two or more autoimmune or immune-based conditions may occur in the same patient. Autoantibodies most frequently found are either organ-specific or non-organ-specific, such as rheumatoid factor, antinuclear antibodies, antineutrophil cytoplasmic (cANCA), or antineutrophil perinuclear antibodies (pANCA), the last two been associated with various vasculitides. Interferon regulatory factor-1 (IRF-1) mRNA expression was found 10-folds increased in MDS patients with autoimmune manifestations, in sharp difference to those without, and to normal controls. It was therefore suggested that absence of IRF-1 expression may be a protective mechanism preventing autoimmunity in MDS [21]. However, from the prognostic point of view although patients with autoimmune manifestations have similar overall survival compared to patients without those with higher IRF-1 expression have longer survival [22].

There is no agreement whether autoimmune manifestations influence prognosis. This is because the severity of autoimmune diseases and conditions, supervened by a MDS, may be substantially diverse and prevent their evaluation as an additional prognostic factor. The majority of retrospective studies tend to demonstrate a survival advantage for patients not exhibiting (auto)immune abnormalities as compared to those who did [23]; however, other studies did not show any difference [9]. In a Japanese study, patients with immune abnormalities had more frequent infections, faster leukemic transformation, and shorter survival. Autoimmune diseases usually respond partially or temporarily to immunosuppressive treatment, but they may relapse and follow the basic disease activity [18]. In other instances they may persist throughout the course of the MDS and demand unaffordable corticosteroid doses to be controlled. In any case, autoimmune diseases remit permanently with allogeneic stem cell transplantation. Remission of autoimmune manifestations has been associated with improved survival, although in some studies it may accelerate evolution to AML. Furthermore, achievement of remission and return to the MDS stage may induce relapse of the autoimmune condition and in general the manifestation of autoimmunity follows the dysplastic phase and disappear during evolution to AML [24].

In the largest retrospective epidemiologic and prognostic analysis of about 1400 patients, 28% exhibited hyper/autoimmune manifestations and the most prominent was hypothyroidism associated with Hashimoto's thyroiditis (12% of the total population or 44% of the autoimmune syndromes), followed by immune thrombocytopenia (12%), rheumatoid arthritis (10%), and psoriasis (7%). Autoimmune conditions were more frequent among females with lower risk disease, and less transfusion dependent. The probability for AML transformation was lower and the median survival significantly higher for patients with autoimmune diseases (60 versus 45 months), and in multivariate analysis, adjusted for age and IPSS, the manifestation of an autoimmune syndrome was an independent favorable prognostic factor [23].

4. Numerical abnormalities of lymphocytes in patients with MDS

4.1. T-lymphocyte abnormalities

Many investigational studies have focused on various parameters of adaptive immunity in MDS. In the majority of patients, peripheral blood lymphopenia, mainly CD4+ cell lymphopenia, and to a lesser degree or at all, CD8+ cell reduction, frequently resulting in reduction or inversion of the CD4/CD8 cell ratio has been recognized. These findings have not been associated with specific FAB subtypes or any other clinical or laboratory feature [10, 20]. Many studies have confirmed the previous findings, particularly in patients with RAEB, and demonstrated severe functional T-cell impairment in terms of sluggish reaction to mitogenic stimuli and increased radiosensitivity, reflecting impaired DNA repair, implying that these defects might impact on patient hematopoiesis [25].

An initial approach for the interpretation of the numerical imbalance of T-cell subsets was that they might be attributed to multiple red blood cell transfusions, since in some early studies a correlation of the severity of T-lymphocyte abnormalities with transfusion intensity was reported [26]. However, it soon became clear that T-lymphocyte imbalance was present already at baseline, before any medical intervention, and therefore this finding might most probably be a disease feature. T cells of MDS patients synthesize lower amounts of the TH1 direction cytokines interleukin-2 (IL-2) and interferon-gamma (IFN-γ), following mitogenic stimulation, respond inadequately to IL-2 and cooperate inefficiently with B lymphocytes in the induction of immunoglobulin production [24–28]. Studies of NK cell function have always reported reduced cytotoxic and cytolytic activity against cellular targets, as well as impaired both complement-dependent (CDC) and antibody-dependent cell-mediated cytotoxicity (ADCC) [27]; however, in many other more recent studies, no abnormality in NK cells has been identified. We have investigated several immune function parameters at baseline on the same population of 81 patients with various MDS subtypes and we have shown that patients with RAEB had more profound CD3+ and CD4+ lymphopenia, and significantly lower and sometimes inverted CD4/CD8 cell ratio. We have also shown that CD3+ and CD8+ cell lymphopenia were associated with more frequent infections, higher AML evolution rate, and shorter overall survival [28]. A Japanese group confirmed decreased CD8+ cells in RA patients and inverted bone marrow CD4/CD8 cell ratio, with increased activated CD8+CD11α+ cells in all patients. RAEB patients had decreased marrow total T cells and all MDS patients had decreased marrow CD4+CD45RA+ naïve- and increased CD4+CD45RO+ memory T-helper cells, probably indicating impaired immune surveillance permitting the undisturbed evolution of the dysplastic clone. The prognostic significance of the numerical T-cell abnormalities on the above-mentioned issues was confirmed by other groups [19, 29]. Evaluation of lymphocyte subsets in bone marrow biopsies with specific immunostaining has not demonstrated any quantitative or qualitative T- and NK-cell abnormality, but only revealed increased B lymphocytes in patients with higher risk disease and it has been suggested that identification of >3% B lymphocytes in the marrow biopsy is an adverse prognostic feature [30].

FAB	Reaction		Total Erythema (mm) / Positive Antigens (mean)	Composite score	*p*
	(+/-)	(+) %			
RA	8/12	66.7	11.9/3.00	18.2 ± 2.7	0.160
RARS	4/10	40.0	8.6/2.40	12.1 ± 1.9	**0.003**
RAEB	10/16	62.5	11.2/2.43	16.1 ± 2.2	**0.029**
RAEBt	2 / 8	25.0	6.3/2.25	10.7 ± 1.5	**0.002**
CMML	5 / 8	62.5	8.8/2.87	14.8 ± 0.7	**0.022**
Total	29/54	53.7	9.8/2.59	14.8 ± 1.0	0.0003
Controls	16/18	88.9	17.4/4.11	25.8 ± 2.4	

Notes: Results of the skin reaction to the Multitest CMI test, consisting of 7 common antigens (Tetanus, Diphtheria, Tuberculin, Candida, Trichophyton, Streptococcus, Proteus): patients with MDS as one group exhibited significantly reduced composite score, compared to healthy controls, matched for age and gender. Significant differences were found for all FAB MDS categories, with the exception of RA (unpublished data).Bold letters indicate statistically significant differences.

Table 2. Results of the skin reaction to Multitest CMI® in patients with MDS

Patients with MDS-RA and with aplastic anemia exhibit Th1 and Tc1 polarization of their immune activation [31]. Later this was confirmed also for patients with refractory cytopenia with multilineage dysplasia (RCMD) and was correlated with very high serum and marrow IFN-γ and tumor necrosis factor-α (TNF-α) levels, and high degree of apoptosis. Higher Th1/Th2 and Tc1/Tc2 ratios have been observed in patients with lower risk IPSS and normal karyotype, but not in aneuploid karyotypes. Th1 polarization may not be a uniform finding in MDS patients, but concerns only a subgroup of RCMD with prominent CD8+ lymphopenia [32].

Activated T lymphocytes do not belong to the dysplastic/leukemic clone and express HLA-DR, CD25, CD45RO, and CD57, but not CD28 and CD62L. This antigenic profile is independent of disease subtype, prognostic classification, kind of cytogenetic abnormality, or any other feature [33]. Interestingly, both patients with lower risk MDS and those with aplastic anemia have increased T-lymphocyte counts and B lymphocytopenia compared to patients with high-risk MDS and to controls, but lower risk MDS patients exhibit stronger and uniform Th1/Tc1 polarization than those with aplastic anemia [34]. Moreover, bone marrow NK T-cell infiltrates express the activated effector T-cell phenotype CD8+CD57+CD28−CD62L− and the NK C-lectin-family receptors NKG2D and CD244. These infiltrates represent oligoclonal expansions of autoreactive T cells, as this can be demonstrated by TCR clonality assays and are more prominently identified in the bone marrow than in the peripheral blood [35].

MDS patients also exhibit impairment of delayed cutaneous T-cell hypersensitivity, as this can be demonstrated with various skin patch tests, challenging reaction to common antigens. Most importantly, they may lose immunologic memory against potentially important antigens, such as tuberculin and *clostr. tetani* anatoxin, the clinical consequence of which is unclear [36]. **Table 2** resumes the results from our study of skin reactions to the multitest CMI® in 54 patients with MDS compared to 20 controls (unpublished data).

Further understanding of the immune dysregulation of MDS was achieved through investigation of the regulatory T cells (T-regs). T-regs are a specific subset of helper T cells, inducing immune tolerance and moderating the intensity of immune reactions. Many autoimmune and neoplastic diseases are associated with T-reg impairment, favoring uncontrolled immune activation and attenuation of immune surveillance against tumor growth. An increase of polyclonal/nonclonal T cells in higher risk MDS, and a significant correlation of T-reg number, with the percentage of marrow blasts, the IPSS and progression to AML has been reported [37]. T-regs, characterized as CD4+ CD25^{high}+FOXP3+ or CD4+CD25^{high}+CD127^{low} cells, were found increased in lower risk MDS but they were not correlated with any known disease feature or lab finding [38]. Investigation of the T-reg kinetics, function, and trafficking has revealed that in early MDS, peripheral blood and marrow T-regs are normal in number but dysfunctional, exhibiting lower CXCR4 expression and impaired marrow homing. In contrast, at late MDS or at leukemic transformation, T-regs increase and become functional and migrating. Effective treatment partially restores the number, but disease relapse is again associated with T-reg expansion. Thus, T-regs may share a pathophysiological role in MDS, since impaired suppressor function results in autoimmune phenomena, whereas in more advanced stages, their expansion favors clonal development and leukemic transformation [39]. It has been suggested that absolute number of a T-reg subpopulation, the "effector regulatory T cells," characterized as CD4+FOXP3+CD25+CD127^{low}CD45RA−CD27− cells, could be used as a prognostic factor in lower risk MDS predicting severity of anemia, AML transformation, and overall survival [40].

Other interesting T-cell subsets are the IL-17 producing helper T cells, the so-called Th17 cells and the Th22 cells. Th17 cells were found substantially increased in patients with lower risk MDS and their number was inversely correlated with that of T-regs. T-regs, although suppressive for other T-cell populations, do not affect Th17 cell number. Thus, the Th17/T-reg cell ratio has been found very high in lower risk disease and has been proposed as a marker of "effective" immunosuppression, high degree of apoptosis, and higher risk for autoimmunity, as well as an indicator for application of immunosuppressive treatment [41]. In contrast, helper T cells producing IL-22 (Th22 cells), involved in the pathogenesis of inflammatory reaction and autoimmunity, were found increased in patients with advanced MDS and their number was correlated with the mRNA levels of proinflammatory cytokines [42].

Finally, peripheral blood $T_{\gamma\delta}$ lymphocytes, possessing a TCR with rearranged gamma/delta chains, and particularly $V_{\gamma 9}V_{\delta 2}$ T cells, the major $T_{\gamma\delta}$-cell subset, which represent an important subpopulation for antitumor activity, were found reduced in patients with MDS and the reduction was greater in patients exhibiting autoimmune manifestations. Although $T_{\gamma\delta}$ cells were not clonal, they reacted poorly to IL-2, and bromohalohydrin, a specific mitogen for these cells, induced mitogenic responses in only 60% of the MDS studied, unrelated to any specific disease feature. However, when activated, they exerted normal antileukemic effects against leukemic blasts. Therefore, the impaired number and function of this T-cell subpopulation may play a role in clonal expansion and disease progression of MDS [43].

4.2. B-lymphocyte abnormalities

Although B lymphocytes in MDS patients do not demonstrate the spectrum of abnormalities detected in T cells, since their production and function is governed by T cells, their aberration actually reflects the functional integrity of T cells. Information for B lymphocytes is fewer and often conflicted. In many studies, decreased proportion and peripheral blood absolute B lymphocytopenia, frequently accompanied by hypogammaglobulinemia and recurrent infections has been reported [27, 44]. These findings are mostly confined to patients with lower risk disease and are associated with T-lymphocyte imbalance and reduced numbers of bone marrow B cells and B-cell precursors.

Analysis of the marrow CD34+ cell differentiation toward B lymphocytes in patients with low-risk MDS has revealed low expression of B-lineage differentiation genes and reduced production of B-cell precursors, a finding proposed to be used as a hallmark of low-risk disease [45]. An additional factor contributing to B lymphocytopenia is that bone marrow B-, but not T lymphocytes, exhibit increased apoptosis, similar to that observed in nonlymphoid cells. Increased B-cell apoptosis could not be considered a clonal "property," since it was found neither in leukemic nor in normal marrows [44]. This was also confirmed on trephine biopsies of patients with high-risk MDS only, and the percentage of B lymphocytes was inversely correlated with prognosis [30]. Bone marrow flow cytometry analysis has shown increased proportion of CD34+CD45^{low} B-cell precursors in patients with RA and RARS, and lower values in those with RAEB, whereas in AML B-cell precursors were not found at all, probably reflecting differentiation incapability of the CD34+ cells. Indeed, an inverse correlation of CD34+CD45^{low}+ B cells with marrow blasts and a positive one with hemoglobin was found. Abnormal expression pattern of B-cell differentiation antigens, with hypoexpression of CD79α and TdT has also been reported, implying a possible role of the MDS marrow microenvironment in the maturation process of B lymphocytes [46].

Regarding the origin of B- and T lymphocytes, available data are again conflicting. In the majority of clonal studies, neither T- nor B lymphocytes or NK cells were found to originate from the dysplastic clone. Some studies have shown clonal origin of the B lymphocytes in a proportion of MDS patients, and in a Japanese study, the majority of patients with RA and those with immunological abnormalities exhibited clonal B lymphocytes [47]. Clonal origin was also found in 5% of the CD20+/CD22+ B cells of patients with trisomy 8. By using interphase FISH on sorted marrow cells, 13% of the CD5+CD19+ lymphocytes were clonal, implying that a part of the B lymphocytes in some patients may be clonal and that these cells may contribute to the manifestation of immune abnormalities [48].

B lymphocytes of MDS patients express low number of HLA-DR molecules (HLA class-II antigens) and are either deficient of EBV receptors or they carry abnormal Fc_{γ} and C3d receptors, which cannot be used by EBV viral particles to enter and activate B cells. B-lymphocyte cultures produce increased amounts of IL-6 and IL-10, following mitogenic stimulation. IL-6 is overproduced even without mitogenic stimuli. Finally, B lymphocytes of patients manifesting immune abnormalities have lower number of cell surface Fas ligand receptors, a finding possibly indicating their resistance to apoptosis.

Not surprisingly several quantitative serum γ-globulin and immunoglobulin abnormalities have been described in MDS patients, such as polyclonal hyper-γ-globulinemia, monoclonal M-spikes, or hypo-γ-globulinemia. Monoclonal components have been found significantly higher than in normal age-matched population [49]. It has been suggested that dysplastic monocytes might exert unspecific immune stimulation on B- and T lymphocytes through increased IL-1 production favoring the development of monoclonal B-cell populations and producing M-spikes.

Investigating the significance of serum protein electrophoresis in 158 patients, we noticed a normal pattern in 36% (mainly in RA and RARS) and only in 8% of CMML. A normal baseline pattern was associated with longer survival, independently of the IPSS and FAB classification. An acute phase reaction (alpha2-globulins >10 g/l) was seen in 17% at baseline, developed in additional 24% in the course of the disease, but in 80% of the patients transformed to AML and was associated with shorter survival. Hypo-γ-globulinemia was found in 6%, mainly RARS, was not related to frequent infections, and in RAEB it was associated with decreased marrow cellularity, deeper cytopenias, and longer survival. Polyclonal hyper-γ-globulinemia was found in 41% of patients (particularly RAEB-t, CMML) and monoclonal proteins in 16 cases (10%) more commonly in CMML and 2.5 times more frequently than in a control population of similar age. An additional 18% of the patients exhibited discrete M-components among polyclonal spectrum of γ-globulins. This finding has not yet been described and its significance is unclear [50].

4.3. NK cell abnormalities

Patients with MDS exhibit severe functional NK-cell impairment, but sometimes also numerical abnormalities. Cytotoxic NK-T cells, phenotypically characterized as CD3+CD8+CD16+, are usually normal or decreased but IFN-γ production is normal or increased. NK cells, characterized as CD3–CD8–CD11b+HNK1+ CD56+CD57+ cells, have been found normal, rarely decreased, but sometimes even increased [51]. The NK activity of MDS patients is almost always decreased compared to healthy controls [27, 51], although immunophenotypically NK cells are indistinguishable. In general, CD8+ T-cell function and the defective NK activity in MDS have been strongly and inversely correlated with bone marrow blast cell percentage, marrow cellularity, and serum sIL-2R levels [51]. Alloantigen- or mitogen-induced cell-mediated cytotoxicity [27] as well as IFN-α and IL-2 production following NK cell activation is also impaired and the preincubation of NK cells with IFN-α may partially increase NK activity [52]. There are conflicting data regarding the origin of NK cells. By using FISH on FACS-sorted cells of patients with monosomy 7, monosomic signs in CD3–CD56+ cells were detected in 3 out of 4 [53]. In another study, between 20 and 50% but not all the NK cells were clonal, demonstrating a kind of "chimerism" by clonal and nonclonal NK cells in the majority of patients.

Many groups investigated whether IFN-α treatment could induce blast/clonal cell clearance, through augmentation of the NK activity. In one study on 38 patients with RAEB, following 3-month treatment with IFN-α, NK activity and NK cell number and function was increased, but these alterations were not associated with any meaningful clinical response. NK cells exhibited normal tumor cell binding capacity, but inability of releasing cytotoxic factors, possibly suggesting intrinsic functional defects [52]. Another group did not confirm any quantitative defect and found normal expression of the activating receptors NKp46, NKp30, and NKG2D, but a depressed cytolytic activity. Incubation with IL-2 upregulated the NKp46 expression, but did not enhance NK-cell cytotoxicity but induced higher rate of apoptosis [53]. A strong correlation of the NK activity with higher IPSS, abnormal karyotype, excess of blasts and marrow hypercellularity, and downregulation of the NKG2D receptor has also been reported [54]. The Nordic MDS study Group showed that decreased expression of DNAM1 and NKG2D receptors on marrow NK cells was inversely correlated with blast percentage and suggested that DNAM1 plays a pivotal role in NK-mediated cell killing [55].

IL-12, alone or combined with IL-2, induces variable and unpredictable response to NK cells. Some patients (mainly with RA) exhibit a response closer to normal, while others respond poorly. The combination of IL-2 and IL-12 increases IFN-γ and TNF-α production in a synergistic way. IL-12 alone is not so stimulatory, and the combination of IL-2+IL-12 generates stimulation, similar to that obtained by IL-2 alone. Indeed, priming of peripheral blood mononuclear cells (PBMC) with IL-12 increased their cytotoxicity against autologous leukemic blasts to almost normal levels and significantly reduced WT1 mRNA expression, used as a marker of residual leukemic burden, except in patients with overt, high-bulk AML. Thus, *ex vivo* priming of cytotoxic NK-T and NK cells could be used as a tool, targeting residual disease, following systemic chemotherapy [56].

In a study from Düsseldorf, the authors recognized a small subgroup of high-risk patients, with almost absent peripheral blood NK cells, but intact populations of NK T cells. A larger subgroup with normal number but poor function of NK cells was characterized by reduced intracellular granzyme-B and perforin levels. This subgroup restored almost completely NK-cell function, following mitogen or cytokine stimulation. NK cells were mainly immature but exhibited normal mature/activated ($CD56^{bright}$+CD107+) immunophenotype and a restricted repertoire of KIR receptors. It is therefore suggested that the dysfunctional NK cells lead to inefficient/insufficient immune surveillance and clonal expansion [57]. The Pittsburgh Group reported different marrow frequencies of NK and NK T cells in MDS and AML. In MDS they did not find numerical impairment of the NK-cell population, but a significant decrease in mature $CD56^{dim}CD16+CD57^{bright}$ cells, which had great prognostic significance for survival [58]. Other groups have reported increased intracellular granzyme-B levels in the NK cells of MDS patients [59].

5. Serum cytokine profiles

The immune-activated status of MDS patients lead to overproduction and elevated serum levels of many cytokines. We were the first group to report elevated serum soluble interleukin-2 receptors (sIL-2R) and tumor necrosis factor-α levels in 42 MDS patients confirming an abnormal immune stimulatory status. Although the difference in TNF-α levels between early and advanced MDS was not significant, patients with advanced MDS had significantly higher serum sIL-2R levels compared to those with early MDS [60]. *In vivo* treatment with rhGM-CSF or high-dose IL-3 further increases sIL-2R levels, which are associated with higher marrow cellularity and blast cell percentage, faster AML evolution, and shorter survival. These findings possibly reflect quantitative and qualitative abnormalities of the CD8+ and NK-cell subsets, resulting in ineffective T-B cell communication and impaired NK-cell function, since sIL-2R antagonizes the cellular receptor in IL-2 uptake, restricting T-cell activation [61]. sIL-2R levels are negatively correlated with T- and NK-cell counts and positively with adverse events occurring in the course of lower risk patients for whom sIL-2R levels are an independent adverse prognostic factor.

Serum IL-6 levels were found elevated in the majority of MDS patients and serum GM-CSF levels in less than half of them, although these cytokines were undetectable in normal subjects. Higher IL-6 concentrations were found in patients with advanced subtypes, were inversely correlated with the severity of the anemia and positively with peripheral blood and bone marrow blast cell percentages, and may increase further following chemotherapy. IL-6, IL-7, MCSF, TGFβ, and IL-1β are constitutively produced by marrow stromal cells of patients with MDS and AML, but not from stromal cells of normal subjects, and IL-6 gene transcription could be induced by exogenous addition of IL-1β confirming a cytokine network dysregulation [62]. Serum IL-8 levels were also found elevated, but they dropped under chemotherapy or during remission.

A Dutch group measured serum levels of seven cytokines in 75 MDS patients and found detectable levels of G-CSF in the majority of them, and increased IL-3 and IL-6 levels in a minority of patients but not in controls [63]. Serum TNF-α levels have been correlated with the severity of anemia, poor performance status, leucocytosis and monocytosis, higher β2-microglobulin and lower albumin levels, liver and renal impairment, and shorter survival [62–64]. TNF-α levels <10 pg/ml have been associated with achievement of higher remission rate and longer PFS Progression Free and overall survival, whereas lower TNF-α and IL-1β levels could predict response to treatment with erythropoietin [64]. Thus, TNF-α represents the most important circulating and measurable cytokine, from the pathogenetic and the prognostic point of view. In general, serum levels of type-1 cytokines (IL-1β, IL-7, IL-8, IL-12, RANTES, and IFN-γ) [64, 65] are found elevated in lower risk MDS, whereas inhibitory factors (IL-10, sIL-2R) are elevated in higher risk disease.

The group of Mayo Clinic evaluated plasma levels of 30 different cytokines in 78 patients, and showed that although levels of 19 cytokines differed significantly from controls, in multivariate analysis, only levels of IL-6, IL-7, and CXCL10 had independent prognostic value for survival. Indeed, patients with normal levels of all these three cytokines had a median survival of 76 months compared to only 25 months for patients with elevated levels of at least one of them. For IL-6 levels in particular, a strong association with inferior leukemia-free survival, independent from other prognostic factors, was found [66].

Finally, a Spanish group, among other findings, demonstrated an inverse correlation of the CD3+, CD4+, and CD8+ populations with age, as well as an inverse correlation of serum IL-10 levels with the number of CD8+ cells, disease progression, and overall survival [67]. In another study, investigating the association of IL-10 gene polymorphisms with the development and the features of MDS, the highly IL-10-expressing genotype *-592 CC* was associated with more severe anemia and poorer survival compared to non-IL10-expressing genotypes, thus confirming a significant prognostic role for IL-10 [68].

6. Functional immunoregulatory abnormalities of T lymphocytes

6.1. Mixed lymphocyte reactions (MLRs): basic information

A basic property of the immunocompetent cells is the recognition of the "self" and the orchestration of an immune response against the "nonself" or the "altered self," and when self-recognition is impaired, an autoimmune disorder emerges. An initial interpretation for the frequent autoimmune disorders and other immune abnormalities of MDS patients was that they might probably reflect clonal origin of B- and T lymphocytes. Later, however, it was demonstrated that, in the majority of cases, B- and T lymphocytes are nonclonal, but T-lymphocyte abnormalities may influence disease course. Various T-lymphocyte subsets exert complex immunoregulatory activities on other T-cell populations, B lymphocytes, and monocytes. Mixed lymphocyte cultures are performed with the coculture of a pure T-cell population (responder cells), upon which a kinetically inactive, but cell-surface intact, non-T cell population (stimulant cells) affects, thus generating a mixed lymphocyte reaction. MLRs represent dynamic *in vitro* models for the study of various cellular interactions and of the immunoregulatory mechanisms developed between different immunocompetent cell populations. When the stimulant and the responder cell population stem from the same subject, the model is called *autologous MLR* (AMLR), whereas when the stimulant population stems from another subject the model is called *allogeneic MLR* (Allo-MLR). AMLR and Allo-MLR constitute practical tools for the investigation of various diseases and conditions with an underlying immune-based pathogenesis or pathophysiology.

The proliferative reaction (MLR) is mediated through recognition of structural antigenic domains of the cell surface of non-T cells, and particularly HLA class-II antigens. The stimulating capacity of the non-T-cell population is abrogated when cell membrane structure is destroyed, either following mechanical stress or treatment with proteolytic enzymes. Moreover, the stimulatory capacity is not a soluble factor and non-T- or B-lymphocyte supernatants do not retain any stimulatory activity on T lymphocytes [69], whereas preincubation of the non-T-cell population with anti-HLA-DR monoclonal antibodies completely abrogates the AMLR and substantially depresses the Allo-MLR. The stimulatory potential of other membrane determinants on the MLRs was identified in a similar way. Such molecules are HLA class I (HLA-A, -B, and -C) for the Allo-MLR, CD3-Ti complex for any type of MLR, and probably additional minor antigenic determinants of the MHC. Stimulating capacity of the non-T-cell population is dependent on the various mononuclear cell constituents included. B lymphocytes are stronger stimulants than NK cells and null lymphocytes. Activated B lymphocytes, surface IgM(+) B lymphocytes, and B lymphoblasts are better stimulants than resting- and IgM(−) B lymphocytes, and this property is independent of their content in EBV-DNA or the origin from a mitogen-enriched culture. The role of monocytes is contradictory, since inactive monocytes enhance autologous reactivity, whereas the admixture of monocytes in the responder T-cell population results in severe impairment of both AMLR and Allo-MLR.

MLRs share the characteristic features of an orchestrated immune reaction showing immunologic memory and specificity. When T lymphocytes, previously exposed to autologous non-T cells and obtained the seventh day of culture, are re-exposed to the same non-T-cell population, they demonstrate their peak proliferation earlier, on the third day of culture (secondary AMLR), thanks to previously engrafted immunologic memory. The same has been confirmed for the Allo-MLR, because when in the secondary culture the allogenic stimuli are different, then different responder T-cell population is activated and the reaction shows the kinetic of the primary MLR. There are different autoreactive and alloreactive T-cell populations. The number of alloreactive T cells is 5–40 times higher than autoreactive, and represents 1/400–1/150 of the total peripheral blood T lymphocytes, whereas autoreactive constitute 1/5000–1/2200 of them.

The basic function of the MLRs is the production of suppressor "activity" or of suppressor/cytotoxic T cells. The main part of the responder population are CD4+ helper/inducer T lymphocytes and treatment of this population with an anti-CD4 monoclonal antibody, practically abrogates all types of MLR. Conversely, treatment with an anti-CD8 antibody quantitatively decreases the strength of both types of MLR. Thus, from the relative content of the two major T-cell subpopulations AMLR has two different phases. Responder CD4+ T lymphocytes undergo a proliferative reaction upon sensation of autologous signals (self-MHC antigens: autoreactive T cells). CD4+ cell proliferative reaction is peaked on the third and fourth day of the culture, when helper T-cell population dominates. This reaction is followed by a secondary activation of the suppressor CD8+ T cells, which is quantitatively stronger, is peaked on the sventh and eighth day of the culture and inhibits any further proliferation of the autoreactive T cells. This serially fulfilled lymphocyte reaction is mediated through the production of IL-2 by the CD4+ T cells. In the Allo-MLR the responder population (alloreactive T cells) is activated through the recognition of the MHC alloantigens and is consisted of both helper and suppressor T lymphocytes. Allo-MLR is always stronger than AMLR. Deficiency

http://dx.doi.org/10.5772/64618

of AMLR and of Allo-MLR has been reported in various diseases and conditions, a list of which is provided in **Table 3**.

Connective tissue disorders	Autoimmune diseases
Rheumatoid arthritis	Immunohemolytic anemia
Still's disease	Immune thrombocytopenic purpura
Systemic Lupus Erythematosus	Henoch-Schoenlein puprpura
Dermatomyosistis/polymyositis	Insulin-dependent diabetes mellitus
Sjogren's syndrome	Hashimoto's thyroiditis
Ankylosing spondylitis	Chronic active hepatitis
	Inflammatory bowel disease
Infectious diseases	Primary biliary cirrhosis
Infectious mononucleosis	Myasthenia gravis
Chronic mucocutaneous candidiasis	Multiple sclerosis
Acquired immunodeficiecy syndrome	Arthropathic psoriasis
Chronic Hepatitis C	
Chronic periodontitis	**Allergic diseases and conditions**
	Allergic asthma
Neoplastic diseases	Atopic dermatitis
Breast cancer	Hay fever
Lung cancer	Food allergy
Colon cancer	
Head and neck cancer	**Various diseases and conditions**
Gastric cancer	Sarcoidosis
Bladder cancer with schistosomiasis	Down's syndrome
Kaposi's sarcoma	Congenital immunodeficiency
Myelodysplastic syndromes	Idiopathic portal hypertension
	Ataxia-telangiectasia
Lymphoproliferative disorders	Congenital hyper-IgM syndrome
Chronic lymphocytic leukemia	Mixed cryoglobulinemia
Hairy cell leukemia	Hemophilic patients treated with fVIII concentrates
Hodgkin's lymphoma	Transplanted patients
B-cell non-Hodgkin's lymphoma	Patients in chronic hemodialysis
Peripheral T-cell lymphoma	Advanced age
Multiple myeloma	

Table 3. Diseases with an abnormal autologous mixed lymphocyte reaction.

Besides the immunoregulatory cell circuits, generated following "autorecognition" in the AMLR, helper and suppressor T lymphocytes exert regulatory function in normal hematopoiesis. T lymphocytes obtained at the early phase of the AMLR (third day) have promoting activity on the formation of early (bursts) and late erythroid colonies (CFU-E) and this activity is similar to that obtained by PHA-activated T lymphocytes. This activity, initially termed *Burst Promoting Activity,* is attributed to the production of various hematopoietic cytokines and particularly interleukin-3. Following the development of suppressor activity for dampening autologous reaction on the seventh culture day, this activity also induces suppression of development of immature erythropoietic and other progenitor cells, similar to that generated from activated lymphocytes following prolonged antigenic stimulation, as this happens in chronic infections, inflammatory conditions, connective tissue diseases, and in aplastic anemia. In these situations activated suppressor T lymphocytes produce suppressive cytokines, and particularly but not exclusively IFN-γ.

Cytotoxic activity, generated in the MLRs, is also directed against autologous and allogeneic B lymphocytes, monocytes, and cells with an altered antigenic profile, either neoplastic or not. Generation of cytotoxic activity against tumor cells as a result of immune activation is of tremendous clinical significance. In AMLR and Allo-MLR the neoplastic cells may represent the stimulant cell population, whereas responder populations might be both the suppressor/cytotoxic CD3+CD16+ NK-T cells and the CD3-CD16+CD56+ NK cells. Activation of these populations results in increased proliferation and the adoption of an activated profile. Thus, cytotoxic T cells generated in AMLR may play an important role in antitumor surveillance [70].

6.2. Autologous and allogeneic MLRs of patients with myelodysplastic syndromes

AMLR and Allo-MLR were found significantly reduced on 12 MDS patients and the amount of IL-2 produced during these reactions was severely depressed. Exogenous addition of IL-2 partially restored the strength of the reactions, which, however, continued to be substantially reduced compared to normal controls. To investigate which cell population was primarily affected, the authors compared the strength of Allo-MLR by using allogeneic non-T cells from both normal controls and other MDS patients against T cells from MDS patients. They also tested Allo-MLR of T lymphocytes from healthy controls against non-T cells obtained either from normal subjects or from MDS patients. Allo-MLR of T cells from MDS patients was substantially improved with the use of normal allogeneic non-T cells, but did not reach the normal range. Conversely, Allo-MLR of T cells from normal subjects was severely deficient when stimulant non-T cells had been obtained from MDS patients compared to the reaction against non-T cells from normal subjects. Therefore, it appears that in MDS there is an impaired stimulating capacity of the non-T-cell population consisting of B lymphocytes, monocytes, and immature myeloid cells [26]. Almost concurrently the presence of "leukemia-inhibitory activity" (LIA) of peripheral blood non-T cells of MDS patients mainly obvious in patients with an excess of blasts, but also in some patients without an excess of blasts (RA-RARS) was reported. Moreover, the majority of the patients without an excess of blasts, whose serum contained LIA, evolved quickly to RAEB/AML. This "activity" of higher risk MDS patients could be eluted from culture of PBMC in FCS-enriched media with the addition of GM-CSF and IL-4 [71]. Cells responsible for the induction of suppression/inhibition of cell growth are clonal macrophages, transformed in culture to "giant macrophages" or dendritic cells. The mediator of suppression was a soluble factor, other than IFN-γ or TNF-α, identified as acidic isoferritin [72].

We investigated the MLRs in 20 MDS patients in paired experiments with sex- and age-matched controls at baseline, before the administration of any interventional treatment. To express the strength of reactions we used the *Stimulation Index*, i.e., the ratio of the incorporated ^{3}H-thymidine in the MLR divided by the incorporated ^{3}H-thymidine in an unstimulated culture of equal number of purified CD3+ T lymphocytes. Patients with MDS exhibited severely impaired AMLR in all experiments with a median value almost half as that of the controls, without overlapping values, and the difference between the two groups was statistically very significant ($p < 0.000001$). Patients with RAEB showed that the most attenuated reactions were significantly weaker than the remaining patients [73]. Cumulative results are shown in **Table 4**.

FAB group	N	(Mean ± SEM) cpm	(Mean ± SEM) S.I.	p	AMLR patient/AMLR control
RA	4	2068 ± 205	2.64 ± 0.33	**0.0023**	0.58 ± 0.09
RAS	5	2301 ± 206	2.77 ± 0.18	**0.0012**	0.63 ± 0.06
RAEB	8	1837 ± 310	1.90 ± 0.07	**<0.0001**	0.40 ± 0.03
CMML	3	2562 ± 177	3.39 ± 0.21	**0.0413**	0.51 ± 0.08
All patients	20	2108 ± 154	2.49 ± 0.15	**<0.0001**	0.51 ± 0.04
Controls	20	4396 ± 404	5.31 ± 0.32		
RAEB vs. other MDS pts (S.I.): 1.90 ± 0.07 vs. 2.88 ± 0.16				**0.0004**	

Table 4. Results of the autologous mixed lymphocyte reaction in patients with MDS (counts per min and stimulation index, S.I.) Bold letters/numbers indicate statistically significant differences.

To evaluate the capability of the stimulant cell population, Allo-MLR was performed against non-T cells originating either from another MDS patient or from a healthy control. Moreover, to evaluate the capability of the responder cells, Allo-MLR of the healthy controls was performed against non-T cells from MDS patients or from other controls. In all cases, Allo-MLR against normal non-T cells was substantially higher, and on average threefold as strong as AMLR and Allo-MLR against "dysplastic" non-T cells was weaker, but always stronger than AMLR of the same person. The difference between these two types of controls' Allo-MLR was significant (S.I.: 7.90 ± 0.89 versus 14.12 ± 1.59, $p = 0.0035$, unpublished data). When compared to controls, Allo-MLR of MDS patients was significantly impaired in all comparisons (S.I.: 4.53 ± 0.41 versus 14.12 ± 1.59, $p = 0.000014$, unpublished data). Significant difference was maintained in the comparison of Allo-MLR between healthy controls and patients with RA, RARS, and RAEB separately, whereas CMML patients exhibited the less, and RAEB patients the most attenuated reactions, significantly weaker than the remaining MDS. In paired analysis, alloreactivity of MDS patients was always weaker than that of the corresponding control and the ratio Patient's Allo-MLR/Control's Allo-MLR was always <1 (median 0.36, range 0.06–0.58). Among MDS patients, "dysplastic" origin of the non-T cells did not further impair the already depressed alloreactivity. However, even in this Allo-MLR the difference between patients and controls was still significant (S.I.: 3.64 ± 0.21 versus 7.90 ± 0.89, $p = 0.026$) [73]. Results of the Allo-MLR are shown in **Table 5**.

	Normal non-T cells				Dysplastic non-T cells			
FAB Group	**N**	**× ±SEM**		**p**	**N**	**× ±SEM**		**p**
		cpm	**S.I.**			**cpm**	**S.I.**	
RA	4	3562 ± 334	4.79 ± 0.64	**0.020**	3	2532 ± 407	3.01 ± 0.23	n.s.
RAS	5	4569 ± 702	5.86 ± 0.87	**0.021**	4	3859 ± 685	4.89 ± 1.16	n.s.
RAEB	8	2643 ± 328	3.04 ± 0.25	**< 0.000**	7	1865 ± 563	2.21 ± 0.49	n.s.
CMML	3	4215 ± 695	5.93 ± 0.62	0.070	1	3380	4.47	–
All Pts	20	3544 ± 312	4.53 ± 0.41	**< 0.0001**	15	2697 ± 389	3.63 ± 0.21	**0.040**
Controls	20	11,355 ± 1459	14.12 ± 1.59		12	6558 ± 869	7.90 ± 0.89	
RAEB vs. all other MDS (S.I.)			3.04 ± 0.29	**<0.001**			5.52 ± 0.47	**0.001**

Table 5. Allogeneic mixed lymphocyte reaction in patients with myelodysplastic syndromes – counts per min and stimulation index (S.I.) Bold letters/numbers indicate statistically significant differences.

Similar results were obtained by the Czech group who found significantly decreased MLRs with lower TNF-α and IFN-γ production in the supernatants of patients with RA compared to the MLRs of RARS patients. They also found less affected the allo-MLR against normal non-T cells, and identified as more defective the second (effector) phase of the reaction [74]. Therefore, in the MLRs of MDS patients there is an impairment of both the responder (T cells) and the stimulant population (non-T cells). The responder population reacts poorly to autologous and allogeneic stimuli and exhibits a profile of immune tolerance, which is clearer in the high-risk patients. Moreover, the stimulant population provides insufficient stimuli for reaction to the T cells, since it also depresses the alloreactivity of normal T lymphocytes. The possible, if any, clinical consequences of these findings are practically unknown or remain only speculative.

6.3. Pathogenesis of immune dysregulation in MDS: immune abnormalities or immune adaptation?

6.3.1. Autoreactivity against the clone: Autologous progenitor cell/T-lymphocyte reaction (APLR)

"Inhibitory activity" derived from serum and PBMC culture's supernatants of MDS patients has earlier been described and associated with poor prognosis [71]. Normal PBMC inhibit autologous hematopoietic cell colony formation in short-term cultures, as did also PBMC of patients with RA, but they induced a clear inhibitory activity later on day 10. Responsible cells are probably cytotoxic T and NK cells, which may react against the clone and suppress the growth of clonal cells at early stages of the disease. If this suppressor function develops early and is effective, clonal growth may be arrested. Nevertheless, NK cells of MDS patients usually exhibit impaired function and sometimes are clonal. However, since suppressor activity is achieved through various soluble cytokines and mainly through TNF-α, it is not quite specific and may also affect nonclonal cells, resulting in hematopoietic suppression, as this is observed in hypoplastic MDS and aplastic anemia. Indeed, lymphocyte culture supernatants from MDS patients exert suppressive activity on the growth of normal hematopoietic progenitors [75].

This form of cytotoxicity was also identified in high-risk MDS and in AML, and was attributed to possible infection of leukemic cells by an oncogenic virus. However, viral infection is not necessary for the generation of an immune reaction, since clonal cells contain and sometimes express on their membrane many abnormal or mutated proteins, possibly representing neoantigens capable to induce lymphocytotoxic reactions by CD8+ T cells. Autoantigens are hardly found in MDS and may only be speculative but have been identified in some other marrow failure syndromes, such as aplastic anemia and paroxysmal nocturnal hemoglobinuria. As possible antigens, the Wilms Tumor protein (WT1), moesin, a cytoskeleton protein, KIF20B (kinesin), desmoplakin, and proteinase-3, an enzyme of blast-cell granules, have been indicated [76]. T lymphocytes of some MDS/AML patients stimulated *in vitro* with WT1 and proteinase-3 were polarized toward TH1 direction with the production of IFN-γ and the enrichment of their cytoplasm with granzyme B [77]. Moreover, patients expressing defined proteinase-3 aplotype generate stronger allogeneic lymphocytotoxic reactions following allogeneic hematopoietic stem-cell transplantation (GVL effect).

A challenging hypothesis is that the adaptive immunity may rather "react" than be impaired following various cellular interactions, and this immune "reaction," or at least such cellular interactions, might be a part of the pathogenesis of MDS. This "reaction" also may represent a defensive mechanism of the immune system against the dysplastic/neoplastic clone and is orchestrated specifically against clonal bone marrow cells. Specific CD8+ suppressor/cytotoxic T cells recognizing progenitor cells with trisomy 8 have been identified in MDS patients with this abnormality. Clonal inhibition is achieved via MHC class I recognition and through induction of FAS-mediated apoptosis [78]. The possible contributing role of an altered marrow microenvironment in the development of such immune alterations is also tempting.

The presence of increased number of immunocompetent T lymphocytes with an activated cytotoxic immunophenotype CD8+CD25+CD28-CD57+ has been reported in the marrows of patients with aplastic anemia and MDS. These cells do not to directly influence the severity of peripheral blood cytopenias [79]. In our study on 41 patients, the percentage of activated marrow suppressor/cytotoxic T lymphocytes was inversely correlated with marrow cellularity and blast cell percentage, and positively with Fas antigen expression on CD34+ clonal progenitor cells [80]. The cytotoxic reaction against marrow CD34+ cells of MDS patients has a well-defined signal transduction pathway in the T cells and can be augmented *in vitro* with the exogenous addition of IL-2 [81]. The strength of this reaction has not been associated with any TNF-α-, IL-10-, or lymphotoxin gene polymorphism, although as it is well-known that these polymorphisms appear to influence the severity of acute GVHD, following allogeneic hematopoietic stem-cell transplantation [82].

We also investigated the behavior of the clonal CD34+ progenitors as stimulant population in mixed cultures with autologous T lymphocytes as responder cells, in other words the immune reaction when T cells are in close contact with clonal stem cells. We compared this type of reaction (autologous progenitor cell mixed lymphocyte reaction—APLR) with the classical types of MLRs. APLR reflects the strength of the immune reaction against the clone in a background of established relative immune tolerance. We tested APLR in 20 MDS patients and 10 healthy controls. We noticed significant differences in the strength of the reaction between patients and controls, as well as between the various subtypes of MDS. Results are shown in **Table 6**. Among normal subjects APLR was rather a mild proliferative reaction, less than half strong as AMLR and about six- to sevenfold weaker than Allo-MLR. Among MDS patients, APLR was significantly stronger than in controls ($p = 0.048$, unpublished data, see **Table 6**). Stimulation index ranged between 1.8 and 26.0 in patients, and between 1.4 and 3.0 in controls. Thus, APLR was the only MLR in which MDS patients exhibited stronger reactions than controls and with high variability [83]. In particular, patients without excess of blasts had APLR similar to normal subjects, whereas patients with RAEB showed significantly stronger reactions. Specifically, a subgroup of four RAEB patients exhibited very strong reactions with a SI >10, significantly higher than the remaining MDS patients, although the same patients developed weak responses against autologous and allogeneic non-T cell stimuli. As mentioned earlier, in all healthy controls the ratio APLR/AMPR was always <1. In patients with RA or RARS this ratio was around 1 but in some of them higher than 1, whereas in patients with RAEB, APLR/AMLR ratio was substantially higher than 1. Thus, the three subject groups tested with MLRs (low-risk MDS, high-risk MDS, and controls) could be compartmentalized in three different areas in the plot (see **Figure 1**).

FAB Group	N	cpm (Mean ± SEM)	Stim. Index (Mean ± SEM)	p	APLR pt/APLR control
RA	4	2334 ± 382	2.88 ± 0.41	0.173	1.21 ± 0.11
RAS	5	2365 ± 385	2.77 ± 0.18	0.109	1.34 ± 0.13
RAEB	8	7502 ± 1194	10.35 ± 2.46	**0.001**	3.92 ± 0.74
CMML	3	3488 ± 556	4.55 ± 0.25	**<0.001**	1.43 ± 0.12
All patients	20	4582 ± 735	6.09 ± 1.27	**0.048**	2.39 ± 0.85
Controls	10	1866 ± 308	2.21 ± 0.31		
RAEB	8	7502 ± 1194	10.35 ± 2.46		
Other MDS	12		3.26 ± 0.95	**0.004**	

Table 6. Autologous progenitor cell mixed lymphocyte reaction (APLR) Counts per min and stimulation index Bold letters/numbers indicate statistically significant differences.

Our results have been confirmed by Chamuleau et al., who demonstrated increased non-MHC-restricted autologous cytotoxicity against clonal marrow precursors in eight patients with lower risk MDS, possibly indicating immune surveillance against clonal expansion although they have not provided clinical data on its significance [59]. Suppression may not be restricted against the dysplastic clone and may also affect nonclonal (normal) hematopoiesis. Lymphocyte-depleted long-term bone marrow cultures from patients with lower risk MDS also generated some nonclonal hematopoietic colony growth, which was abrogated when T lymphocytes were present in the culture system [82]. Autologous lymphocytes were particularly cytotoxic in patients with hypoplastic MDS, trisomy 8, or bearing the DR15 allele [84]. The suppressive role of autologous T lymphocytes has been very nicely demonstrated in a patient with MDS and cyclic hematopoiesis, in whom, the percentage of marrow CD3+ lymphocytes was inversely correlated with neutrophil and platelet count during the various phases of ineffective hematopoiesis [85].

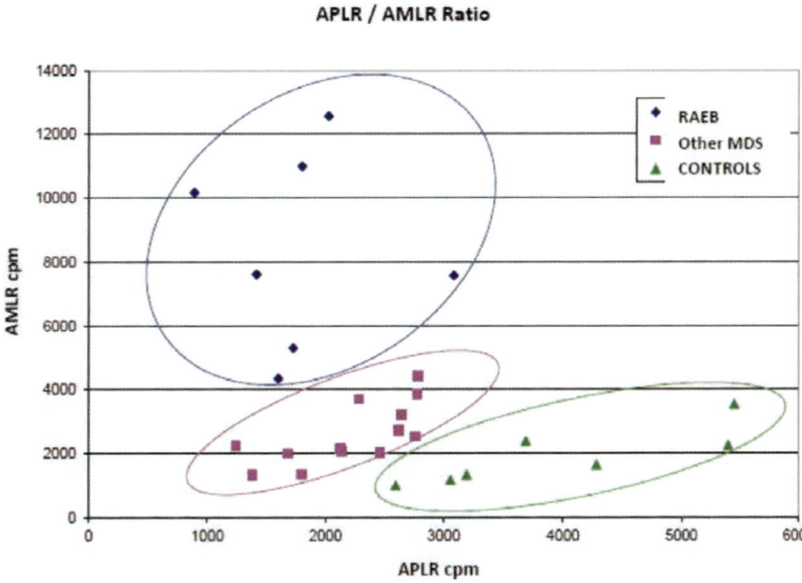

Figure 1. Correlation of AMLR to APLR in each subject tested with MLRs. By correlating AMLR to APLR an almost complete, discrete compartmentalization of the three main subject groups was found. Normal controls exhibited higher AMLR than APLR, patients with lower risk MDS had lower, both types of MLRs, whereas patients with an excess of marrow blasts showed impaired AMLR and very increased APLR.

6.4. The role of clonal hematopoietic cells in the induction of immune dysregulation

The strong MLR against autologous clonal CD34+ progenitors observed in patients with RAEB was inversely correlated with marrow cellularity. All four patients with a strong APLR had marrow cellularity of <35% and marrow blast cell percentage of 5–10% (RAEB-1). These patients, although severely pancytopenic and transfusion dependent, had a delayed evolution to AML or they did not progressed at all. In two of them who progressed, marrow cellularity was increased and in a new APLR, performed at the time of AML progression, lymphocyte activation against autologous blasts had been abrogated [86]. Thus, it appears that lymphocyte activation in patients with RAEB is rather inversely correlated with leukemic burden, but immunologic memory for this reaction is maintained and patients who lose their immune activation during leukemic transformation may regain it following the achievement of remission. Moreover, maintenance of remission is completely dependent on the presence of autologous cytotoxicity against leukemic cells, mainly exerted by NK cells. This cytotoxic reaction is disappeared upon relapse of the leukemia [87]. Unfortunately, immune activation against clonal cells is not the rule and T cells in MDS (particularly $T_{\gamma\delta}$ cells) may respond poorly, if not at all, even following IL-2 stimulation, despite normal IL-2R expression, demonstrating impaired immune surveillance against the clone [51]. Indeed, the Czech group did not find any significant lymphocyte activation in eight out of nine patients tested and confirmed the nonclonal origin of the T cells [71].

Clonal dendritic cells can also induce T-cell stimulation in AML. Proliferative reaction against these cells is high but results in the generation of cytotoxic T lymphocytes with low activity against autologous or allogeneic nonleukemic targets [88]. Dendritic cells of MDS patients in Allo-MLR systems are poor stimulators for both normal and MDS-derived T cells, indicating an impaired antigen presenting capacity. These cells, generated from CD34+ cells, although immunophenotypically normal, were significantly decreased as were also the populations or circulating myeloid- and plasmacytoid-derived dendritic cells, confirming ineffective "dendritopoiesis" [89] and produce less IL-12 and more IL-10 in response to LPS and IFN-γ showing qualitative and quantitative defects of cytokine production.

Blast cells exert direct suppressor activity on the activation, TH1 polarization and proliferation of T lymphocytes. This activity is mediated through protein substances transcribed via the NF-AT and NF-kB signals by inhibition of transition from G_0 to G_1 phase [90]. Upon NK cells, leukemic cells induce impaired killing capacity, reduced TNF-α and IFN-γ production, reduced CD107α degranulation, downregulation of the NKp46- and upregulation of the NKG2A receptor expression, effects directed via IL-10, and favoring clonal escape and expansion [91]. In other instances, however, blast cells induce lymphocyte activation, as previously described, with the production of IL-2, IL-4, IL-10, IL-13, and IFN-γ. Lymphocyte culture supernatants, when further activated with IL-2, generate strong cytotoxic LAK and NK cells inducing lysis of autologous and allogeneic leukemic cells [92]. In the majority of cases, immune effector function of NK-T and NK cells, observed in some patients with MDS, are abolished on leukemic transformation.

7. Immunopathogenetic aspects of myelodysplastic syndromes

From the pathogenetic point of view it appears that an initial, harmful event (viral, drug, irradiation, etc.), affecting the pluripotent hematopoietic stem cell compartment in the bone marrow, may antigenically alter a minor population of these cells. Even when the consequences of the harmful event are negligible and maturation and differentiation processes might remain almost intact, it is possible that an immunologic reaction could be initiated. This reaction is directed against the even minimally modulated hematopoietic progenitor cell population. Indeed, the strength of the autologous cytotoxic immune reaction, frequently accompanying the emergence of a dysplastic clone, is not related to the complexity/severity of the cytogenetic abnormalities, and a minor genetic damage may induce a strong reaction. Conversely, complex chromosomal aberrations and other gross genetic damage, leading to hematopoietic failure, may induce a weak or not any immune reaction. This reaction may be less specific and may also generate cytotoxicity, not only against the affected cells, but also to the unaffected/normal hematopoietic progenitors, inducing apoptosis and resulting in stem-cell depletion and hematopoietic failure. Soluble factors (cytokines) released by the activated lymphocytes might also harm accessory/stromal cells. This cascade of events usually leads to aplastic anemia. When the initial harmful event induces deeper genetic damage in a pluripotent stem cell and this cell, although genetically altered, succeeds in escaping from apoptotic cell death may generate an abnormal (dysplastic) clone. Clonal cells continue to trigger the immunocompetent cells, but the latter although activated cannot eliminate the clonal cells, which continue to escape, gradually expand, and suppress the unaffected/normal stem cell compartment through at least two mechanisms:

(1) Immune effector cytotoxic cells can destroy more easily the nonclonal/normal progenitor cells as a result of clonal cell escape from the immune attack.

(2) Secondary genetic alterations occurring gradually provide growth advantage to the clonal cells.

Thus, immune activation may perpetuate and when cytotoxic activity is ineffective and incapable to eliminate clonal cells, it becomes an "immunologic abnormality." The more effective the immune activation, the higher the degree of apoptosis induced, affecting more and more marrow cellularity and creating a syndrome mostly similar to aplastic anemia. Therefore, the decreased marrow cellularity observed in some marrow failure syndromes might be considered an "adverse event" of an effective immune reaction capable to restrict the growth of the abnormal/mutated/genetically altered clonal cell population. On rare occasions, the intensive immune activation, augmented by an infection or a blood transfusion, may be capable to completely eradicate the dysplastic clone leading to spontaneous complete remission even after evolution to AML. In contrast, when immune activation is ineffective, clonal expansion and evolution continues unimpededly until the stage of AML. At this stage, either passively, due to high "antigenic burden," or actively, through mechanisms, induced by the leukemic cells, immune tolerance or immune paralysis is established abrogating further immune reaction [93]. In rare instances, even after evolution, immune activation may be maintained and result in an oligoblastic/hypoplastic AML. Conversely, when immune activation is abolished early or when the dysplastic/neoplastic clone achieves in earning immune tolerance, the evolution might be uneventful and lead to a hypercellular AML.

About 10–15% of MDS patients at initial presentation have a hypoplastic marrow (cellularity ≤30%). These patients exhibit more severe cytopenias, various degrees of trilineage dysplasia, more prominent immune abnormalities, and usually a normal karyotype or single chromosomal abnormalities. Although hypoplastic MDS share many similarities with aplastic anemia, different molecular mechanisms of marrow damage have been identified between them and other/nonhypoplastic MDS. Among them development of oligoclonal expansion of cytotoxic T lymphocytes, overexpression of TRAIL- and Fas ligand-induced apoptosis, underexpression of Flice-like inhibitory protein long isoform (FLIPL), and increased production of IFN-γ and TNF-α are included. Patients with hypolastic MDS have more stable clinical course and lower evolution rates in relation to patients with nonhypoplastic disease of the same FAB/WHO categories. They show good response to treatment with corticosteroids, cyclosporine-A, antithymocyte globulin, or alemtuzumab, and to various combinations of the above. Overall survival varies and if patients will not succumb to a severe infection, they may retain a prolonged leukemia-free survival [94, 95].

Suppressor/cytotoxic autoimmune reactions are more frequently identified among lower risk MDS, have specificity against the pluripotent or an early committed, usually erythropoietic progenitor cell, and are associated with higher degree of marrow apoptosis. In the majority of cases, the autoimmune process includes the production of specific antierythroblastic antibodies without the positivity of direct antiglobulin test. The production of such IgG autoantibodies can be provoked *ex vivo* following antigenic stimulation [96]. These patients show higher caspace-3 activity and lower TNF-α and IL-4 production. Analysis of the total IgM and IgG antibody repertoire in 10 MDS patients without prominent autoimmune disease or known autoantibody and in 10 healthy controls revealed different patterns of antibodies against self-antigens in MDS patients from those of controls, and patterns of IgG antibodies had distinct profiles implying disturbed self-recognition related to pathogenetic mechanisms of the disease [97].

Increased marrow apoptosis is a dominant feature of MDS and affects all hematopoietic cell compartments from the more immature-undifferentiated to the mature and recognizable cells. The apoptotic rate of CD34+ cells in normal subjects has been calculated at about 1%, whereas in MDS, it ranges from 3 to 15%. Higher apoptotic rate is usually found in patients with early MDS and in few patients with an excess of blasts [98]. Apoptotic rate may vary in the same patient at different time points reflecting also the evolution of mutational status of the clonal cells. Specific cytogenetic abnormalities, such as trisomy 8 have been associated with higher degree of apoptosis. Apoptosis is a multifactorial process in MDS with a possible contribution of the immune effector cells. Clonal cells' death could create abnormal structures with potentially (auto)antigenic properties and apoptosis can represent the causative factor of the initiation of autologous cytotoxic immune reaction. Indeed, increased apoptotic cell rate has been associated with higher marrow cytotoxic T-cell infiltration and in many instances by oligoclonal T cells in MDS patients, who also express the TIA-1 antigen on their hematopoietic cells [99]. The proapoptotic marrow microenvironment triggers stromal cells to produce IL-32, which in turn induces further TNF-α transcription, thus establishing a vicious cycle. IL-32 expression has been found many folds higher in the stromal cells of MDS patients, rendering this cytokine a specific stromal cell marker for MDS [100].

Although immune activation plays the dominant pathogenetic role for the generation of marrow failure in aplastic anemia, in MDS this cannot be easily identified in every individual patient. In other words, it is not identifiable which part of the hematopoietic failure results from the clonal disorder *per se* and which is attributed to the immune activation. This fact could explain, at least in part, why there is not a uniform response rate to the immunosuppressive treatment and this rate may vary widely in different series of patients, irrespective of FAB or WHO category, cytogenetics, and the severity of the cytopenias [101].

8. Immunosuppressive/immunomodulating treatment applied to patients with MDS

Corticosteroids are the most widely used immunosuppressive treatment administered to patients with MDS and autoimmune diseases [17, 20]. Response rates vary broadly and the required dose depends on the type of autoimmune disease, MDS subtype, chronicity of the condition, and other factors. Although symptom resolution may be fast, autoimmune disease may relapse during tapering, demanding higher doses, which may not be tolerable by elderly patients. Thus, corticosteroids usually lead to partial or transient response and second-line treatment with other agents is necessary. Steroids may also benefit hematopoiesis, improving cytopenias and reducing RBC transfusion needs. Responses are mainly seen in patients with lower risk IPSS, with a specific profile, but also by some patients with RAEB [102] and may be long-lasting and maintained with small maintenance steroid doses.

Cyclosporin-A (Cy-A) is the second more widely used immunosuppressive agent and has also been used in combination with cytotoxic chemotherapy as a modulator of multidrug resistance, which is commonly found in higher risk MDS and in AML following MDS. Cy-A is effective even at lower doses, aiming to achieve serum levels lower than those desirable in aplastic anemia and in allogeneic stem cell transplantation and therefore is well-tolerated and induces durable remissions [103, 104]. Retrospective evaluation of 50 patients showed a hematological improvement and particularly an erythroid response in 60%. Better response was achieved by patients with hypoplastic marrow, favorable karyotype, or carrying the DRB1*1501 allele [105]. The NIH group has reported more frequent expression of the HLA-DR2/HLA-DR15 allele in patients with MDS and aplastic anemia compared to a control population and an association of the expression of this allele with a favorable response to immunosuppression [106]. Cy-A added to T-lymphocyte cultures decreases IFN-γ- but not Fas-L production and lead to abrogation of the inhibitory activity of the supernatant on hematopoietic colony formation. However, the growth of secondary colonies continues to be decreased due to low number of pluripotent CD34+ progenitors.

Probably the most effective immunosuppressive treatment is antithymocyte globulin (ATG), which has been given to MDS patients with any marrow cellularity [101, 104]. Hematopoietic improvement is achieved following elimination of the autoreactive cytotoxic T cells and may result in restoration of the dysplastic marrow and peripheral blood morphology. In many instances cytogenetic complete remission has also been reported, whereas in others, hematologic remission is not accompanied by cytogenetic remission. In these cases, most probably immune activation mainly suppresses nonclonal hematopoiesis without significantly disturbing the dysplastic clone. Finally, rapid evolution to AML or increase of marrow blasts despite hematological improvement has occasionally been reported following treatment with Cy-A or

ATG [107]. In these cases, immune activation may effectively suppress clonal cells and its abrogation has favored the unimpeded clonal expansion and evolution. Mofetil mycophenolate (MMF) or alemtuzumab can be used when corticosteroids and/or Cy-A are ineffective or contraindicated, or when severe adverse effects emerge, but the experience with these agents is limited. The main drawback of immunosuppression is that combined with the usually coexisting neutropenia substantially increases the risk for common and opportunistic infections, even when all prophylactic measures are applied. Cy-A, in particular, may further impair previously existed renal failure and may induce various adverse events as a result of pharmacodynamic interactions to patients concommittantly treated with many other drugs.

Immune-stimulating treatment, targeting NK-/NK-T cells and aiming to generate cytotoxic T-cell activity and eliminate the dysplastic clone, has been associated with rather disappointing results. A promising message is that newer immunomodulating drugs, such as lenalidomide, appear to increase NK T cells and improve their function, including cytokine production, although this is not the major mechanism of action of the drug [108]. Hypomethylating agents, currently used particularly in higher risk patients, when effective and leading to complete response may also benefit autoimmune or hyperimmune clinical syndromes associated with MDS. It has also been suggested that 5-azacytidine has an independent immune-modulating activity and that remissions of the auto-/hyperimmune syndrome may occur independently of the induction of hematological and cytogenetic response, and might also be effective in cases in which other immunosuppressive treatments have been proved ineffective [109].

The injudicious use of immunosuppressive treatment in MDS may become a trench knife [110]. Patients exhibiting overactive immune response, but clonal hematopoiesis, even when sharing a hypoplastic bone marrow, might need even more effective immune activation to wear down the dysplastic clone. Similarly, patients with an established clonal disease, but without any immune activation, could potentially gain benefit with the administration of immune stimulation in an effort to eliminate the clone. On the other hand, abrogation of an overactive immune stimulation should be attempted when this activation suppresses primarily the residual normal/nonclonal hematopoiesis and minimally disturbs the development of the abnormal/dysplastic clone. When immune activation/reaction status cannot be identified and/or quantified, in the middle of established dysplastic hematopoiesis, a course of moderately strong immunosuppressive treatment with corticosteroids and/or cyclosporine could be administered, and in cases of a favorable response, careful tapering of the drugs should be tested in an effort to maintain the obtained response.

Author details

Argiris Symeonidis* and Alexandra Kouraklis-Symeonidis

*Address all correspondence to: argiris.symeonidis@yahoo.gr

Hematology Division, Department of Internal Medicine, University Hospital of Patras, Patras, Greece

References

[1] Fianchi L, Leone G, Posteraro B et al. Impaired bactericidal and fungicidal activities of neutrophils in patients with myelodysplastic syndrome. Leuk Res. 2012;36:331–333. DOI: 10.1016/j.leukres.2011.11.012.

[2] Tatsumi G, Watanabe M, Kaneko H, Hirata H, Tsudo M. Multiple splenic abscesses in two patients with myelodysplastic syndrome. Intern Med. 2012;51:1573–1577. DOI: 10.2169/internalmedicine.51.7267.

[3] Yamaguchi N, Ito Y, Ohyashiki K. Increased intracellular activity of matrix metalloproteinases in neutrophils may be associated with delayed healing of infection without neutropenia in myelodysplastic syndromes. Ann Hematol. 2005;84:383–388. DOI: 10.1007/s00277-0040965-5.

[4] Oren H, Ucar C, Gülen H, Duman M, Irken G. Autoimmune hemolytic anemia occurring with myelodysplastic syndrome: report of a pediatric case and review of the literature. Ann Hematol. 2001;80:540–542. DOI: 10.1007/s002770100332.

[5] Jaeger U, Panzer S, Bartram C et al. Autoimmune-thrombocytopenia and SLE in a patient with 5q-anomaly and deletion of the c-fms oncogene. Am J Hematol. 1994;45:79–80. DOI: 10.1002/ajh.2830450112.

[6] Kuroda J, Kimura S, Kobayashi Y, Wada K, Uoshima N, Yoshikawa T. Unusual myelodysplastic syndrome with the initial presentation mimicking idiopathic thrombocytopenic purpura. Acta Haematol. 2002;108:139–143. DOI: 10.1159/000064703

[7] Houwerzijl EJ, Blom NR, van der Want JJ, Vellenga E, de Wolf JT. Megakaryocytic dysfunction in MDS and idiopa-thic thrombocytopenic purpura is in part due to different forms of cell death. Leukemia 2006;20:1937–1942. DOI: 10.1038/sj.leu.2404385.

[8] Symeonidis A, Kouraklis A, Patsouris E, Kittas C, Zoumbos N. Coexistence of chronic myelomonocytic leukemia and peripheral T-cell lymphoma in a patient presented with autoimmune thrombocytopenia and monoclonal hyper-γ-globulinemia. Haema 1999;2:31–36.

[9] Billström R, Johansson H, Johansson B, Mitelman F. Immune-mediated complications in patients with myelodysplastic syndromes: clinical and cytogenetic features. Eur J Haematol. 1995;55:42–48. DOI: 10.1111/j.1600-0609.1995.tb00231.x.

[10] Gupta R, Soupir CP, Johari V, Hasserjian RP. MDS with isolated del-20q: an indolent disease with minimal morphological dysplasia and frequent thrombocytopenic presentation. Br J Haematol. 2007;139:265–268. DOI: 10.1111/j.1365-2141.2007.06776.x.

[11] Peker D, Padron E, Bennett JM et al. A close association of autoimmune-mediated processes and autoimmune disorders with chronic myelomonocytic leukemia: observation from a single institution. Acta Haematol. 2015;133:249–256. DOI: 10.1159/000365877.

[12] Kim KJ, Kwok SK, Park YJ, Kim WU, Cho CS. Low C3 levels is associated with neutropenia in a proportion of patients with myelodysplastic syndrome: retrospective analysis. Int J Rheum Dis. 2012;15:86–94. DOI: 10.1111/j.1756-185X.2012.01704.x.

[13] Kulasekararaj AG, Kordasti S, Basu T, Salisbury JR, Mufti GJ, du Vivier AW. Chronic relapsing remitting Sweet syndrome—a harbinger of myelodysplastic syndrome. Br J Haematol. 2015;170:649–656. DOI: 10.1111/bjh.13485.

[14] Saif MW, Hopkins JL, Gore SD. Autoimmune phenomena in patients with myelodysplastic syndromes and chronic myelomonocytic leukemia. Leuk Lymphoma. 2002;43:2083–2092. DOI: 10.1080/1042819021000016186.

[15] Diebold L, Rauh G, Jäger K, Löhrs U. Bone marrow pathology in relapsing polychondritis: high frequency of myelodysplastic syndromes. Br J Haematol. 1995;89:820–830. DOI: 10.1111/j.1365-2141.1995.tb08420.x.

[16] Coha B, Fustar-Preradovic L, Sekelj S, Sekelj A. Total hearing loss and blindness caused by relapsing polychondritis and myelodysplastic syndrome. Eur Arch Otorhinolaryngol. 2007;264:1517–1519. DOI: 10.1007/s00405-007-0387-9.

[17] Marisavljevic D, Kraguljac N, Rolovic Z. Immunologic abnormalities in myelodysplastic syndromes: clinical features and characteristics of the lymphoid population. Med Oncol. 2006;23:385–391. DOI: 10.1385/MO:23:3:385.

[18] Okamoto T, Okada M, Mori A, Saheki K, Takatsuka H, Wada H. Correlation between immunological abnormalities and prognosis in myelodysplastic syndrome patients. Int J Hematol. 1997;66:345–351.

[19] Giannouli S, Voulgarelis M. A comprehensive review of myelodysplastic syndrome patients, with autoimmune diseases. Expert Rev Clin Immunol. 2014;10:1679–1688. DOI: 10.1586/1744666X.2014.970181.

[20] Mekinian A, Grignano E, Braun T et al. Systemic inflammatory and auto-immune manifestations associated with myelodysplastic syndromes and chronic myelomonocytic leukemia: a French multicentre retrospective study. Rheumatology (Oxford) 2016;55:291–300. DOI: 10.1093/rheumatology/kev294.

[21] Giannouli S, Tzoanopoulos D, Ritis K, Kartalis G, Moutsopoulos HM, Voulgarelis M. Autoimmune manifestations in human myelodysplasia: a positive correlation with interferon regulatory factor-1 (IRF-1) expression. Ann Rheum Dis. 2004;63:578–582. DOI: 10.1136/ard.2003.012948.

[22] Pinheiro RF, Metze K, Silva MR, Chauffaille Mde L. The ambiguous role of interferon regulatory factor-1 (IRF-1) immunoexpression in myelodysplastic syndrome. Leuk Res. 2009;33:1308–1312. DOI: 10.1016/j.leukres.2009.03.008.

[23] Komrokji RS, Kulasekararaj A, Al Ali NH et al. Autoimmune diseases and myelodysplastic syndromes. Am J Hematol. 2016;91:E280-283 DOI: 10.1002/ajh.24333.

[24] Tabata R, Tabata C, Omori K, Nagai T. Disappearing myelodysplastic syndrome-associated hemolytic anemia in leukemic transformation. Int Arch Allergy Immunol. 2010;152:407–412. DOI: 10.1159/000288294

[25] Knox S, Greenberg B, Anderson R, Rosenblatt S. Studies on T-lymphocytes in preleukemic disorders and acute nonlymphocytic leukemia: in vitro radiosensitivity, mitogenic responsiveness, colony formation and enumeration of lymphocytic subpopulations. Blood 1983;61:449–455.

[26] Ayanlar-Batuman O, Shevitz J, Traub U et al. Lymphocyte interleukin-2 production and responsiveness are altered in patients with primary myelodysplastic syndromes. Blood 1987;70:494–500.

[27] Kerndrup G, Meyer K, Ellegaard J, Hockland P. NK cell activity and antibody dependent cellular cytotoxicity in primary myelodysplastic syndromes. Leuk.Res. 1984;8:239–247.

[28] Symeonidis A, Kourakli A, Katevas P et al. Immune function parameters at diagnosis in patients with myelodysplastic syndromes: correlation with FAB classification and prognosis. Eur J Haematol. 1991;47:277–281. DOI: 10.1111/j.1600-0609.1991.tb01571.x.

[29] Iwase O, Aizawa S, Kuriyama Y, Yaguchi M, Nakano M, Toyama K. Analysis of bone marrow and peripheral blood immunoregulatory lymphocytes in patients with myelodysplastic syndrome. Ann Hematol. 1995;71:293–299. DOI: 10.1007/BF01697982.

[30] Hilbe W, Eisterer W, Schmid C et al. Bone marrow lymphocyte subsets in myelodysplastic syndromes. J Clin Pathol. 1994;47:505–507. DOI: 10.1136/jcp.47.6.505.

[31] Tsuda H, Yamasaki H. Type I and type II T-cell profiles in aplastic anemia and refractory anemia. Am J Hematol. 2000;64:271–274. DOI: 10.1002/1096-8652(200008)64:4<271::AID-AJH6>3.0.CO;2-C.

[32] Hamdi W, Ogawara H, Handa H, Tsukamoto N, Murakami H. Clinical significance of Th1/Th2 ratio in patients with myelodysplastic syndrome. Int J Lab Hematol. 2009;31:630–638. DOI: 10.1111/j.1751-553X.2008.01090.x

[33] Meers S, Vandenberghe P, Boogaerts M, Verhoef G, Delforge M. The clinical significance of activated lymphocytes in patients with myelodysplastic syndromes: a single centre study of 131 patients. Leuk Res. 2008;32:1026–1035. DOI: http://dx.doi.org/10.1016/j.leukres.2007.10.004

[34] Li X, Xu F, He Q, Wu L, Zhang Z, Chang C. Comparison of immunological abnormalities of lymphocytes in bone marrow in myelodysplastic syndrome (MDS) and aplastic anemia (AA). Intern Med. 2010;49:1349–1355. DOI: 10.2169/internalmedicine.49.3477

[35] Epling-Burnette PK, Painter JS, Rollison DE et al. Prevalence and clinical association of clonal T-cell expansions in myelodysplastic syndrome. Leukemia 2007;21:659–667. DOI: 10.1038/sj.leu.2404590

[36] Symeonidis A, Kouraklis A, Katevas P, Zoumbos N. Impaired cutaneous hypersensitivity in patients with myelodysplastic syndromes. 14th Meeting Int. Soc of Hematology, Stoccholm, 30.8–4.9.1997, Abstr. P-278, p. 130.

[37] Kordasti SY, Ingram W, Hayden J et al. CD4+CD25high Foxp3+ regulatory T cells in myelodysplastic syndrome. Blood 2007;110:847–850. DOI: 10.1182/blood-2007-01-067546.

[38] Fozza C, Longu F, Contini S et al. Patients with early-stage myelodysplastic syndromes show increased frequency of CD4+CD25+CD127(low) regulatory T cells. Acta Haematol. 2012;128:178–182. DOI: 10.1159/000339498.

[39] Kotsianidis I, Bouchliou I, Nakou E et al. Kinetics, function and bone marrow trafficking of CD4+CD25+FOXP3+ regulatory T cells in myelodysplastic syndromes. Leukemia 2009;23:510–518. DOI: 10.1038/leu.2008.333.

[40] Mailloux AW, Sugimori C, Komrokji RS et al. Expansion of effector memory regulatory T cells represents a novel prognostic factor in lower risk myelodysplastic syndrome. J Immunol. 2012;189:3198–3208. DOI: 10.4049/jimmunol.1200602.

[41] Kordasti SY, Afzali B, Lim Z et al. IL-17-producing CD4(+) T cells, pro-inflammatory cytokines and apoptosis are increased in low risk myelodysplastic syndrome. Br J Haematol. 2009;145:64–72. DOI: 10.1111/j.1365-2141.2009.07593.x.

[42] Shao LL, Zhang L, Hou Y et al. Th22 cells as well as Th17 cells expand differentially in patients with early-stage and late-stage myelodysplastic syndrome. PLoS One 2012;7:e51339. DOI: 10.1371/journal.pone.0051339.

[43] Kiladjian JJ, Visentin G, Viey E et al. Activation of cytotoxic $T_{\gamma\delta}$-cell receptor lymphocytes in response to specific stimulation in myelodysplastic syndromes. Haematologica 2008;93:381–389. DOI: 10.3324/haematol.11812.

[44] Amin HM, Jilani I, Estey EH et al. Increased apoptosis in bone marrow B lymphocytes but not T lymphocytes in myelodysplastic syndrome. Blood 2003;102:1866–1868. DOI: http://dx.doi.org/10.1182/blood-2003-01-0221.

[45] Sternberg A, Killick S, Littlewood T et al. Evidence for reduced B-cell progenitors in early (low-risk) myelodysplastic syndrome. Blood 2005;106:2982–2991. DOI: http://dx.doi.org/10.1182/blood-2005-04-1543.

[46] Ribeiro E, Matarraz S, Santiago M et al. Maturation-associated immunophenotypic abnormalities in bone marrow B-lymphocytes in myelodysplastic syndromes. Leuk Res. 2006;30:9–16. DOI: http://dx.doi.org/10.1016/j.leukres.2005.05.019

[47] Okada M, Okamoto T, Takemoto Y, Kanamaru A, Kakishita E. Function and X chromosome inactivation analysis of B-lymphocytes in myelodysplastic syndromes with immunological abnormalities. Acta Haematol. 2000;102:124–130. DOI: 10.1159/000040985.

[48] Billstrom R, Johansson B, Strömbeck B et al. Clonal CD5+ B lymphocytes in myelodysplastic syndrome with systemic vasculitis and trisomy 8. Ann Hematol. 1997;74:37–40. DOI: 10.1007/s002770050253.

[49] Mufti GJ, Figes A, Hamblin TJ, Oscier DG, Copplestone JA. Immunological abnormalities in myelodysplastic syndromes: I. Serum immunoglobulins and autoantibodies. Br J Haematol. 1986;63:143–147. DOI: 10.1111/j.1365-2141.1986.tb07504.x.

[50] Symeonidis A, Kouraklis-Symeonidis A, Onoufriou A, Zoumbos N. Prognostic significance of serum protein electro-phoresis pattern changes in patients with myelodysplastic syndromes. Leuk Res. 21 (suppl. 1): S18, abstr. 66, 1997. DOI: 10.1016/S0145-2126(97)81280-5.

[51] Demeter J, Schmid M, Vargha P, Porzsolt F. Correlation of elevated plasma soluble IL-2R levels with defective NK and CD8+ T-cells in myelodysplastic syndromes: is it part of a spectrum? Leuk Res. 1995;19:583–584. DOI: http://dx.doi.org/10.1016/0145-2126(95)00021-F.

[52] Kiladjian JJ, Bourgeois E, Lobe I et al. Cytolytic function and survival of NK cells are severely altered in myelodysplastic syndromes. Leukemia 2006;20:463–470. DOI: 10.1038/sj.leu.2404080

[53] Eliopoulos GD, Coulocheri SA, Eliopoulos AG et al. Mechanisms accounting for the impaired natural-killer cell activity in refractory anemia with excess of blasts. Eur J Haematol. 1992;48:237–243. DOI: 10.1111/j.1600-0609.1992.tb01800.x.

[54] Epling-Burnette PK, Bai F, Painter JS et al. Reduced natural killer (NK) function associated with high-risk myelodysplastic syndrome (MDS) and reduced expression of activating NK receptors. Blood 2007;109:4816–4824. DOI: http://dx.doi.org/10.1182/blood-2006-07-035519.

[55] Carlsten M, Baumann BC, Simonsson M et al. Reduced DNAM-1 expression on bone marrow NK cells associated with impaired killing of CD34+ blasts in myelodysplastic syndrome. Leukemia 2010;24:1607–1616. DOI: 10.1038/leu.2010.149.

[56] Pan L, Ohnishi K, Zhang WJ et al. In vitro IL-12 treatment of peripheral blood mononuclear cells from patients with leukemia or myelodysplastic syndromes: increase in cytotoxicity and reduction in WT1 gene expression. Leukemia 2000;14:1634–1641. DOI: 0887-6924/00.

[57] Hejazi M, Manser AR, Fröbel J et al. Impaired cytotoxicity associated with defective natural killer cell differentiation in myelodysplastic syndromes. Haematologica 2015;100:643–652. DOI: 10.3324/haematol.2014.118679.

[58] Aggarwal N, Swerdlow SH, TenEyck SP, Boyiadzis M, Felgar RE. Natural killer cell (NK) subsets and NK-like T-cell populations in acute myeloid leukemias and myelodysplastic syndromes. Cytometry B Clin Cytom. 2015. DOI: 10.1002/cyto.b.21349.

[59] Chamuleau ME, Westers TM, van Dreunen L et al. Immune mediated autologous cytotoxicity against hematopoietic precursor cells in patients with myelodysplastic syndrome. Haematologica 2009;94:496–506. DOI: 10.3324/haematol.13612.

[60] Zoumbos N, Symeonidis A, Kourakli A, Katevas P, Matsouka P, Perraki M, Georgoulias V. Increased levels of soluble interleukin-2 receptors and tumor necrosis factor in serum of patients with myelodysplastic syndromes. Blood 1991;77:413–414.

[61] Seipelt G, Ganser A, Duranceyk H, Maurer A, Ottmann OG, Hoelzer D. Induction of soluble IL-2 receptor in patients with myelodysplastic syndromes undergoing high-dose IL-3 treatment. Ann Hematol. 1994;68:167–170. DOI: 10.1007/BF01834361.

[62] Wetzler M, Kurzrock R, Estrov Z, Estey E, Talpaz M. Cytokine expression in adherent layers from patients with myelodysplastic syndrome and acute myelogenous leukemia. Leuk Res. 1995;19:23–34. DOI: http://dx.doi.org/10.1016/0145-2126(94)00059-J.

[63] Verhoef GE, De Schouwer P, Ceuppens JL, Van Damme J, Goossens W, Boogaerts MA. Measurement of serum cytokine levels in patients with myelodysplastic syndromes. Leukemia 1992;6:1268–1272.

[64] Musto P, Matera R, Minervini MM et al. Low serum levels of tumor necrosis factor and interleukin-1β in myelodysplastic syndromes responsive to recombinant erythropoietin. Haematologica 1994;79:265–268.

[65] Tsimberidou AM, Estey E, Wen S, Pierce S, Kantarjian H, Albitar M, Kurzrock R. The prognostic significance of cytokine levels in newly diagnosed acute myeloid leukemia and high-risk MDS. Cancer 2008;113:1605–1613. DOI: 10.1002/cncr.23785.

[66] Pardanani A, Finke C, Lasho TL, Al-Kali A, Begna KH, Hanson CA, Tefferi A. IPSS-independent prognostic value of plasma CXCL10, IL-7 and IL-6 levels in myelodysplastic syndromes. Leukemia 2012;26:693–699. DOI: 10.1038/leu.2011.251.

[67] Lopes MR, Traina F, Campos Pde M et al. IL10 inversely correlates with the percentage of CD8+ cells in MDS patients. Leuk Res. 2013;37:541–546. DOI: 10.1016/j.leukres.2013.01.019.

[68] Kasamatsu T, Saitoh T, Minato Y et al. Polymorphisms of IL-10 affect the severity and prognosis of myelodysplastic syndrome. Eur J Haematol. 2016;96:245–251. DOI: 10.1111/ejh.12577.

[69] Opelz G, Kiuchi M, Takasugi M, Terasaki PI. Autologous stimulation of human lymphocyte subpopulation. J Exp Med. 1975;142:1327–1333.

[70] Schwartzentruber D, Topalian S, Mancini M. Specific release of granulocyte-macrophage colony stimulating factor, tumor necrosis factor-α and IFN-γ by human tumor-infiltrating lymphocytes after autologous tumor stimulation. J Immunol. 1991;146:3674.

[71] Cukrova V, Neuwirtova R, Cermak J, Malaskova V, Neuwirt J. Leukocyte-derived inhibitory activity in patients with myelodysplastic syndrome. Blut 1987;55:165–171.

[72] Ohmori M, Ueda Y, Masutani H, Hirama T, Anzai N, Yoshida Y, Okuma M. Myelodysplastic syndrome (MDS)-associated inhibitory activity on haematopoietic progenitor cells: contribution of monocyte-derived lipid containing macrophages (MDLM). Br J Haematol. 1992;81:67–72. DOI: 10.1111/j.1365-2141.1992.tb08173.x.

[73] Symeonidis A, Zoumbos N. Defective autologous and allogeneic mixed lymphocyte reaction in patients with primary myelodysplastic syndromes. Leuk Res. 1991;15(suppl. 1):29. DOI: 10.1016/0145-2126(91)90436-W

[74] Cukrova V, Neuwirtova R, Dolezalova L et al. Defective cytotoxicity of T lymphocytes in myelodysplastic syndrome. Exp Hematol. 2009;37:386–394. DOI: 10.1016/j.exphem.2008.11.001.

[75] Kerndrup G, Hokland P. Natural killer cell-mediated inhibition of bone marrow colony formation in refractory anaemia (preleukaemia): evidence for patient-specific cell populations. Br J Haematol. 1988;69:457–462. DOI: 10.1111/j.1365-2141.1988.tb02398.x.

[76] Alahmad A, Preuss KD, Schenk J et al. Desmoplakin and KIF20B as target antigens in patients with paroxysmal nocturnal haemoglobinuria. Br J Haematol. 2010;151:273–280. doi: 10.1111/j.1365-2141.2010.08345.x

[77] Scheibenbogen C, Letsch A, Thiel E et al. CD8 T-cell responses to Wilms tumor gene product WT1 and proteinase 3 in patients with acute myeloid leukemia. Blood 2002;100:2132–2137. DOI: http://dx.doi.org/10.1182/blood-2002-01-0163.

[78] Sloand EM, Mainwaring L, Fuhrer M et al. Preferential suppression of trisomy 8 compared with normal hematopoietic cell growth by autologous lymphocytes in patients with trisomy 8 MDS. Blood 2005;106:841–851. DOI: http://dx.doi.org/10.1182/blood-2004-05-2017.

[79] Kook H, Zeng W, Guibin C, Kirby M, Young NS, Maciejewski JP. Increased cytotoxic T cells with effector phenotype in aplastic anemia and myelodysplasia. Exp Hematol. 2001;29:1270–1277. DOI: http://dx.doi.org/10.1016/S0301-472X(01)00736-6.

[80] Symeonidis A, Karakantza M, Kouraklis A, Zoumbos N. Activated marrow CD8+ T-lymphocytes influence marrow cellularity, Fas antigen expression on CD34+ cells and disease progression in patients with myelodysplastic syndromes (MDS). Blood 2001;98:276b, abstr. 4841.

[81] Torelli GF, Guarini A, Palmieri G, Breccia M, Vitale A, Santoni A, Foa R. Expansion of cytotoxic effectors with lytic activity against autologous blasts from acute myeloid leukemia patients in complete haematological remission. Br J Haematol. 2002;116:299–307. DOI: 10.1046/j.1365-2141.2002.03277.x.

[82] Baumann I, Scheid C, Koref MS, Swindell R, Stern P, Testa NG. Autologous lymphocytes inhibit hemopoiesis in long-term culture in patients with myelodysplastic syndrome. Exp Hematol. 2002;30:1405–1411. DOI: http://dx.doi.org/10.1016/S0301-472X(02)00968-2.

[83] Symeonidis A, Lafi T, Zoumbos N. Immune regulation of hematopoiesis in myelodysplastic syndromes: increased proliferation of T cells in response to isolated autologous progenitor cells. Blood 1990;76 (suppl. 10):325a.

[84] Zheng Z, Feng X, Xiao L, Qianqiao Z, Qi H, Lingyun W. Removal of autologous activated CD4-positive T lymphocytes also results in increased colony-forming units in patients with low and intermediate-1 risk MDS. Eur J Haematol. 2011;86:47–56. DOI: 10.1111/j.1600-0609.2010.01535.x.

[85] Abe Y, Hirase N, Muta K et al. Adult onset cyclic hematopoiesis in a patient with myelodysplastic syndrome. Int J Hematol. 2000;71:40–45.

[86] Symeonidis A, Kourakli A, Zikos P et al. Hypoplastic refractory anemia with excess of blasts (RAEB). A distinct subtype with specific features and good prognosis. 12th Meeting of ISH, 1993; abst. No 8, page 6.

[87] Lowdell MW, Craston R, Samuel D et al. Evidence that continued remission in patients treated for acute leukemia is dependent upon autologous NK cells. Br J Haematol. 2002;117:821–827. DOI: 10.1046/j.1365-2141.2002.03495.x.

[88] Woiciechowsky A, Regn S, Kolb HJ, Roskrow M. Leukemic dendritic cells generated in the presence of FLT3 ligand have the capacity to stimulate an autologous leukemia-specific cytotoxic T cell response from patients with acute myeloid leukemia. Leukemia 2001;15:246–255. DOI: 0887-6924/01.

[89] Micheva I, Thanopoulou E, Michalopoulou S, Kakagianni T, Kouraklis-Symeonidis A, Symeonidis A, Zoumbos N. Impaired generation of bone marrow CD34-derived dendritic cells with low peripheral blood subsets in patients with myelodysplastic syndrome. Br J Haematol. 2004;126:806–814. DOI: 10.1111/j.1365-2141.2004.05132.x.

[90] Buggins AG, Milojkovic D, Arno MJ, Lea NC, Mufti GJ, Thomas NS, Hirst WJ. Microenvironment produced by acute myeloid leukemia cells prevents T cell activation and proliferation by inhibition of NF-kappaB, c-Myc, and pRb pathways. J Immunol. 2001;167:6021–6030. DOI: 10.4049/jimmunol.167.10.6021.

[91] Stringaris K, Sekine T, Khoder A et al. Leukemia-induced phenotypic and fun-ctional defects in NK cells predict failure to achieve remission in AML. Haematologica 2014;99:836–847. DOI: 10.3324/haematol.2013.087536.

[92] Costello RT, Mallet F, Chambost H, Sainty D, Arnoulet C, Gastaut JA, Olive D. Acute myeloid leukaemia triggering via CD40 induces leukocyte chemoattraction and cytotoxicity against allogenic or autologous leukemic targets. Leukemia 2000;14:123–128.

[93] Schui DK, Singh L, Schneider B, Knau A, Hoelzer D, Weidmann E. Inhibiting effects on the induction of cytotoxic T lymphocytes by dendritic cells pulsed with lysates from AML blasts. Leuk Res. 2002;26:383–389. DOI: http://dx.doi.org/10.1016/S0145-2126(01)00141-2

[94] Serio B, Risitano A, Giudice V, Montuori N, Selleri C. Immunological derangement in hypocellular myelodysplastic syndromes. Transl Med UniSa. 2014;8:31–42.

[95] Symeonidis A, Kouraklis A, Polychronopoulou S et al: Reduced risk of leukemic transformation and prolonged survival for patients with hypoplastic myelodysplastic syndromes. Leuk Res. 2003;27(suppl 1):S67–S68. DOI: http://dx.doi.org/10.1016/S0145-2126(03)00046-8.

[96] Barcellini W, Zaninoni A, Imperiali FG, Boschetti C, Colombi M, Iurlo A, Zanella A. Anti-erythroblast auto-immunity in early myelodysplastic syndromes. Haematologica 2007;92:19–26. DOI: 10.3324/haematol.10546.

[97] Stahl D, Egerer G, Goldschmidt H, Sibrowski W, Kazatchkine MD, Kaveri SV. Altered self-reactive antibody repertoires are a general feature of patients with myelodysplastic syndrome. J Autoimmun. 2001;16:77–86. DOI: 10.1006/jaut.2000.0459.

[98] Tsoplou P, Kouraklis-Symeonidis A, Thanopoulou E et al. Apoptosis in patients with myelodysplastic syndromes: differential involvement of marrow cells in "good" versus "poor" prognosis patients and correlation with apoptosis-related genes. Leukemia 1999;13:1554–1563.

[99] Pülhorn H, Herrmann M, Harms H, Jung A, Baumann I. Apoptotic cells and clonally expanded cytotoxic T cells in bone marrow trephines of patients with myelodysplastic syndrome. Histopathology 2012;61:200–211. DOI: 10.1111/j.1365-2559.2012.04209.x.

[100] Marcondes AM, Mhyre AJ, Stirewalt DL, Kim SH, Dinarello CA, Deeg HJ. Dysregulation of IL-32 in myelodysplastic syndrome and chronic myelomonocytic leukemia modulates apoptosis and impairs NK function. Proc Natl Acad Sci U S A 2008;105:2865–2870. DOI: 10.1073/pnas.0712391105.

[101] Molldrem JJ, Leifer E, Bahceci E et al. Antithymocyte globulin for treatment of the bone marrow failure associated with myelodysplastic syndromes. Ann Intern Med. 2002;137:156–163. DOI:10.7326/0003-4819-137-3-200208060-00007

[102] Ten Oever J, Kuijper PH, Kuijpers AL, Dercksen MW, Vreugdenhil G. Complete remission of MDS RAEB following immunosuppressive treatment in a patient with Sweet's syndrome. Neth J Med. 2009;67:347–350.

[103] Park SJ, Han CW, Lee JH, Eom HS, Lee SH, Jeong DC, Lim JH. Cyclosporine A in the treatment of a patient with immune thrombocytopenia accompanied by myelodysplastic syndrome and nephrotic syndrome. Acta Haematol. 2003;110:36–40. DOI: 10.1159/000072413

[104] Jonásova A, Neuwirtová R, Cermák J et al. Cyclosporin A therapy in hypoplastic MDS patients and certain refractory anaemias without hypoplastic bone marrow. Br J Haematol. 1998;100:304–309. DOI: 10.1046/j.1365-2141.1998.00551.x

[105] Sauntharararajah Y, Nakamura R, Nam JM et al. HLA-DR15 (DR2) is overrepresented in myelodysplastic syndrome and aplastic anemia and predicts a response to immunosuppression in myelodysplastic syndrome. Blood 2002;100:1570–1574.

[106] Selleri C, Maciejewski JP, Catalano L, Ricci P, Andretta C, Luciano L, Rotoli B. Effects of Cy-A on hematopoietic and immune functions in patients with hypoplastic MDS: in vitro and in vivo studies. Cancer 2002;95:1911–1922. DOI: 10.1002/cncr.10915

[107] Olnes MJ, Sloand EM. Targeting immune dysregulation in myelodysplastic syndromes. JAMA 2011;305:814–819. DOI: 10.1001/jama.2011.194

[108] Chan AC, Neeson P, Leeansyah E et al. Testing the NKT cell hypothesis in lenalidomide-treated myelodysplastic syndrome patients. Leukemia 2010;24:592–600. DOI: 10.1038/leu.2009.279

[109] Frietsch JJ, Dornaus S, Neumann T et al. Paraneoplastic inflammation in myelodysplastic syndrome or bone marrow failure: case series with focus on 5-azacytidine and literature review. Eur J Haematol. 2014;93:247–259. DOI: 10.1111/ejh.12311

[110] Steensma DP, Dispenzieri A, Moore SB, Schroeder G, Tefferi A. Antithymocyte globulin has limited efficacy and substantial toxicity in unselected anemic patients with myelodysplastic syndrome. Blood 2003;101:2156–2158. DOI: http://dx.doi.org/10.1182/blood-2002-09-2867.

Chapter 3

Disorders Mimicking Myelodysplastic Syndrome and Difficulties in its Diagnosis

Lale Olcay and Sevgi Yetgin

Additional information is available at the end of the chapter

http://dx.doi.org/10.5772/64422

Abstract

Myelodysplastic morphology of blood cells can be encountered not only in myelodysplastic syndrome (MDS) but also in nonclonal disorders like viral, bacterial, parasitic infections, juvenile rheumatoid arthritis, polyarteritis nodosa, immune thrombocytopenic purpura (ITP), iron deficiency anemia, megaloblastic anemia, dysgranulopoietic neutropenia, congenital neutropenia, cases with microdeletion 22q11.2, malignant lymphoma, after administration of granulocyte colony stimulating factor, chemotherapy, steroids, smoking, alcohol, posttransplantation, copper deficiency also, together with or without cytopenia. Absence of cytogenetic abnormality in 50–70% of cases with MDS, some overlapping morphological and/or pathophysiological features make it challenging to differentiate between MDS and other diseases/disorders like aplastic anemia, refractory ITP, copper deficiency. Transient genetic abnormalities including monosomy 7 in megaloblastic anemia; increased immature myeloid cells in bone marrow of cases with copper, vitamin B12, or folic acid deficiency in the setting of cytopenia and dysmorphism may also lead to the misdiagnosis of MDS. On the other hand, there are also cases of transient MDS. In this chapter, a literature is be presented to draw attention of the readers on the disorders that mimic MDS. Additionally, our personal experiences are also be shared. Awareness of disorders mimicking MDS may prevent over- or underdiagnosis of MDS.

Keywords: secondary myelodysplasia, cell death, cell cycle, transient MDS, apoptosis, rapid cell senescence

1. Introduction

Myelodysplastic syndromes (MDS) are clonal stem cell disorders characterized by ineffective hematopoiesis in bone marrow and cytopenias in peripheral blood. It is heterogeneous reflected by a number of subgroups with different characteristics both in adulthood and childhood [1–11].

A single diagnostic parameter specific to MDS has not been discovered yet, and a considerable number of patients with MDS lack chromosomal abnormality [1, 4]. Currently, the diagnosis of MDS is mainly dependent on quantitative and qualitative dysplastic abnormalities [5]. Establishment of special characteristics of dysplasia like the number of dysplastic cell lines, the percentage of the dysplastic cells, and characteristic megakaryocytes as in del(5q) syndrome are critical in order to be able to assess which subgroup of MDS the patient fits according to the World Health Organization (WHO) classification. Because uni- or multilineage dysplasia may be the only criterion that differentiates the subgroups refractory cytopenia with unilineage dysplasia (RCUD) and refractory cytopenia with multilineage dysplasia (RCMD) [1, 5, 6, 10, 11]. Additionally, for the lineage to be considered as dysplastic, at least 10% of the lineage should display displastic findings [1, 2, 5, 6, 8, 10, 11] both in adulthood and childhood MDS.

	Dyserythropoiesis	Dysgranulopoiesis	Dysmegakaryopoiesis
Peripheric blood	-Anisocytosis -Poikilocytosis -Basophilic stippling	-Nuclear hypolobulation (pseudo-Pelger-Huet cells) -Cytoplasmic hypo/agranulation -Blasts	-Platelet anisocytosis -Giant platelets
Bone marrow	-Nuclear budding Irregular nuclear edges Internuclear bridging -Karyorrhexis -Multinuclearity -Nuclear hyperlobulation -Binuclearity -Megaloblastic changes -Ring sideroblasts -Vacuolization -Periodic acid-Schiff positivity -Cytoplasmic inclusions Incomplete -Hemoglobinization -Fringed cytoplasm -Cytoplasmic bridging	-Anisocytosis -Nuclear hypolobulation (pseudo-Pelger-Huet cells) -Nuclear hypersegmentation -Irregular hypersegmentation -Bizarre nuclear shapes -Decreased granules -Agranularity -Pseudo Chediak Higashi granules -Auer rods	-Micromegakaryocytes -Nuclear hypolobulation -Large monolobular forms -Small binucleated elements -Dispersed nuclei -Degranulation

Table 1. Recent definitions of morphological features of myelodysplasia (adulthood) [2, 5].

http://dx.doi.org/10.5772/64422

Nearly half of which is constituted by refractory cytopenia of childhood (RCC) [4]. Minimal diagnostic criteria for childhood MDS require fulfillment of at least two of the following criteria: sustained, unexplained cytopenia (neutropenia, thrombocytopenia, or anemia); at least bilineage morphologic myelodysplasia; acquired clonal cytogenetic abnormality in hematopietic cells; increased blast count (>5%) [3].

	Dyserythropoiesis	Dysgranulopoiesis	Dysmegakaryopoiesis
Abnormality	-Megaloblastic changes[1] -Lobulated nuclei in erythroblasts (kidney-shaped, bilobulated, multilobulated, bizarre irregular nuclear profile) -Multinuclearity (two or more distinctly separated nuclei of the same or of different sizes) -Cytoplasmic granules or inclusions[2]	-Bizarre nuclear shape[3] -A- or hypogranularity[4] -Nuclear/cytoplasmic (N/C) asyncrony[5] -Pseudo-Pelger anomaly[6]	-Micromegakaryocytes[7] -Small binucleated megakaryocyte[8] -Megakaryocyte with small round separated nuclei[9] -Megakaryocytes with nonlobated round nucleus[10]

[1]Megaloblastic changes: At least 1.5 times the size of a normal poly- or orthochromatic erythroblast with coarse condensation of chromatin and an increased nuclear-to-cytoplasmic ratio or orthochromatic erythroblasts with decreased nuclear-to-cytoplasmic ratio and at least double the size of a normal erythrocyte of the same maturational state.
[2]Cytoplasmic granules or inclusions: Presence of granules or nuclear fragments that can be definitely differentiated from ribosomal RNA.
[3]Bizarre nuclear shape: Abnormal nuclear shape, including irregularly lobulated nuclei of segmented granocytes with chromatin clumping or large twisted bands, large bands or metamyelocytes, multinuclearity (two distinctly separated neutrophilic bands or segmented nuclei).
[4]A- or hypogranularity: Neutrophilic or azurophilic granules should be markedly or completely absent and the cytoplasm of mature neutrophilic granulocytes has to stain pale blue/gray or translucent in the Romanowsky-Giemza stain. All maturation stages except blast cells should be affected.
[5]Nuclear/cytoplasmic (N/C) asyncrony: Mature neutrophilic granulocytes and metamyelocytes with basophilic cytoplasm and myelocytes with neutrophilic cytoplasm.
[6]Pseudo-Pelger anomaly: Mature granulocytes with either a centrally located round to ovoid nucleus (monolobated type) or two round nuclei of similar size connected by a slender chromatin bridge (bilobated type).
[7]Micromegakaryocytes: Mononucleated megakaryocyte with a size comparable to that of a promyelocyte or less, lacking features of a blast cell.
[8]Small binucleated megakaryocyte: Small megakaryocyte with the size of a micromegakaryocyte or slightly larger, with two round well-separated nuclei.
[9]Megakaryocyte with small round separated nuclei: Megakaryocytes of any size with multiple, at least three, round separated nuclei.
[10]Megakaryocytes with nonlobated round nucleus: Megakaryocytes of normal or reduced size with a nonlobated round nucleus and a mature granular cytoplasm.

Table 2. Morphological features of myelodysplasia (childhood-EWOG-MDS Group, 2005) [13].

The unilineage dysplasia in RCUD of adult MDS should have lasted for at least 6 months if no clonal cytogenetic abnormality is found and/or ring sideroblasts are less than 15% [12], so for these patients a repeated bone marrow examination is recommended after a 6 months' observation [5].

The dysplastic changes have been standardized in childhood [13, 14] and adulthood MDS [2, 5, 15, 16] (**Tables 1–4**) being restricted to three lineages as erythroid, granulocytic, and megakaryocytic lineages. Although monocytes are rarely affected in MDS, their presence rather is associated with CMML and AML [5].

	Dyserythropoiesis	Dysgranulopoiesis	Dysmegakaryopoiesis
Abnormality	-Abnormal nuclear lobulation -Multinuclear cells -Nuclear bridges	-Pelger-Huet cells -Hypo- or agranularity -Giant bands (in severe neutropenia, this criteria may not be complied)	-Megakaryocytes with variable size and separated nuclei or round nuclei (absence of megakaryocytes does not rule out RCC)

Table 3. Morphological features of myelodysplasia in refractory cytopenia of childhood (RCC) (WHO, 2008) [14].

Dyserythropoiesis	Dysgranulopoiesis	Dysmegakaryopoiesis
-Polychromasia	Neutrophilic lineage	-Megakaryocyte fragments
-Cleaves in nuclear membrane	-Macropolycyte (PMNL >14 μm)	-Giant granules in thrombocyte
-Pyknosis	-Ring nucleus	-Bothryoid nucleus in megakaryocytes
-Gigantism	-Increase in nuclear chromatin clumping	-Hypogranulation in megakaryocytes
-Punctate basophilia	-Nuclear sticks	
	-Vacuolated cytoplasm	
	-Increased granules/giant granules	
	-Hypergranular promyelocytes	
	-Increased apoptotic forms	
	Eosinophilic lineage	
	-Ring nuclei	
	-Charcot-Leyden crystals in nucleus	
	-Basophilic granules	

Table 4. Other parameters for myelodysplasia that were suggested previously but had not been included in the recent guidelines [15, 16].

On the other hand, myelodysplastic findings in blood cells arise due to any challenge during the course of normal differentiation and therefore these changes can be encountered not only in clonal disorders like MDS (primary myelodysplasia), but also in various nonclonal disorders affecting bone marrow like viral, bacterial, parasitic infections [17–27], autoimmune disorders (juvenile rheumatoid arthritis, polyarteritis nodosa, systemic lupus erythematosis, immune thrombocytopenic purpura) [17, 28–32], hemophagocytic histiocytosis (HLH), nutritional problems (malnutrition, iron deficiency anemia, megaloblastic anemia, copper deficiency, vitamin D deficiency, hyper vitaminosis A) [27, 33–43], neutropenia (congenital dysgranulopoietic, congenital severe, idiopathic) [32, 44, 45], inherited disorders [27, 46, 47], malign lymphoma [48], due to effects of drugs and toxins [17, 27, 49–54], during posttransplantation period [27, 55], and other reasons [27] also and called "secondary myelodysplasia" [27]. These findings are neutrophils with nuclear shape, hypoagranulation, abnormal nuclei, cytoplasm and granulation, anisocytosis, poikilocytosis, microspherocytes, giant thrombocytes, lymphocytes with cytoplasmic protrusions and vacuoles, monocytes with dysmorphic nuclei, cytoplasmic vacuoles and cytoplasmic protrusions, chromatin clumping, nucleocytoplasmic asyncrony, interchromatin bridges between erythroid precursors, oligonuclear megakaryocytes, naked megakaryocyte nuclei and cytoplasm, most of which have been included in the dysplasia criteria in MDS of childhood [13, 14], and adulthood [2, 15, 16].

While MDS is potentially preleukemic, disorders with secondary myelodysplasia are not neoplastic or preleukemic and are reversible when the underlying factor is removed [27].

Such cases with additional cytopenia in one or more cell lines, due to transient suppression of hematopoiesis may erroneously lead the physician to the diagnosis of MDS, especially when no cytogenetic abnormality can be attained. Additionally, assessment of morphological abnormalities in MDS is still not completely objective [56], in spite of that a number of dysmorphic findings were simplified, categorized [2, 13–16] and cut-off values were established [5]. This situation is valid especially for low-risk MDS cases without excess blasts and any detectable cytogenetic abnormalities. Additionally, necessity to wait without definite diagnosis and therefore therapy for at least 6 months in cytopenia cases with unilineage dysplasia [5, 12] is distressing for the patient and the family.

On the other hand, it is also challenging to differentiate cases which present as ordinary aplastic anemia, refractory immune thrombocytopenic purpura (ITP) [31], chronic neutropenia [44, 45] from MDS [4, 9, 14, 57–60]. Transient MDS or MDS-like disorders with or without [61–70] chromosomal abnormalities, acute myeloblastic leukemia (AML) cases with low blast cell count [71] should also be considered for accurate diagnosis. Additionally, it should not be forgotten that autoimmune disorders may also be a component of MDS itself [72–74] and there may be cases complying the criteria of other MDS subtypes like idiopathic cytopenia of undetermined significance (ICUS), idiopathic dysplasia of undetermined significance (IDUS) [5, 7, 58].

This chapter reviews on these diagnostic problems, in the following order:

- Nonclonal disorders which present as dysplasia and cytopenia
- Cases with hypoplastic bone marrow mimicking hypocellular MDS
- Transient chromosome abnormalities in the setting of cytopenia/spontaneous remission in MDS
- Mutations in the elderly and other cases
- Acute myeloblastic leukemia
- ICUS-IDUS
- Autoimmune disorders
- Common features in pathogenesis

- Differential diagnosis
- Conclusion and future recommendations

2. Nonclonal disorders which present as dysplasia and cytopenia

2.1. Viral and bacterial infections

In a pilot and unpublished study that we carried on in our clinic, we compared the dysmorphic parameters in the neutrophils of patients with viral (n:6; infections: rubella, rubeola, viral eruption of unknown origin, Ebstain Barr virus infection), bacterial (n:7; infections: preseptal cellulitis, urinary infection, tonsillitis, maxillary sinusitis, lymphadenitis, otitis media) infections and those of healthy controls. We found that the neutrophil diameter of those with bacterial infections; the percentage of pseudo Pelger-Huet cells and irregular distribution of granules in both viral and bacterial infections; the percentage of chromatin clumping in viral diseases were higher than the control. These findings showed that nonspecific infections can also give rise to dysmorphic findings in neutrophils.

In another study, we reported that those with bacterial diseases additionally displayed comparable diameter, macropolycyte (neutrophils with diameter >14 μm) percentage, bizarre nucleus, irregular distribution of granules with those of pretreatment ITP who also displayed myelodysplasia [17].

Striking dyserytropoiesis was reported in tuberculosis [27]. Several viral infections which closely mimick MDS will be delineated below.

2.1.1. Parvovirus infection

In the literature, there are cases of parvovirus infection, with [19–21] or without [22] immunodeficiency or chronic hemolytic anemia which transiently or chronically mimicked MDS or dyserythropoietic anemia [22]. Among them the two [19, 20] are of note.

The reported case of Hasle et al. [19] was an 8-year-old, previously healthy boy who admitted to the hospital with severe anemia, moderate thrombocytopenia, and granulocytopenia and a 2 weeks' history of intermittent fever. Physical examination was normal except for pallor. Bone marrow was hypercellular with marked erythroblastopenia and maturation arrest of the erythropoietic cell line. No giant pronormoblast and hemophagocytosis was noted. Dysplasia in myeloid and megakaryocytic lineage was evident. He had increased immunoglobulin (Ig) M, low IgG, slightly decreased natural killer (NK) cells which reduced during follow-up; impaired in vitro proliferation of blood mononuclear cells on stimulation.

The patient was assumed as MDS and was administered prednisolon, androgenic steroid, cyclophosphamid and cyclosporine, IgG infusion and frequent blood transfusions and developed hemochromatosis and hepatosplenomegaly. Thrombocytopenia deepened; hemoglobin transiently normalized. Parvovirus antibody studies revealed negative but when polymerase chain reaction technique became available, serum samples of the previous two years of the disease course and bone marrow smears were found positive for parvovirus infection.

http://dx.doi.org/10.5772/64422

The reported case of Baurmann et al. [20] was a 36-year-old, previously healthy woman who admitted to the hospital with fever, pancytopenia, and atypical lymphoid cells with dysplastic hematopoietic changes. She had frank splenomegaly, slightly increased bilirubin, lactate dehydrogenase (LDH), negative Coombs test. Since the bone marrow was hypocellular with multiple abnormal megakaryocytes, absence of erythropoiesis and 15% blasts carrying monocytic and histiocytic characteristics, she was diagnosed as MDS-refractory anemia with excess blasts (RAEB). A second bone marrow aspiration performed 6 days after admission revealed hypercellularity, no excess of blasts, erythropoietic hyperplasia with giant proerythroblasts, megakaryocytes which were in normal number but still dysplastic.

Parvovirus antibodies and DNA were positive while the serologic tests for other viruses were negative. Reticulocytosis, spherocytes, increased osmotic fragility test, and persistent subclinical hemolysis indicated at transient aplastic crisis mimicking MDS-RAEB due to parvovirus infection in the setting of hereditary spherocytosis.

2.1.2. *Cytomegalovirus (CMV) infection*

Miyahara et al. [23] reported a 41-year-old, previously healthy man who developed severe thrombocytopenia with myelodysplastic changes of bone marrow and multiple autoimmune abnormalities, low CD4/CD8 ratio following CMV infection. The bone marrow aspiration was hypocellular with decreased megakaryocytes, atypical lymphocytes, and trilineage dysplasia. After a short-course prednisolone therapy, he improved.

It was suggested that direct CD34+ multipotent stem cells were infected with CMV giving rise to injury to the bone marrow cells. The inhibitory effect of cytokines [tumor necrosis factor alpha (TNF-α), interferon gamma (IF-)] produced by CMV-infected leukocytes and stromal cells on hematopoiesis and autoimmunity might have been responsible for myelodysplastic changes and thrombocytopenia.

2.1.3. *Human immunodeficiency virus (HIV) infection*

At the time of primary infection, transient pancytopenia, lymphocytosis, increased hematogones, increase in CD8+ lymphocytes, isolated autoimmune thrombocytopenia, anemia, reticulocytopenia, neutropenia, trilineage myelodysplasia both in the peripheral blood and bone marrow were reported. Megakaryocytes which were in normal or increased numbers showed apparent naked nuclei and were occasionally dysplastic [18]. Dysplastic findings were found increased and erythropoiesis became megaloblastic during antiretroviral therapy.

2.1.4. *Hepatitis C virus (HCV) infection*

HCV-infected patients frequently had varying degrees of bone marrow dysplasia and patients with pancytopenia were those who had the most frequent bone marrow abnormalities. In the cohort of HCV-infected patients, those with hematopoietic malignancy also existed [24]. However, bone marrow was a site where HCV replicated extrahepatically which contributed to the etiology of HCV-associated neutropenia and thrombocytopenia. Peripheral clearance or consumption of platelets might have increased in HCV infection also [75, 76] like in other abnormalities in infections [77].

2.1.5. Virus infections in MDS

It should not be forgotten that more than 50% of patients with myelodysplasia and chronic myeloproliferative diseases showed elevated antibody titers against viruses like EBV and HHV-6 [78].

2.2. Parasitic infections

2.2.1. Visceral leishmaniasis

Yaralı et al. [25] reported seven cases with leishmaniasis all of whom had pancytopenia, dysplasia in erythroid myeloid, and megakaryocytic lineages. The all qualitative and quantitative findings disappeared after 2 months' therapy.

The authors postulated that increased TNF-α which was shown to be associated with increased macrophages, increased oxidized pyrimidine nucleotides, decreased glutathione concentration and presumably reduced clearance of free oxygen radicals might be responsible for myelodysplasia in visceral leishmaniasis, and other hematological findings.

Dhingra et al. [26] also reported 18 cases with leishmaniasis who had various combinations of cytopenia with increased bone marrow cellularity. Trilineage myelodysplasia (22%), bone marrow fibrosis (16.6%), hemophagocytosis (11.1%), and increased iron stores (33.3%) were evident.

It was thought that infected bone marrow stromal macrophages with leishmania, selectively enhanced myelopoiesis by granulocyte macrophage colony stimulating factor (GM-CSF) and TNF-α overproduction, giving rise to hypercellularity and trilineage myelodysplasia. Increased iron stores were attributed to cytokine overproduction which also led to anemia.

2.2.2. Others

Secondary myelodysplasia due to plasmodium falciparum and *P. vivax* infection was also reported [27].

2.3. Autoimmune disorders

2.3.1. Juvenile rheumatoid arthritis (JRA)

Yetgin et al. [28] reported myelodysplasia in 17 patients with JRA, none of whom had received iron, corticosteroids, immunosuppressive drugs, or any transfusions, and none had acute infection or gross bleeding. Bone marrow of all cases revealed normal along with abnormal maturation at different levels, like left shift, along with trilineage dysplasia, the most prominent dysplasia being in myeloid lineage. Increased bone marrow cellularity, fatty changes, erythroid hypoplasia, myeloid and mild-moderate megakaryocytic hyperplasia were detected. They all had anemia, mostly being microcytic; the most had leukocytosis and thrombocytosis.

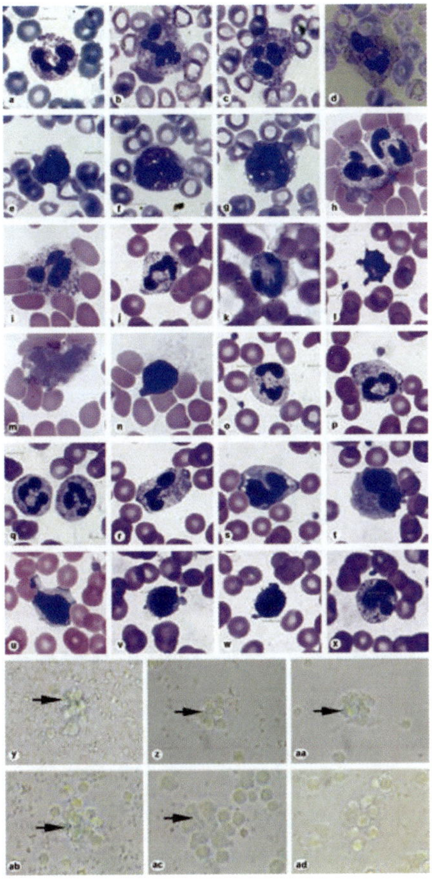

Figure 1. Dysmorphic hematological features of the peripheric blood smears of the patient ASİ with chronic ITP (a–g), patient MEY with JRA (h–n), patient TÇ with JRA (o–x). Courtesy of Turk J Med Sci [79]. **Neutrophils**: Macropolycytes (neutrophil > 15 μm) (b, c, h, i), hypersegmentation (c), cytoplasmic vacuoles (a), hypogranulation (d, o), cytoplasmic protrusions with or without granules (h, k), irregular distribution of granules (a, c, j), abnormal nuclei with nucleic protrusions (q, r), neutrophils with long chromatin between the nuclei (j, o), pseudo Pelger-Huet cells (o, p) **Lymphocytes**: Cytoplasmic protrusions (e, n, u, v, w). Basophils: Centralization of granules (f), abnormal nuclei and hypogranulation (x). **Monocytes**: Abnormal nuclei (g, s, t), cytoplasmic vacuoles (g, s), cytoplasmic protrusion (g). **Platelets**: Big or giant platelets (l, m) **β-gal staining photographs of the patients**. Patient TÇ JRA (y), patient MBY with JRA (z), patient KÇ with SLE (aa), patient HA with acute ITP (ab), patient ASİ with chronic ITP (ac), control (ad) (×100).

The score of myelodysplastic peripheral blood findings but not those of bone marrow correlated significantly with CRP and ferritin.

It was postulated that abnormally regulated cytokines and other local intracellular messengers by cellular immune system lead to alterations of the microenvironment of bone marrow giving rise to the myelodysplastic features (**Figure 1**).

On the other hand, clinicians should keep cautious since rheumatoid arthritis and other rheumatoid disorders may present as a part of immune abnormalities in MDS also [72–74].

2.3.2. *Polyarteritis nodosa (PAN)*

Yetgin et al. [29] reported a child with hematopoietic dysplastic characteristics in an 11-year-old girl with PAN. While her blood smear revealed occasional trilineage dysplasia, her bone marrow displayed moderate cellularity, fatty changes, and trilineage dysplasia in addition to blast and blast-like mononuclear cells. She received therapy of methyl prednisolone and cyclophosphamide and all of the hematologic abnormalities were found to have resolved after 6 months. It was suggested that these dysplastic findings were associated with the primary inflammatory process and increased cytokines.

2.3.3. *Systemic lupus erythematosis (SLE)*

Voulgarelis et al. [30] reported bone marrow biopsy and aspiration findings of 40 SLE cases in comparison with 10 MDS-refractory anemia (RA) cases. The patients had mono-bi- or trilineage cytopenia. The bone marrows were hyponormocellular with increased erythroid and megakaryocytic lineages in the majority of cases. All patients had dyserythropoiesis and dysmegakaryopoiesis. Dysmyelopoiesis was less striking with a left shifting. While the rate of dyserythropoiesis and dysmegakaryopoiesis were similar in patients with SLE and MDS-RA (100% vs 100%), the features of bone marrow biopsy specimens differed in that normo-hypercellularity and abnormal localization of immature progenitors (ALIP) aggregates were less but bone marrow necrosis was higher in SLE. Dilated sinuses (20%) were seen in SLE while no dilated sinus was noted in MDS-RA (0%). Increased reticulin, striking stromal edema, lack of inflammatory vascular damage and lack of microvascular obstruction by thrombus plugs, aggregates of T and B lymphocytes with polyclonal immunoglobulin expression were other striking features of SLE [30]. Specific lupus erythematosus (LE) cells (neutrophils containing a round, amorphous mass of purple, degraded nuclear material) were reported to be rarely seen when the bone marrow aspirate is anticoagulated and spreading of films were delayed [27]. These findings showed that bone marrow was a main target in SLE.

In SLE, it was shown that bone marrow fibroblasts could not produce enough hematopoietic growth factors and stromal cells of SLE patients failed to support allogenic progenitor cell growth in culture leading to defective hematopoietic microenvironment and altered cytokine expression. Additionally, autoreactive lymphocytes in the bone marrow of SLE patients might have directly caused immune destruction of both stromal cells and hematopoietic cells and indirectly affected them via releasing pro-inflammatory cytokines like TNF-α [35]. Secondary dysplastic changes in autoimmune diseases, in particular SLE, were demonstrated to closely mimick those in HIV [27] (**Figure 1**).

	MDS (RCC, RCUD, RCMD with unilineage cytopenia as thrombocytopenia)	Chronic ITP
Increased platelet destruction	-Present (peripheral) [81]	-Present (intrasplenic) [82]
Thrombocyte life span	-Short [81, 91]	-Short [82]
Thrombocyte production rate	-Decreased [81, 91]	-Decreased/normal [82]
Micromegakaryocytes	-Present [83]	-Present [84]
Naked megakaryocyte nuclei and megakaryocyte emperipolesis	-Present (more prominent) [31]	-Present (less prominent) [31]
Other dysplastic changes	-Present [14, 31]	-Present [17, 79]
Megakaryocyte apoptosis	-Only in micromegakaryocytes [31, 83] -Necrosis-like programmed cell death (mature + immature MKs) [81]	-Stage 3 megakaryocytes (apoptosis/ paraapoptosis) [82] -No apoptosis [85]
Apoptosis in other cell lines	-Apoptosis in all cell lines [86, 87]	-Lymphocytes: Resistant to apoptosis [88] -Granulocytes: No increased apoptosis [89]
Thrombocyte microparticles (TMPs)	-Present (TMPs/thrombocyte > normal) [90]	-Present (TMPs/thrombocyte > normal both in acute and chronic ITP) [90]
Response to splenectomy	-Response in several patients with different rates* [91, 92]	-Sustained response (70–80%) [93]

*Complete thrombocyte response in 50% (at 3 months) and 33% (at 12–54 months) of patients with short thrombocyte lifespan (<3.5 days), no transfusion requirement, but sustained neutropenia [91, 92].

Table 5. Characteristics of chronic ITP and MDS with unilineage cytopenia as thrombocytopenia (RCC subgroup of childhood MDS and RCUD, RCMD in adulthood MDS).

2.3.4. *Immune thrombocytopenic purpura*

In a previous study, we established neutrophil and eosinophil dysmorphism and increased macropolycytes in patients with acute and chronic ITP before treatment, in comparison with normal children. Several dysplastic features increased at the end of mega dose steroid (methyl prednisolone 30 mg/kg/day × 3 days followed by 20 mg/kg/day for the consecutive 4 days) therapy but decreased within 1–4 weeks after therapy was stopped. Hyperdiploidy in neutrophils which developed during steroid therapy normalized 7 days after therapy was stopped [17]. Dysplastic features were noted in other cell lines too [79].

These findings suggested that not only an intrinsic megakaryocyte proliferative defect giving rise to deficient platelet production were present in refractory chronic ITP patients but a defect before or at the level of colony forming unit-granulocyte-erythroid-monocyte-megakaryocyte (CFU-GEMM) also. The antiplatelet antibodies and the increased cytokines in ITP [80] might have been effective at this level (**Figure 1**).

2.3.4.1. Differentiation between MDS (refractory thrombocytopenia) and chronic ITP

Myelodysplastic syndrome with isolated thrombocytopenia (RCC subgroup of childhood MDS and RCUD, RCMD, MDS-U subgroups of adulthood MDS) can be masqueraded as refractory chronic ITP and the accurate diagnosis may be challenging due to close similarities between the two entities like decreased life span, decreased production rate in thrombocytes, increased thrombocyte destruction, presence of dysplastic findings in myeloid and megakaryocytic cell lines including micromegakaryocytes, naked megakaryocyte nuclei and megakaryocyte emperipolesis; and additionally megakaryocyte apoptosis, platelet microparticles and good response to splenectomy in several patients [17, 31, 81–93] (**Table 5**).

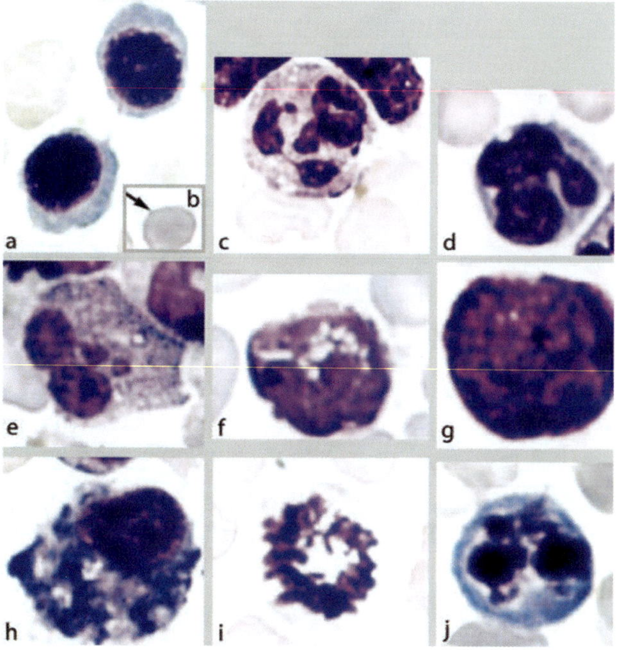

Figure 2. Myelodysplastic findings in a patient with MDS (refractory thrombocytopenia). Courtesy of Ped Hemat Oncol [31]. **Erythroid serie**: Interchromatin bridge between erythroblasts (a), spherocytes (b). **Neutrophilic serie**: Bizarre nucleus, nuclei with striking chromatin clumping, abnormal projections, cytoplasm with irregular distribution of granules and vacuoles (c), nucleocytoplasmic asyncrony (c, d). **Eosinophilic serie** with micronuclei, cytoplasmic vacuolation, cytoplasm with both eosinophilic and basophilic granules (e). **Monocytic serie** with cytoplasmic vacuoles (f). **Blast-like cells** (g). **Histiocytic serie**: Sea-blue histiocyte (h). **Mitotic cells**: Mitosis in an unknown cell (i). **Apoptotic cells** with condensed and fragmented nuclei and condensed cytoplasm (j).

Thrombocyte microparticles per thrombocyte were reported more than normal in both disorders [90] and the both can benefit from splenectomy although with different success rates [91–93]. Two of these characteristics can be used to differentiate between the two entities. The first is that, while megakaryocyte apoptosis in ITP starts at stage 3 (mature) megakaryocyte level [82] (or apoptosis does not take place in megakaryocytes of ITP patients [85], megakaryocyte apoptosis in MDS is detected in micromegakaryocyte level [31, 83]. The second is that while apoptosis takes place in myeloid, lymphoid, and monocytic cell lines in MDS [86, 87], no increase in apoptosis (in granulocytes and lymphocytes) on the contrary resistance to apoptosis (in lymphocytes) [88, 89] were reported in ITP (**Table 5**). We followed a patient with RCC that mimicked therapy resistant chronic ITP, who developed intracranial hemorrhage twice but underwent a successful bone marrow transplantation [31] (**Figures 2–4**).

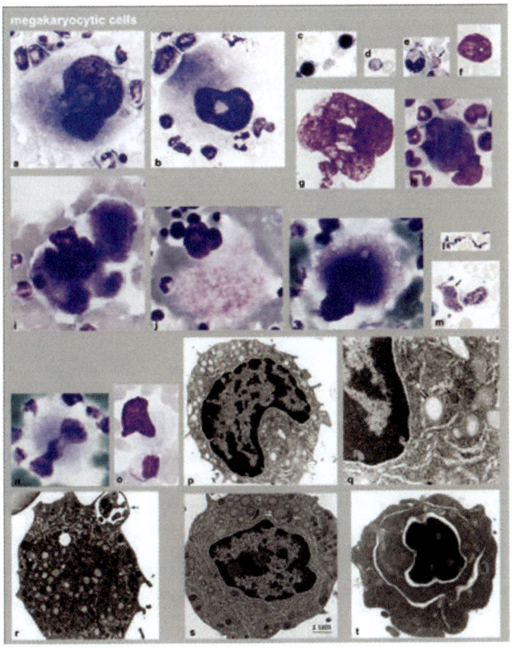

Figure 3. Dysmorphism in megakaryocytic serie, in a patient with MDS (refractory thrombocytopenia). Courtesy of Ped Hemat Oncol [31]. **Evaluation by light microscopy**: Mononuclear megakaryocytes (a, b), megakaryocyte with ring-shaped nucleus (b), megakaryocytes with nuclei that are being extruded out of the cell (i–k, o), the cytoplasm which is lobulated (i), basophilic and condensed (i, k), naked megakaryocyte nuclei (f–h) with abnormal nuclear shape (g–i), macroplatelets (c–e, m), dysmorphic platelets (e, l, m) are seen (×100). **Evaluation by transmission electron microscopy**: Stage I megakaryocyte with large, oval, and intended nucleus and a cytoplasm containing abundant ribosomes and granules. Demarcation system of membranes and granules are abundant in cytoplasm, all of which indicates nucleocytoplasmic asyncrony. The granules were identified as azurophilic granules (single arrow) and unidentifiable, large, oval, and electron lucent, abnormal granules (double arrow) (×10,000) (p) and lots of free ribosomes, azurophilic (single arrow) and abnormal unidentifiable, large, oval, electron lucent granules (double arrow) with demarcation membranes in the cytoplasm of the same cell (×27,800) (q). A megakaryocyte that shows abundant demarcation membranes, ribosomes, and granules. The granules are heterogenous as to both size and electron density. A phagosome (emperipolesis) is also seen (×12,930) (r). A stage I megakaryocyte with double nucleoli and abundant demarcation membranes, abundant azurophilic (single arrow) and unidentifiable, large, oval, electron lucent abnormal granules (double arrow) (s). Apoptotic stage I megakaryocyte that shows a condensed nuclear fragment and condensed cytoplasm, but mitochondria, mitochondrial crystae, and demarcation membranes are still intact (×16,700) (t).

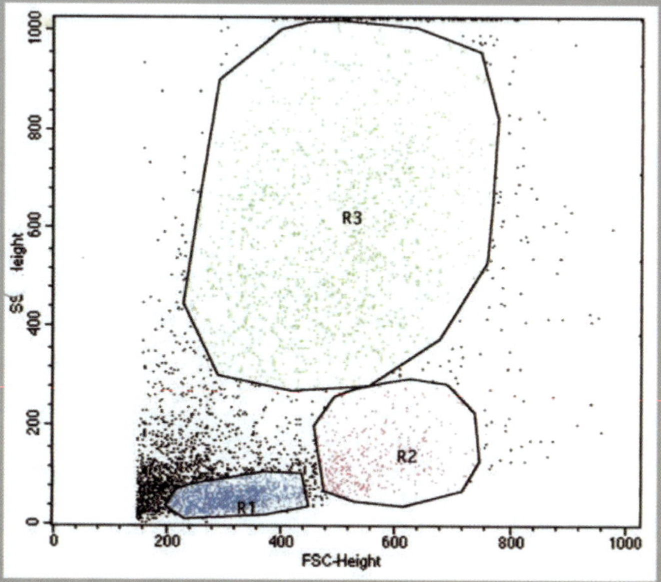

	R1	R2	R3
CD95	1.37 (Control: 32.27)	0.0 (Control: 87.94)	0.07 (Control: 92.80)
Annexin	23.24 (Control: 0.32)	30.26 (Control:6.21)	11.67 (Control: 0.11)
Bcl-2	0.0 (Control: 0.00)	0.0 (Control: 0.46)	4.26 (Control: 0.00)

Figure 4. Fas, annexin and bcl-2 values in lymphocytes (R1), monocytes (R2), granulocytes (R3) from the bone marrow of the child with MDS (refractory thrombocytopenia), established by flow cytometry (Coulter Elite). Courtesy of Ped Hemat Oncol [31].

2.3.5. *Autoimmune neutropenia*

Although chronic idiopathic and autoimmune neutropenia are considered as benign disorders, it was reported that the bone marrow of these patients displayed dyserythropoiesis by 55% and they transformed to clonal hematological diseases including NK expansion, hairy cell leukemia, myelomonocytic leukemia, and MDS (RCUD, RCMD) within 30 months, with a rate up to 6.5%. Therefore, these patients should be closely followed up [32].

2.4. Hemophagocytic lymphohistiosis (HLH, hemophagocytic syndrome)

All patients whom we followed in our clinic due to primary or secondary HLH had myelodysplastic features in addition to cytopenia involving at least two cell lines. The common

http://dx.doi.org/10.5772/64422

findings in the bone marrow were erythroid hyperplasia, chromatin bridges between erythroid precursors, multiple nuclei in erythroblasts, mild megaloblastic changes, vacuoles in erythroblasts, myeloid precursors and monocytes, sometimes in thrombocytes; hypogranulation in neutrophil myelocytes, micromyelocytes, irregular distribution of cytoplasmic granules, large and sometimes hybrid granules in eosinophils; anisocytosis in thrombocytes including giant thrombocytes, naked megakaryocyte cytoplasm, megakaryocyte emperipolesis, oligomononuclear megakaryocytes. These changes were probably due to the cytokine storm that played the major role in the pathogenesis of HLH (**Figure 5**).

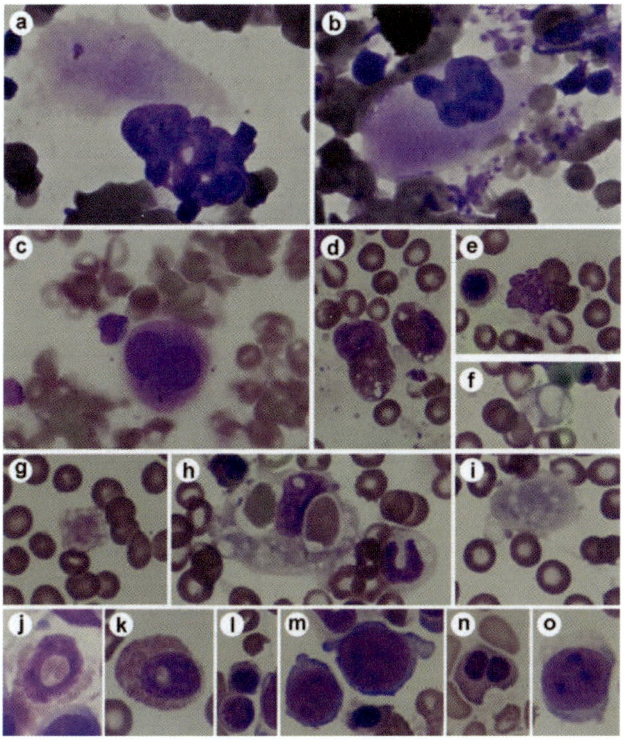

Figure 5. Myelodysplastic bone marrow findings of two patients with secondary (a, b) and primary (c–o) hemophagocytic histiocytosis (HLH) (personal archives). Megakaryocytes with mononuclear nuclei that have irregular edges and condensed cytoplasm are seen just after (a) and during (b) the process of extruding the nuclei out of the cell, developing naked megakaryocyte cytoplasm and nucleus (a). Bilobed erythroid precursor (c), eosinophil myelocytes with cytoplasmic vacuolation and rare basophilic granules, cytoplasmic protrusion (d), a naked nuclei of an unknown cell (e), cells or formations with heterogenous morphology consisting of numerous vacuoles with various sizes (f, g, i), indistinguishable from abnormal trombocytes and detached cytoplasm of hemophagocyting histiocyte (h), hypogranulated and vacuolated band (h), ringed nuclei in eosinophilic myelocytes (j, k), internuclear chromatin bridge (slightly dim) (l), cytoplasmic protrusions in basophilic erythroblasts (m), bilobed normoblast (n), cytoplasmic vacuolation in a proerythroblast (o) (vitamin B12, folic acid, Cu, Zn levels were normal).

2.5. Nutritional deficiencies

2.5.1. Malnutrition

Mono-, bi-, pancytopenia, and hematopoietic dysplasia were reported in patients with malnutrition, who were generally deficient in iron, vitamin B12, folate, and trace elements also. Bone marrow cellularity was reduced with normoblastic dyserythropoiesis. Giant metamyelocytes, vacuolation in erythroid and granulocytic precursors, abnormal sideroblasts including ring sideroblasts [27], hemophagocytosis, necrotic cells, and rarely dysmegakaryocytosis were reported.

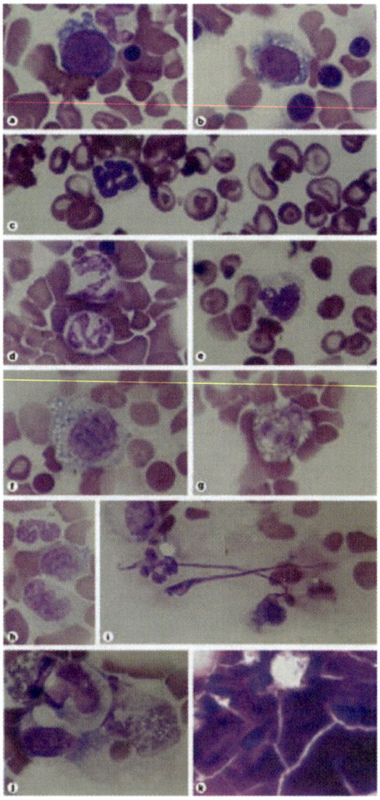

Figure 6. Myelodysplastic bone marrow findings of a child with malnutrition and gelatinous transformation (personal archives). Basophilic erythroblasts with cytoplasmic protrusions (a) and vacuoles (b), agranular neutrophil (c, i) with numerous cytoplasmic vacuoles and hypersegmented nucleus (c), hypoagranular neutrophils with hypolobulated nuclei with abnormal protrusions, mild chromatin clumping (d, h), eosinophil with abnormal nucleus, irregular distribution of granules (g), eosinophilic band with few basophilic granules distributed irregularly (j), vacolated monocytes (e, j) and histiocytes (f), degenerating histiocytes (j), hypha and amorphous material representing the gelatinous material (i, k).

In anorexia nervosa, severe diseases with cachexia and starvation, acantocytosis in the peripheral blood, hypocellularity with/without "gelatinous transformation" were noted. In gelatinous transformation, the fat cells in the bone marrow are lost, and hematopoietic cells are replaced by extracellular matrix material composed of acid mucopolysaccharide rich in hyaluronic acid is detected [18, 33]. All the reported cases had anemia, leukopenia ± thrombocytopenia [33, 34], rarely only anemia [35] (**Figure 6**).

Trilineage dysplasia in peripheric blood of iron deficient patients were reported, being higher than the control group. In addition, microspherocytes which were observed in 20% of iron-deficient patients were not noted in the control group [36]. Leukopenia and thrombocytopenia may accompanied these changes as iron deficiency deepened, making the differential diagnosis between iron deficiency anemia and MDS more difficult. Alcantara et al. [94] showed that iron supported 11 genes in phorbol myristate acetate-induced HL-60 cell lines which were involved in critical cell decision points to pursue a differentiation or cell death pathway.

Additionally, increased erythropoietin in iron deficiency anemia might also have activated hematopoietic lineages. Presence of microspherocytes was attributed to a putative involvement of Rac1 and Rac2 GTPase, also known as Ras-related C3 botulinum toxin substrates 1 and 2 GTPase deficiency which reportedly altered actin assembly in red cells in mice. Further factors like cellular metabolic enzyme changes, cell growth and differentiation, and gene expression regulation might have been involved in the pathogenesis [36].

On the other hand, leukemia cases who were under chemotherapy and had myelodysplastic features were shown to have hypochromic macrocytes and increased serum iron and ferritin levels and increased soluble transferrin receptor implying at a disturbance in utilizing iron (functional iron deficiency) [49].

2.5.2. Megaloblastic anemia

See Section 4.2.

2.5.3. Copper deficiency

Copper is a cofactor of a number of enzymes (cuproenzymes) including those important for hematologic system like hephaestin, seruloplasmin (ferroxidases) and others like cytochrome *c* oxidase, superoxide dismutase 1, extracellular superoxide dismutase, and zyklopen, a new member of the vertebrate multicopper ferroxidase family

Pregnant and lactating women, premature infants, those with malabsorption, inflammatory bowel diseases, celiac disease, long lasting diarrhea, short bowel syndrome, those under total parenteral nutrition, or nutrition through jejunal tube, those who underwent gastric resection, bariatric surgery; Wilsons' disease patients who consumed copper-depleting drugs, conditions with excess zinc are under risk of copper deficiency [37–41].

The most important problem in copper deficiency lays in its diagnosis. It may be misdiagnosed as MDS or underdiagnosed. The time which lapses until appropriate diagnosis is made was reported as approximately 1 year. Early diagnosis is important since therapy after neurological symptoms have developed is difficult [40].

On the other hand, it is of note that 11 out of 32 MDS patients were found to have copper deficiency [95].

The most striking hematologic findings in copper deficiency are mono-, bi-, and pancytopenia [39–41]. Anemia which is the most common hematologic finding (97.5%) in copper deficiency is generally normochromic or macrocytic but rarely microcytic, being dependent on the severity of the deficiency. When the activity of copper-dependent enzymes decrease, iron absorption is expected to be impaired, iron transport across intestinal cells be decreased, conversion of ferrous iron to the ferric form which is necessary for transport of iron by transferrin be impaired, conversion of ferric iron to ferrous iron which is necessary for incorporation of iron into the protoporphyrin molecule during hemoglobin synthesis be inadequate. The latter defect gives rise to both formation of ring sideroblasts and possibly erythrocyte membrane defect due to low levels of antioxidant zinc/copper dismutase activity necessary to convert superoxide-free radicals to hydrogen peroxide [37, 39]. However, the mechanism of anemia is not fully understood [37].

	Copper deficiency	MDS
Vacuolization	-In erythroid + myeloid lineages [39]	-In erythroid lineage [39]
Dysmegakaryopoiesis (nuclear lobulation and abnormal sizes)	-Not present [39] -Present [37]	-Generally present [2, 5, 14, 39]
Dysplasia	-No [39] -Bilineage [38] -Three lineage dysplasia [37]	-Unilineage: RCUD; RARS (erythroid) -Two or more lineages (RCC, RCMD; MDS-U) [2, 5, 14, 39]
Increased hematogones	-Present [37]	-Absent [39]
Other	-Left shift in myelopoiesis -Reduced terminally differentiated myeloid cells, myeloid arrest [39] -Erythroid arrest at proerythro blast stage [37]	-Erythroid hyperplasia (generally) [15] -Myeloid arrest or left shift (generally in RAEB) [96]
Ring sideroblast	-Present [37–39]	-Present only in RARS subgroup [2, 5]

Table 6. Bone marrow findings in copper deficiency in comparison with MDS.

Leukopenia in copper deficiency is together with neutropenia which was reported to be the most frequent and earliest manifestation of copper deficiency [41]. The neutrophils in peripheric blood smear are dysplastic. Impaired and delayed maturation, differentiation and regeneration of hematopoietic precursor cells, increased destruction of myeloid precursors in the bone marrow, defective neutrophil egress from the bone marrow, shortened life-span of neutrophils, and presence of antibodies to neutrophils are the possible etiologic factors for neutropenia [39, 41].

The bone marrow is generally hypercellular [40] with increased myeloid and/or erythroid precursors mimicking myeloid and erythroid arrest, vacuolization in erythroid and myeloid precursors, increased iron stores, prominent ring sideroblasts, plasma cells in which hemosiderin is incorporated, increased hematogones [37] with [37, 38], without [39] myelodysplasia. In MDS, generally erythroid hyperplasia [15] is encountered. Myeloid arrest or left shift in granulopoiesis is seen generally in RAEB subgroup of MDS [96]. Characteristics of MDS and copper deficiency are summarized in **Table 6**.

2.5.4. Vitamin D deficiency

Vitamin D has both proliferating and differentiating effect on hematopoiesis [42]. The bone marrow taken from infants with vitamin D deficiency rickets and anemia showed early signs of myelofibrosis with increase of reticulin which was reversed by vitamin D treatment [97]. Anemia, thrombocytopenia, hepatosplenomegaly, hypocellularity and increased osteoblast count in bone marrow, and hematopoietic precursors in spleen aspirates were striking. Hypochromia, macrocytosis, tear drop cells, young myeloid elements along with nucleated red blood cells were evident [98]. Dysdifferentiation due to its deficiency might have been aggravated by coexistent malnutrition in many of several patients.

2.5.5. Hypervitaminosis A

An infant with hypervitaminosis A reportedly had eversible severe anemia, thrombocytopenia, and dyserythropoiesis. It was shown that in overdoses, vitamin A strongly inhibited the proliferation of multipotent hematopoietic cell line and bone marrow mesenchymal stem cells, through upregulating $p21^{Cip1}$ and $p27^{Kip1}$, cyclin-dependent kinase inhibitors [43].

2.6. Severe congenital neutropenia (SCN)

We, previously detected hematopoietic dysmorphism in congenital neutropenia, their non-neutropenic parents and one sibling, irrespective to the neutropenia mutation that the patients had [45, 99]. All the tested patients were negative for molecular genetics of MDS and were normal in conventional cytogenetics. Apoptosis of lymphocytes, granulocytes [45, 99], and monocytes [45], of both patients and parents and rapid cell senescence (RCS) in leukocytes of a few patients and their mothers were established [45, 99]. A substantial portion of cases had clinical or laboratory evidence of hemorrhagic diathesis and low NK and CD4+ cells.

These findings showed that pluripotent stem cells were involved in SCN irrespective to the genetic defect and non-neutropenic family members were also affected ([45, 99], study in submission) and congenital neutropenia and MDS shared the same death types and involved pluripotent stem cells.On the other hand, it should not be forgotten that MDS can present as isolated neutropenia (RCC, as refractory neutropenia). In our clinic, we followed a 4-year-old girl who was admitted to our hospital for chronic neutropenia, but the genetic evaluation revealed trisomy 8 and a complex karyotype; while the molecular genetic studies for congenital neutropenia (*HAX1, ELANE, and G6PC3*) were negative (unpublished data).

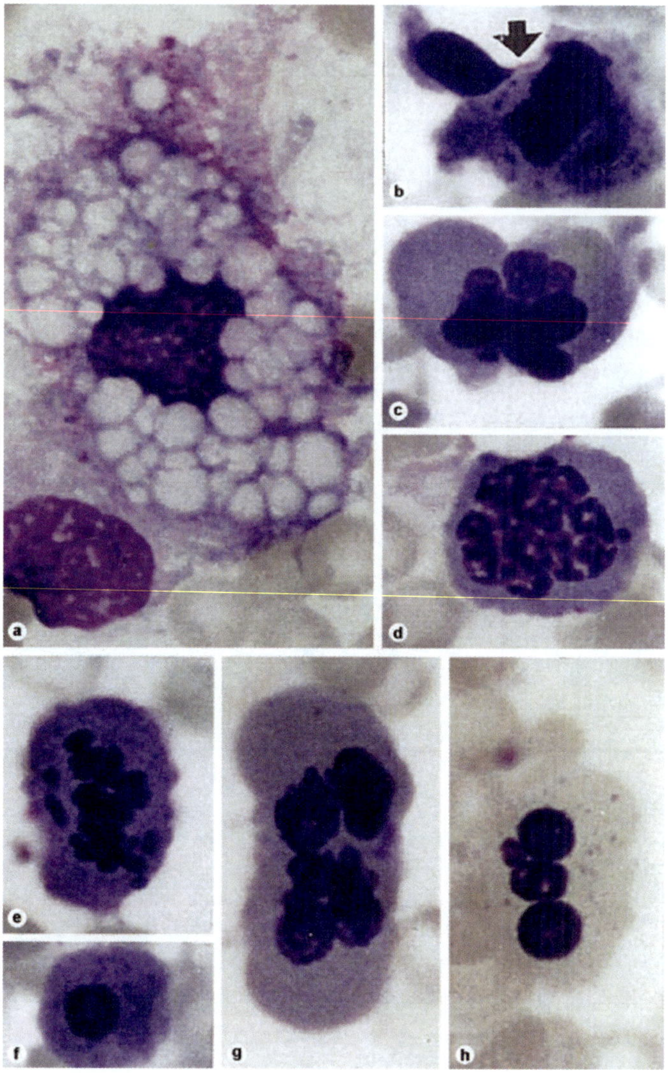

Figure 7. Myelodysplastic bone marrow findings of a 5-year-old patient with ALL who was on chemotherapy and had coexistent autoimmune hemolytic anemia [100] (personal archives). A Gaucher-like histiocyte that is hemophagocytosing a cell (a), internuclear chromatin bridge between two erythroblasts (b) (arrow), multinucleated erythroblasts with various sizes (c, e, g, h), striking megaloblastic changes (d), basophilic stippling (b, e–h).

2.7. Inherited conditions

Özbek et al. [46] reported myelodysplastic features in myeloid and erythroid cell lines, in 20 patients with microdeletion 22q11.2 (del22q11.2) with slight cytopenia. Their smears showed dysmorphism in erythroid and myeloid cell lineages, in addition to a few vacuolated plasmatoid lymphocytes; monocytic cells mimicking hypogranular myelocytes with cytoplasmic vacuoles and protrusions and blast-like cells.

Myelodysplasia scores in the myeloid cells and eosinophils and macropolycyte percentages were higher than those with conotruncal heart defects, viral and bacterial infections, and healthy children. Genes in the deleted region, like human cell division cycle-related (hCDCrel) gene was proposed to be responsible for these changes.

Other inherited conditions which present as dyserythropiesis and anemia are congenital dyserythropoietic anemia, thalassemia, congenital dyserythropoietic porphyria, mitochondrial myopathies, hereditary sideroblastic anemia, homozygous hemoglobin C, heterozygous unstable hemoglobins, some cases with thiamine-responsive anemia with diabetes and deafness, homozygote pyruvate kinase deficiency, stress erythropoiesis like severe hemolytic anemia [100] (**Figure 7**).

Those who present as dysgranulopoiesis with/without neutropenia are mitochondrial cytopaties, myelokathexis, and congenital neutropenia [45]. Those with dysmegakaryopoiesis and thrombocytopenia are inherited thrombocytopenias. Patients with GATA1 mutations have anemia and neutropenia together with trilineage dysplasia [27]. Patients with mevalonc aciduria due to mevalonate kinase deficiency have anemia, thrombocytopenia with/without fluctuation, dysplasia in erythroid and myeloid lineages [47].

2.8. Malignant lymphoma

In non-Hodgkin lymphoma (NHL) and Hodgkin lymphoma (HL) patients, myelodysplasia in granulocytic and erythroid lineages were noted without any marked myelodysplasia in megakaryocytic lineage. The myelodyspastic features were found comparable in patients with and without bone marrow infiltration of lymphoma cells.

The bone marrow was normal or hypercellular, with normal, reduced number of erythroid and increased number of myeloid cells, normal, or increased megakaryocytes; ALIP was not encountered. Reticulin fibrosis was rare (6.1%).

The myelodysplasia in lymphoma was thought to be a reaction to the lymphoma or to result from an impaired bone marrow stem cell [48].

2.9. Effect of drugs and toxins

2.9.1. Chemotherapy

Most of chemotherapeutic and immunosuppressive agents give damage to the bone marrow, inducing megaloblastic dyserythropoiesis in low doses, and hypoplasia in high doses. Drugs that cause megaloblastosis are methotrexate, cyclophosphamide, daunorubicin, doxorubicin, cytarabine, hydroxyurea, azathioprine, and zidovudine [27]. Mycophenolate mofetil is known to cause Pelger-Huet anomaly, abnormal chromatin clumping, detached nuclear fragments in granulocyte lineage. Alemtuzumab was also reported to be associated with increased dysplastic features and virus-related hemophagocytic syndrome [27]. In our experience, the most consistent finding of dysplasia in patients who receive chemotherapy was hypoagranulation of myeloid cells (**Figures 7** and **8**).

We previously showed that leukemia patients displayed hypochromic macrocytes in their peripheric blood due to failure to utilize iron ([49], study in submission). Additionally, serum reticulocyte counts in the beginning of chemotherapy blocks declined significantly in the end of the blocks when erythropoiesis was markedly depressed and were found to have increased significantly at the beginning of the next chemotherapy block when the bone marrow regenerated and erythropoiesis increased [49].

Increased apoptosis, increased hemophagocyting macrophages, erythroid and megakaryocytic regeneration generally preceding granulocytic regeneration, megakaryocytic clustering and ALIP together with myelodysplasia were described after intensive chemotherapy and persisted for months [27]. The infections that the patients could have developed, possibly aggravated the myelodysplasia.

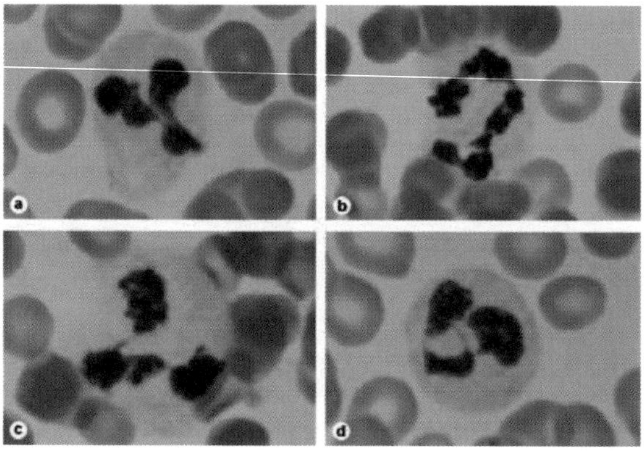

Figure 8. Neutrophils of a pediatric ALL patient while he was on maintenance chemotherapy (a, b), and 6 months after cessation of therapy (c, d) (personal archives). Cytoplasmic agranulation (a–d), large size (a–d), chromatin clumping (b, c), long chromatin string between the nuclear lobes (d) are striking.

On the other hand, these findings closely overlap with those in therapy-related MDS (t-MDS) or therapy-related myeloid neoplasms (t-MN) in the new nomenclature. It was reported that t-MN followed treatment of lymphomas and solid tumors but more rarely leukemias [101]. Appearance of new dysplastic changes after complete remission of leukemia [102] or solid tumors should alert the physician for development of t-MN.

2.9.2. *Steroids*

Steroids give rise to hyperdiploidy, and therefore macropolycytes in neutrophils [17] in addition to abnormal nuclear lobulation (**Figures 9** and **10**).

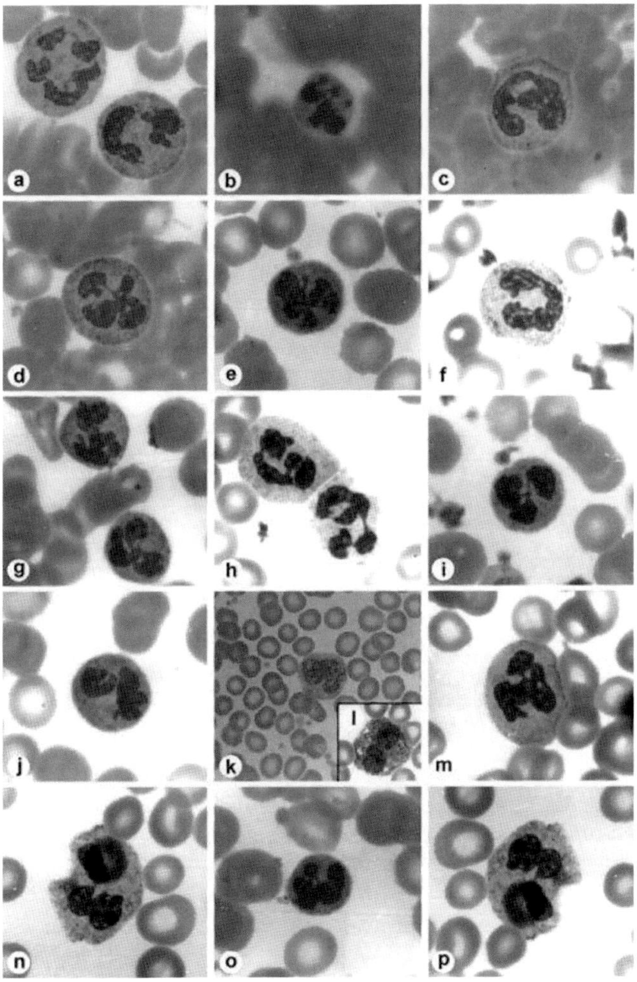

Figure 9. Peripheric blood neutrophils of children who were on high dose or long-term steroid therapy for acute and chronic ITP (personal archives). On the seventh (last) day of mega-dose methyl prednisolone therapy [116] of patient IY (a–g, i, j, l, o) and OI (k); during the phase of tapering down long-term prednisolone therapy of patient YP (n, h, p); 6 months after the last steroid therapy in YP (m). Macropolycytes (neutrophils with >14 μm diameter) in 15–20 μm diameter (a, c, h, m, n, p), pseudo-Pelger-Huet/like cells (a, c, j), chromatin clumping (c, f, k, n, p), bizarre nucleus (b, c, d, e, g, j, o), vacuolated eosinophil with both basophilic and eosinophilic granules (l).

2.9.3. *Alcohol*

Anemia with/without other cytopenias or pancytopenia were reported in alcohol dependent patients. Anemia was normochromic or macrocytic with round macrocytes (unlike oval macrocytes of megaloblastic anemia) [27, 50]. Vacuolated neutrophils, stomatocytes, sometimes target cells were evident. In hemolytic anemia and hyperlipidemia due to alcoholic liver disease, spherocytes, irregularly contracted cells (Zieve's syndrome) were demonstrated [27].

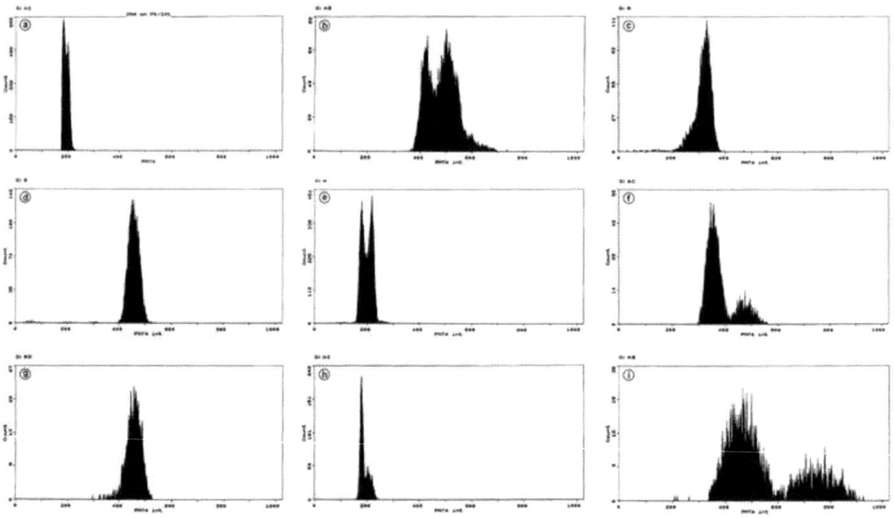

Figure 10. Various cell cycle configurations in patients with myelodysplasia (personal archives). Cell cycle analysis of granulocytic and mononuclear cells of children with acute or chronic immune thrombocytopenic purpura (ITP) before, during and after therapy (a–h), and granulocytes of a non-neutropenic mother of a dygranulopoietic neutropenia patient with dysgranulopoiesis (i). Normal cell cycle of granulocytic cells (G0 phase) (a). Granulocytes of patient YP with chronic ITP while taking oral steroids on different occasions (b, c). Mononuclear cells (d) tested on the same occasion with (c). Granulocytes of patient AT with chronic ITP. Tested 10 days after he received anti-D therapy (e). Granulocytes of IY with acute ITP, before mega dose methyl prednisolone (MDMP) therapy (f, g); 1 week after MDMP therapy ended (h). Granulocytes of non-neutropenic mother of a congenital dysgranulopoietic neutropenia patient who had myelodysplasia (i).

The most striking changes in the bone marrow was in the erythropoietic lineage as erythroid hyperplasia, ineffective erythropoiesis and dysmorphism in erythroid lineage including ring sideroblasts (positive by 75%) and dysmorphic granulopoietic cell lineages. There was no morphologic abnormality in megakaryocytes [50], but the megakaryocytes reportedly increased or markedly decreased [27]. Megaloblastic changes were associated [103] and not associated [50] with folic acid and/or vitamin B12 levels.

Serum iron levels which were elevated in the majority (being the most prominent in those with fatty liver and typical cirrhosis), iron granules in plasma cells [50] macrophages and endothelial cells [27], large numbers of sideroblasts along with ring sideroblasts [50] were other characteristics of alcohol effect. In Zieve's syndrome, excess iron-laden foamy macrophages were encountered [27]. No correlation was found between serum iron and ring sideroblasts in the bone marrow [50].

The normal colonies of all hemopoietic cell lines and cell culture ratios in alcohol-dependent individuals showed that alcohol exerted its toxic effect not on committed stem cells but peripheral cells also [50]. Reversible bone marrow aplasia due to alcohol was also reported [27].

Cytoplasmic vacuolization was reported to be due to inhibition of acetaldehyde dehydrogenase and thus reduced rate of degradation of acetaldehyde.

Alcohol has toxic effect on cell division giving rise to arrest in cell division and multinucleated erythroblasts; direct antifolate effect on nucleic acid metabolism leading to development of megaloblasts. Additionally, it impairs iron utilization giving rise to large number of sideroblasts and ring sideroblasts through disrupting pyridoxine kinase inhibiting delta aminolevulinic acid synthetase which is necessary for heme synthesis [50].

Alcohol-induced hematopoietic abnormalities closely mimick those of MDS-RARS. That alcohol-induced bone marrow damage is always reversible if the patient stops to drink alcohol, and that cell culture of alcohol dependent people show normal colonies of all hematopoietic cell lines are two important points for differentiation between alcohol-induced cell damage and MDS-RARS [50].

2.9.4. Smoking

Moderate leukocytosis being mainly due to neutrophilia and lymphocytosis was reported. Bone marrow biopsies of 32 smokers showed normal or slightly increased cellularity, modest and mild increase in granulopoiesis and erythropoiesis respectively, right shift of granulopoietic cells (the half being mature segmented neutrophils).

The special appearing macrophages with intracytoplasmic small, polygonal corpuscles showing neutrophils were striking. It was postulated that smoking inhibited locomotion of the segmented neutrophils leading to granulocytopoietic hyperplasia and accumulation of mature neutrophils in the bone marrow. These neutrophils were broken-down when they got senescent and were phagocytosed by these macrophages, resulting in "smokers' dysmyelopoiesis" [51].

On the other hand, both smoking and alcohol intake were shown to constitute risk factors for MDS [104].

2.9.5. Arsenic

Arsenic can cause mono-, bi-, and pancytopenia with marked dyserythropoiesis or megaloblastosis. Pancytopenia with trilineage dysplasia in the bone marrow mimicking MDS was reported. Associated symptoms like long-lasting gastrointestinal and neurological symptoms, arsenic in the urine analysis, favorable response to British anti-Lewisite (BAL) help the clinician distinguish between the two entities, although neurological symptoms may progress [27, 52].

2.9.6. *Lead*

Lead poisoning leads to sideroblastic anemia, microcytosis in addition to basophilic stippling and hemolytic anemia [27]. It can mimick MDS.

2.9.7. *Other drugs*

Isoniazid causes sideroblastic anemia. Antibiotiotic linezolid can give rise to vacuolization in elytroid precursors and ring sideroblasts together with anemia or pancytopenia. Chloramphenicol makes mild bone marrow suppression with ring sideroblasts and vacuolation in erythroid and granulocyte precursors. Sodium stibogluconate, prescribed in leishmaniasis causes erythroblast karyorrhexis and severe anemia [27]. Nitrous oxide (laughing gas) which has an anesthetic and recreational use and inactivator of hydroxycobalamin may give rise to megaloblastic anemia and vitamin B12-deficiency related neurological and hematological effects associated with heavy use by healthcare workers who inhalate it in operating rooms or intensive care units [27, 53].

Granulocyte colony stimulating factor (G-CSF) and GM-CSF cause neutrophil vacuolation and dysplastic neutrophils with abnormal lobulation and development of macropolycytes, in addition to neutrophilia, eosinophilia, toxic granulation and blasts in the peripheral blood, the latter mimicking progression of leukemia or MDS [54]. Antiepileptic drugs also can give rise to cytopenia and multilineage dysplasia (personal experience).

2.10. Posttransplantation

Dysplastic findings were demonstrated after solid organ transplantation, like liver, kidney, heart, and lung. Clatch et al. [55] reported bone marrow findings of 17 liver transplantation patients taken before or 1–1288 days after orthotopic liver transplantation (post-OLT) when they developed mono-, pancytopenia or fever. The patients had received cyclosporine A and prednisolone, numerous antibiotics intermittently and a few additionally received Muromonab-CD3 and/or antilymphocyte globulin.

While dysplastic hematopoiesis was completely absent from biopsies of patients with end-stage liver disease obtained before transplantation, significant trilineage dysplasia was a consistent finding in all patients who underwent OLT. Megaloblastic erythropoiesis, the most characteristic finding, macrocytosis, dysynchronous nuclear-to-cytoplasmic maturation and significant nuclear budding or bilobation were striking. Typical megaloblastic changes of the myeloid series were absent. Dysynchronous myeloid maturation, as a left shift giving rise to decreased bands and mature neutrophils, additionally dysmyelopoiesis and dysmegakaryopoiesis were evident [55].

The authors postulated that iatrogenically-induced T-cell dysfunction in transplanted patients which gave rise to alterations in microenvironment, direct pharmacological toxicities and the effects of secondary infections on hematopoietic cells might have had roles in the etiology [55].

After bone marrow or hematopoietic stem cell transplantation, bone marrow was severely hypoplastic and after successful engraftment was achieved, all hematopoietic cells, mostly the erythropoietic cells appeared dysmorphic. During the following months, striking and transient increase in hematogones, mimicking leukemia was observed. During engraftment, bone marrow architecture showed various alterations, some of which were more striking in leukemia patients whose stromal cells had been damaged during previous chemotherapies [27].

Secondary MDS may develop after autologous stem cell transplantation, due to previously damaged stem cells by chemotherapy. Cytogenetic and molecular studies are useful for distinction between secondary MDS and usual secondary myelodysplasia of early posttransplantation [27].

2.11. Other disorders with secondary dysplastic features

Multiorgan failure, autoimmune lymphoproliferative syndrome associated with Fas or Fas ligand deficiency can give rise to secondary myelodysplasia. Hypothermia can lead to sideroblastic anemia with recurrent thrombocytopenia [27].

3. Cases with hypoplastic bone marrow mimicking hypocellular MDS

3.1. Hypoplastic MDS and severe aplastic anemia (SAA)

In childhood MDS, RA (RCC) subgroup constitutes the majority of patients and bone marrow cellularity was reported decreased in nearly 50% [9] and 81% [4] of children with low-grade MDS. On the other hand, hypocellular MDS (H-MDS) in adulthood is encountered in the elderly.

Differentiation between H-MDS/hypocellular RCC and AA may be challenging both in adults and children.

There are many nonhematological factors that can give rise to bone marrow hypoplasia in childhood like any type of infections (vitamin deficiencies, metabolic disorders like mevalonate kinase deficiency, rheumatic disease, mitochondrial deletions (Pearson syndrome)). Moreover, there are many hereditary or nonhereditary hematological disorders that should be differentiated from RCC in the setting of hypoplastic bone marrow like inherited bone marrow failure syndromes [4].

The most recent histopathologic criteria to distinguish RCC from SAA in childhood is presented in **Table 7** [14, 57].

In adulthood, a similar study described standardized criteria to distinguish hypocellular AML from H-MDS and aplastic anemia (AA) (**Table 8**) [59].

	Refractory cytopenia of childhood (RCC)	Severe aplastic anemia (SAA)
Differences	1. Erythroid lineage -Patchy distribution (clusters consist of ≥10 erythroid precursors) -Maturation arrest -Increased mitosis -Increased proerythroblasts (left shift)	1. Erythroid lineage -Missing or a single and small cluster -Clusters consist of <10 erythroid cells -Erythroid cells with maturation
	2. Granulocytic lineage -Marked decrease -Left shift	2. Granulocytic lineage -Missing or marked decrease -Very few clusters of granulocytes with maturation
	3. Megakaryocytic lineage -Marked decrease -Micromegakaryocytes -Dysplastic findings	3. Megakaryocyte lineage -Missing or very few -No dysplastic changes -No micromegakaryocytes
Similarities	1. Lymphoid lineage -May be increased focally or dispersed	1. Lymphocyte lineage -May be increased focally or dispersed
	2. CD34+ cells -No increase	2. CD34+ cells -No increase

Table 7. Histopathologic criteria for differential diagnosis of SAA and RCC [4, 14, 57, 105].

Manifestation	Indicative of
Presence of unequivocal blasts in the peripheral blood	MDS or AML
Hypogranular neutrophils or pseudo-Pelger neutrophils (>10%)	MDS or AML
Presence of >1–20% blasts in the bone marrow + dysplasia	MDS
Dysplasia of either granulocytes or megakaryocytes in the bone marrow (if erythroid hyperplasia is the sole finding, dysplasia in erythroid lineage should be moderate to severe)	Inconsistent with AA
Presence of any abnormal sideroblasts (>5 granules around the nucleus or constituted at least 1/3 of the circumference	Excludes AA
1–2 cm core biopsy demonstrating four to five undistorted fields (×100 magnification)	Reliability in diagnosis
Presence of two or more clusters of immature precursors (being minimum three blast per cluster) in bone marrow biopsy	MDS or AML
Consensus diagnosis required by at least 5/7 participants	Reliability in diagnosis

Table 8. Recommendation for standardized approach to distinguish hypocellular AML from hypocellular MDS and AA [59].

In addition to the parameters listed in **Tables 7** and **8**, presence of ALIP, abnormal localization of megakaryocytes, erythroblast clusters, fibrosis, abnormal karyotype were also reported as parameters to be used to distinguish H-MDS and SAA (**Table 8**) [59]. Nevertheless, further studies are needed to examine the validity of histopathologic approach to hypocellular RCC and AA [60].

3.2. Inherited bone marrow failure (IBMF) disorders in the differential diagnosis of hypocellular RCC

Several children who are diagnosed with hypoplastic RCC, may actually have one of inherited bone marrow failure (IBMF) disorders which have not been diagnosed yet. Hence, 15% of patients diagnosed with hypoplastic RCC and 2, 5, and 10% of patients diagnosed with hypoplastic RCC or aplastic anemia were later diagnosed as Fanconi anemia and heterozygous or homozygous dyskeratosis congenita [4, 9]. Inherited bone marrow failure syndromes with pancytopenia like Fanconi anemia, dyskeratosis congenita, Shwachman Diamond syndrome, amegakaryocytic thrombocytopenia (in progression), and pancytopenia with radio-ulnar synostosis display common manifestations with hypoplastic RCC, such as macrocytosis, elevated HbF, common bone marrow features. Therefore, a careful family and past history, physical examination is essential. Laboratory and molecular studies like chromosome breakage test and telomere length assay should be carried on, since not all children with IBMF syndromes have phenotypic characteristics [4, 9]. These diseases can progress to MDS gaining chromosomal abnormalities specific to MDS and 3q26 segment in Fanconi anemia. However, abnormal clones can also regress in any IBMF syndrome [4].

In childhood, in the setting of hypocellular bone marrow with absence of cytogenetic abnormality [4] or a bone marrow biopsy with topography and cellularity of the local hematopoiesis [9], two bone marrow biopsies at least two weeks apart are necessary [4].

4. Transient chromosome abnormalities in the setting of cytopenia/spontaneous remission in MDS

4.1. Transient MDS with/without chromosomal alterations

Monosomy 7 is an harbinger of poor prognosis and higher risk of transformation to high-risk MDS and AML [4, 61–67, 69, 70] than other chromosomal abnormalities and normal karyotype [4, 105]. The estimated time of progression in children with monosomy 7 was reported as 1.9 years, with a cumulative progression incidence of 80% at the sixth year of diagnosis [4].

In the literature, we found 13 patients who presented with MDS (n:12) or MDS-like features (n:1) and had genetic abnormalities but achieved remission only after symptomatic (n:12) and vitamin B12 and folic acid (n:1) therapies. The patients had abnormalities of chromosome 7 (12 out of 13, as −7, −7q, i7) and 11q23 translocation (1 out of 13), and +21 (1 out of 13, coexistent with −7). Two additional MDS patients (RA, RAEB) with normal karyotype achieved spontaneous remission (**Table 9**).

Spontaneous disappearance of abnormal clones were reported previously in AML, EBV-associated myeloproliferative disorder and Fanconi anemia [65]. Development of cytogenetic abnormality is only one step (first hit) in the progression of malignant clone. In order to gain growth advantage, the transforming cells need other molecular changes within the cells and in the marrow microenvironment (second hit). The cases who attained spontaneous remission suggest that the development of cytogenetic abnormality might have not been supported by the other cellular and microenvironmental changes [65, 66]. Additionally, the mutation may have developed in a hematopoietic cell with limited self-renewal capacity and may not have involved the whole stem cell pool [66]. Two cases of Bader-Meunier et al. [68] suggest that patients with MDS who do not show any chromosomal abnormality can also achieve complete remission (**Table 9**). These cases show that patients who are stable should be closely observed for some time before potentially toxic therapies are started.

Cases	Diagnosis	Age/ sex	Genetic analysis	Management of therapy	Outcome /time elapsed to hematologic /cytogenetic complete remission (hem/cyto rem) (months)	Duration of follow-up after cyto rem attained (months)	Reference
1	De novo MDS†	8/12, M	45,XY,−7 [12]	Transfusions	<2 years (hem + cyto rem)	108 months	[61]
2	De novo MDS†	15/12, M	46,XY [13]/45,XY, −7 [7]	No	8 months (hem + cyto rem)	14 months	[61]
3	t-MDS† (after completing rabdomyo-sarcoma therapy)	10.5, M	46,XY,del (7)(q22q32) [4] (out of 40 metaphases)	No	5 months (hem + cyto rem, hem rem partial)	95 months	[61]
4	t-MDS† (after completing medullo-blastoma therapy)	8/M	46 XY,del(7)(q31q36) [5]/46, XY,+der(1)t(1;7)(p11.2;p11.2), -(3)/46,XY,+dic(1;21) (p11.2;p11.2), −21 [4] and other anomalies	ivIgG and transfusion	4 weeks (hem recovery; cyto rem unknown©)	67 months	[61]
5	RAEB	14/12, M	46,XY [13]/45,XY, −7 [7]	Transfusions /BMT planned	13 months (hem + cyto rem)	21 months	[62]
6	t-MDS† (Spina bifida, ESRF*; AZA therapy**	19, F	45,XY, −7 [5] (out of 62 metaphases)	AZA stopped, transfusions	17 months (hem + cyto rem)	NS♯	[63]
7	t-MDS†*** after completing Hodgkin's disease therapy	15, F	45, XY, −7 [19] (out of 20 metaphases)	NS♯ BMT planned	10 months (hem + cyto rem)	NS♯	[64]
8	t-MDS† (after completing Ewing sarcoma therapy	19, M	46,XY,(11;16)(q23;p13.3) [13] (out of 20 etaphases)	NS♯ BMT planned	12 months (hem + cyto rem)	NS♯	[64]

http://dx.doi.org/10.5772/64422

Cases	Diagnosis	Age/ sex	Genetic analysis	Management of therapy	Outcome /time elapsed to hematologic /cytogenetic complete remission (hem/cyto rem) (months)	Duration of follow-up after cyto rem attained (months)	Reference
9	De novo MDS†	13/12, F	46,XX,i(7)(q10) [3]/46,XX [11]	NS#	10 weeks (hem + cyto rem)	NS#	[65]
10	De novo MDS†	3, M	45, XY, −7 [8] (out of 12 cells)	No BMT planned	30 months (hem + cyto rem)	>80 months	[66]
11	Pancytopenia bilineage dysplasia mimicking de novo MDS‡	7.5, M	Complex karyotype including del(7)(q11) (in 3 out of 21 cells): *58,XY,+2,+3,+6,+inv(7) (p13p22),del(7) (q11),+10,+11[1] * + 15,+17,+18,+19,+20,+22:46, XY,del(7)(q11)[1]* 45,XY, del(7)(q11), −18 [1] (+chromatid, isochromatid breaks)	VB12 and folic acid therapy due to their deficiency	4 weeks (hem + cyto rem)	NS#	[67]
12	RA	8, F	Normal (46,XX) [cell no NS#]	No	Hem rem: NS#	Nearly 72 months	[68]
13	RAEB	3mo, F	Normal (46,XX) [cell no NS#]	No	Hem rem: NS#	Nearly 66 months	[68]
14	Donor cell-derived MDS after cord blood transplantation (+3 mo) for AML secondary to ALL†	4, F	46 XY,-7 [cell no NS#]; full donor chimerism; no genetic abnormality in the cord blood and the donor	Transfusions	Nearly 24 mo (hem + cyto rem)	NS#	[69]
15	Aplastic anemia on intravenous cyclosporine and androgen therapy	21,M	47,XX, −7,+21,+mar [cell no NS]	Drug switched to oral form. Then abnormality disappeared	Hem improvement as transfusion independence; cyto rem	Minimum 6 months	[70]

†The subgroup has not been reported. Probably corresponds to RCC subgroup in childhood and RCMD or MDS-U subgroups in adulthood MDS, according to the WHO 2008 classification.
©Cytogenetic abnormality found sustained on 13th month after hematologic recovery.
*End-stage renal failure.
**The patient received long-term immunosuppressive therapy with cyclosporine (for 19 months), later azacytidine (Aza) (for 6 years).
#Not stated.
***The patient had pancytopenia persisting after the 1st course of Hodgkin's disease therapy.

Table 9. Patients with MDS who achieved remission spontaneously, after supportive or vitamin B12 and folic acid therapy [61–70].

4.2. Vitamin B12 (VB12) and folic acid deficiency and transient chromosome abnormalities which mimick MDS

Vitamin B12 and folic acid deficiencies can present as mono-, bi-, and pancytopenia [106], myelodysplasia, genetic abnormalities like increased frequency of spontaneous chromosome breakage and centromere spreading [107, 108], elongation and despiralization of chromosomes [107], multiple rearrangements and deletions of different chromosomes [108] which can mimick that of MDS (**Table 9**, patient 11) [67].

Many of these chromosomal abnormalities were reported to reduce [107], completely disappear [67, 107, 108] or persist up to 6–12 months after hematological remission was attained [107] after therapy.

These cases show that defective synthesis and repair of DNA which were reversed by VB12 and folate plays role in the pathogenesis of genetic abnormalities in megaloblastic anemia.

Increased immature myeloid cells indistinguishable from myeloblasts in the bone marrow of patients with vitamin B12 and folate deficiency make the differentiation between megaloblastic anemia and MDS more difficult [109].

On the other hand, in our clinics, we have encountered considerable number of patients who had VB12 and/or folic acid deficiency coexistent with MDS or leukemia.

5. Mutations in the elderly and other cases

In more than 10% of healthy people older than 70 years, clonal hematopoiesis is present [10]. Additionally, loss of Y chromosome in hematopoietic cells in association with aging was also reported [1]. Therefore, clinicians should keep reserved when abnormalities in molecular genetics and karyotype are found in the elderly when dysplasia is absent [10].

Mutations like del(20q), +8, −Y have been reported in patients with aplastic anemia or other cytopenic syndromes who were good responders to immunosuppressive therapy and/or no evidence of MDS findings in the follow-up [1].

6. Acute myeloblastic leukemia

6.1. AML with low blast cell count

AML is distinguished from MDS by the percentage of the blasts which is higher than 30% in AML in children (>20% in adults) and lower than 30% (lower than 20% in adults) in MDS. However, patients that have blast cells lower than 30%, but cytogenetic features characteristic of childhood de novo AML [t(8;21), inv(16), t(11;17), t(9;11), i(1)] is designated as AML with low blast cell count (AML-LBC).

Those with AML-LBC were significantly younger than MDS cases (3.7 vs 7.4); their dysplasia score was lower and the response to AML type chemotherapy was higher than that of MDS patients. The authors encountered chloroma only in AML-LBC [71].

6.2. AML with myelodysplasia-related changes (AML-MRC)

In a subgroup of leukemia that was introduced by WHO is AML with myelodysplasia-related changes (AML-MRC) which defines AML arising from previous MDS or MDS/MPN, with an MDS-related cytogenetic abnormality and/or AML with multilineage dysplasia (AML-MLD). This group was reported to have worse overall survival when compared with patients with AML-not otherwise specified [110].

6.3. MDS with myelofibrosis, AML-M7, and other disorders

The blast cell percentage in the bone marrow (>30% in children and >20% in adults) and t(1;22)(p13;q13) differentiated AML-M7 from MDS.

Although hypoplastic MDS with increased reticulin ± collagen fibers is rare in childhood [4], hypoplastic myelofibrosis may be encountered in childhood [111].

7. Idiopathic cytopenia of undetermined significance (ICUS) and idiopathic dysplasia of undetermined significance (IDUS)

Patients with persistent (marked constant) cytopenia(s) involving one of more hematopoietic lineages, for at least 6 months, in the setting of absent multiunilineage dysplasia and cytogenetic abnormality except –Y, +8, del(20q) were suggested to be termed as idiopathic cytopenia of undetermined significance (ICUS) [5, 58, 112–116]. Criteria of cytopenia for diagnosis of both MDS and ICUS according to the 2007 Consensus Group are: Hemoglobin (Hb) <11g/dl and/or neutrophils <1500/mm^3, and/or thrombocytes <100,000/mm^3. The cut off levels for Hb is 10 g/dl, for neutrophils 1800/mm^3 according to WHO and International Working Group on Morphology of MDS (IWGM-MDS) [58, 114].

The terms "ICUS-anemia, ICUS-neutropenia, ICUS-thrombocytopenia, ICUS-bicytopenia, or bi/pancytopenia" were also proposed in which the cut-off levels of cytopenia were the same of those in 2007 Consensus Group, except that of neutropenia which was proposed as <1000/mm^3 [114].

For patients with morphological dysplasia (>10% in a major cell line) with/without karyotypic abnormalities but no or mild cytopenia, idiopathic dysplasia of undetermined significance (IDUS) has been proposed [5, 7]. Criteria of mild cytopenia has been reported as Hb ≥ 11 g/dl, neutrophils ≥ 1500/mm^3, thrombocytes ≥ 100,000/mm^3 [113] (**Table 10**).

Patients with both ICUS and IDUS may progress to overt MDS, MPN, MDS/MPN overlap disease, chronic myelomonocytic leukemia, AML after a variable period. ICUS can also reportedly transform to systemic mastocytosis, non-Hodgkin lymphoma, aplastic anemia [5,

113, 114]. There is no proof that every patient with ICUS or IDUS will develop neoplasia [114]. ICUS was reported to resolve spontaneously also [112]. However, the median overall survival in ICUS group was reported 44.3 months, being shorter than RA but longer than RCMD [116].

	Idiopathic cytopenia of unknown significance (ICUS)	Idiopathic dysplasia of unknown significance (IDUS)
Constant marked cytopenia*	Present [5, 58, 112–116]	Absent [5, 58, 112–116]
Diagnostic criteria of MDS	Absent [5, 58, 112–116]	Absent [5, 58, 112–116]
Diagnostic cocriteria of MDS**,†	Absent [113]; flow cytometric abnormalities: not known [112]	–?
Dysplasia (>10% of cells)	Absent [112–115]	Present [112–116]
Karyotype typical for MDS	Absent but FISH may reveal a very small clone carrying MDS-related cytogenetic defect [113, 114]	Present in a minority [112]
Clonality by HUMARA	In a minority of patients [112] (CCUS)	Not known [112]
Other diseases leading to cytopenia	No [113]	–
Other diseases leading to dysplasia	–	No [113]
Age	Older [113]	Younger [113]
Erythropoietin level	Low [113]	Adequate [113]
Marked reduction in BFU-E	In a minority of patients [112]	In a minority of patients [112]
Ring sideroblasts >15%	Absent [114]	In a majority of patients [114]

*Cytopenia in one or more of hematopoietic lineages lasting for at least 6 months, with Hb <11 g/dl and/or neutrophils <1500/mm^3, and/or thrombocytes <100,000/mm^3.
**Cocriteria of MDS: Colony forming cells and reticulocytes in circulation, abnormal immunophenotyping by flow cytometry, monoclonality of myeloid cells detected by molecular markers or mutations, abnormal gene expression profile by mRNA profiling assays.
†If one or more cocriteria are found, the disorder should be called 'highly susceptive for a clonal myeloid disease/MDS' [113].

Table 10. Diagnostic criteria for ICUS and IDUS [5, 58, 112–116].

On the other hand, recent reports demonstrated that ICUS had a broad spectrum including patients with both nonclonal and clonal hematopoiesis, the latter being called as clonal hematopoiesis of indeterminate potential (CHIP) [112]. Hence, 35% of ICUS patients were found to carry a somatic mutation or chromosomal abnormality indicative of clonal hematopoiesis [117] called clonal ICUS (CCUS).

Differentiation between MDS and ICUS may be challenging. In ICUS, FISH may reveal a very small clone carrying MDS-related cytogenetic defect [113, 114]. Clonal expansion of such a small clone in ICUS and occurrence of slight cytopenia in IDUS in the follow-up, points at an imminent transformation to MDS [58, 113, 114].

These patients should be examined regularly, like in low-risk MDS, from the aspect of hematological findings, karyotype, FISH, flow cytometry, and flow FISH, if available [114].

Reduced number of colony forming unit (CFU) progenitor cells like CFU-granulocyte-macrophage (CFU-GM) and burst-forming unit-erythroid (BFU-E) show impaired bone marrow function in MDS [58]. While BFU-E is markedly reduced in MDS, it is reduced only in a minority of patients with ICUS and IDUS [114]. However, reduced numbers of CFU-GM and BFU-E are also found in aplastic anemia, acute leukemia, and in post chemotherapy conditions, but not in nonclonal cytopenias like vitamin B12 deficiency, autoimmune hemolytic anemia and chronic inflammation [58] (**Table 10**).

Screening for molecular lesions by exome sequencing and other "omics-based techniques" can be used, in order to search clonality. However, these techniques are expensive and not practical [58]. Human androgen receptor gene-based assay (HUMARA) which is promising has restrictions, since it can be used only in females and it is positive in other clonal disorders also [58, 116]. Application of flow cytometric tools are of considerable help [58] (see Section 10). Patients with CCUS can be differentiated from low-risk MDS only by lack of dysplasia [112].

The data about patients with ICUS, CCUS, and IDUS are limited. Future studies will enlighten the pathogenesis of ICUS and IDUS which is not well understood yet.

8. Autoimmune disorders

Patients with chronic immune stimulation and autoimmune disorders have a tendency to develop malignant neoplasias and MDS.

On the other hand, MDS and AML can trigger paraneoplastic syndromes and manifestations including inflammatory paraneoplasia, like seronegative rheumatoid arthritis, Sweets syndrome, hemophagocytic lymphohistiocytosis, pyoderma gangraenosum, cutaneous vasculitis, lupus-like symptoms [72, 73], polychondritis [73], Behçet syndrome, inflammatory bowel disease, cryoglobulins, vitiligo, autoimmune hemolytic anemia, peripheral neuropathy, by 12–19% in adults but in lower frequency in childhood [74].

Relevance of autoimmune disorders with prognosis of MDS is disputable. Their response to immunosuppressive therapy is good [72].

In MDS, not only the stem cells but an inflammatory microenvironment is also involved. Therefore, the inflammatory microenvironment aggravates ineffective hematopoiesis and carcinogenesis/tumorigenesis [72].

The majority of acquired AA and some RCC cases can be considered as T-cell-mediated autoimmune disease, resulting in bone marrow failure [74, 76]. Autoantibodies are detected in both conditions. However, their significance and pathophysiological significance in MDS and SAA is unclear [76].

Relative lymphocytosis, oligoclonal T-cell expansion, elevated cytokine levels are common features of AA and MDS, suggesting a common immune defect in the pathogenesis [72] of adults with low-grade MDS.

Decreased CD4 + FOXP3 + Treg cells, increased NK cells/impaired activity of NK cells, suppression of hematopoietic progenitors by cytotoxic CD8+ cells [72, 74], increased cytokines secreted by bone marrow microenvironment, macrophages (IF-, TNF-α which are pro-apoptotic), increased Th17 cells [interleukin ((IL)-17, IL-23, IL-1, and IL-6] which are cytotoxic to bone marrow precursors, decreased dendritic cells, decreased B cells [72], polyclonal hypo-, hypergammaglobulinemia, C3 hypocomplementemia, altered self-reactive antibody repertoires [74] play role in the pathogenesis, some of which change as to the risk of MDS [72].

Some of these abnormalities overlap with those in autoimmune disorders themselves. The dysmorphic features in autoimmune disorders were delineated previously. Patients with autoimmune disorders should always be suspected for being MDS cases and should be evaluated for pathologic and genetic abnormalities.

9. Common features in pathogenesis

9.1. Cytopenia

Inherited bone marrow failure syndromes, MDS and SAA share the same pathogenetic features for involving a driver mutation, overproduction of cytokines and/or suppression of hematopoiesis through cytokines and deregulation of stem cell niche [76].

MDS and severe aplastic anemia share the same pathogenesis, as to abnormalities in T cells, especially in CD8+ cells; autoimmune manifestations and giving good response to immunosuppressive therapy [76].

9.2. Myelodysplasia in relation to cell cycle and other factors

Myelodysplasia in blood cells arise due to any challenge during the course of normal differentiation in which cells exit the cell cycle and enter G0 phase permanently (**Figure 10a**)

Cell cycle control system depends on cyclically activated cyclin-dependent protein kinases (Cdks) a number of enzymes and other proteins, the most important being cyclins and other genes [118]. Stem cell differentiation is regulated by differentiation specific genes, homeotic genes, tumor suppressor genes, abnormality of which result in restriction in further proliferation giving rise to alteration in normal cell cycle, and dysdifferentiation [119].

Hence, disturbance of expression of iron dependent genes regulating cell cycle in differentiation of hematopoietic cells in iron deficiency (see Section 2.5.2), deletion in human cell division cycle related gene (hCDCrel) in patients with del (22q11.2) are a few examples that lead to aforementioned myelodysplastic findings through genetic abnormalities. That the severity and spectrum of dysmorphic features in myelodysplasia differ according to the underlying secondary or primary pathology like in dysmegakaryopoiesis and thrombocytosis in inv

3(q21q26)/t(3;3)(q21;q26) and 5q-syndrome also reflect the various alterations playing role in different levels of differentiation.

We previously detected various temporary or permanent cell cycle abnormalities in total leukocytes, granulocytes and mononuclear cells from peripheral blood of ITP patients who had received steroids and a child with congenital neutropenia and her non-neutropenic mother all displaying myelodysplasia (**Figure 10**) [17, 45, 99].

The peripheral granulocytes (neutrophils and bands), monocytes, and lymphocytes are expected to be in G0 phase of the cell cycle, since they are terminally differentiated (**Figure 10a**). We interpreted these numerous abnormal cell cycle configurations instead of G0 [99], as an alteration in differentiation, after a stimulus that was sensed as DNA damage, probably through disruption of one or more of these aforementioned enzymes [118]. Increased trilineage apoptosis, a type of cell death in some of these patients [45, 99], all having myelodysplasia are also in accordance of this interpretation.

Overlapping of a number of myelodysplastic features (**Tables 1–4**) closely with those of senescence-like phenotype (SLP) of rapid cell senescence (RCS), another type of cell death, led us to search RCS both in congenital neutropenia [45, 99] and autoimmune disorders (JRA, SLE, and ITP) all having myelodysplasia [17, 28, 30, 31, 79]. We detected that three children with congenital neutropenia and their non-neutropenic mothers [45, 99] and all patients with autoimmune disorders displayed RCS in their leukocytes shown by β-galactosidase (SA-β-gal) positivity [79] (**Figure 1**). In several patients, cell cycle abnormalities accompanied [99] (**Figure 10I**).

The RCS that was detected in autoimmune disorders and those with congenital neutropenia [45] were attributed to increased proinflammatory cytokines and chemokines in autoimmune disorders [79] and congenital neutropenia [45] through giving rise to loss of telomeres by keeping the immune system in a state of low level of activation [79]. Absence of RCS (unpublished data) in iron deficient patients was thought to be due to absence of increase in proinflammatory cytokines, confirming this hypothesis.

Differentiation is controlled not only by intracellular genetic factors but by extracellular factors like extracellular matrix and soluble factors like fibroblast growth factor (FGF), transforming growth factor beta (TGFB), colony stimulating factor-1 (CSF-1), GCSF, GM-CSF, stem cell factor (SCF), Fms-like tyrosine kinase 3 ligand (Flt-3 ligand), ILs as well [119].

The reasons that we previously discussed in secondary myelodysplasia like immune destruction of stromal and hematopoietic cells, inhibitory effects of cytokines and/or other intracellular/extracellular messengers/soluble factors, on the microenvironment and/or hematopoietic cells; decreased differentiation, regeneration and increased clearance of stem cells, reflected by alterations in cell cycle, impairment of heme synthesis and iron utilization also play role in dysdifferentiation.

Therefore, myelodysplasia either primary or secondary is associated with cell death parameters, and cell cycle alterations. It reflects the viability of the cell and can be assumed as a tip of a big iceberg that is an harbinger of a large spectrum of primary (clonal) and secondary (nonclonal) disorders. We think that the criteria of dysplasia should be revised in the definition of MDS and attention should be exercised to find out practical laboratory means to detect clonality.

10. Differential diagnosis

Discrimination between low-risk MDS and disorders mimicking MDS depends on determining whether hematopoiesis is clonal or not.

To assess clonality and dysplasia, flow cytometric evaluation is promising [58, 120, 121]. The minimal requirements to assess dysplasia by flow cytometry have been defined for adulthood low-risk MDS as in the following [120]:

(a) For immature myeloid and monocytic progenitors: Increased percentage of cells in nucleated cell fraction, lack of/decreased/increased expression of CD45, CD34, CD13 + CD33, homogenous under/overexpression of CD117, lack of/increased expression of HLA-DR, asynchronous expression of CD11b, CD15, expression of CD5, CD7, CD19, CD56 which are lineage infidelity markers.

(b) For maturing neutrophils: Decreased percentage of cells as ratio to lymphocytes, sideward light scatter (SSC) as ratio vs SSC of lymphocytes, altered pattern in relationship of CD13 with CD11b and CD13 with CD16, CD15 with CD10 (like lack of CD10 on mature neutrophils).

(c) For monocytes: Decreased or increased percentage of cells, shift toward immature distribution, altered pattern in relationship of HLA-DR with CD11b and CD36 with CD14, homogenous under or overexpression of CD13 and CD33, expression of CD56 as which is a lineage infidelity marker.

(d) Progenitor B cells: Decreased or absent progenitor B cells when enumeration is performed as fraction of total CD34+ based on CD45/CD34/SSC in combination with CD10 or CD19.

(e) Erythroid compartment: Increased percentage of nucleated erythroid cells, altered pattern in relationship of CD71 with CD235a, decreased expression of CD71 and CD36, increased percentage of CD117-positive precursors.

(f) For megakaryocytes: No standard application of flow cytometry has been described for megakaryocytes yet.

World Health Organization recognized more than three flow cytometric aberrancies as indicative of MDS [120]. It was also reported that two or more aberrancies in only the four parameters as increased percentage of CD34+ progenitor cells in bone marrow, decreased number of progenitor B cells within the CD34+ compartment, decreased or increased CD45 expression on myeloid progenitor cells and decreased SSC of neutrophils, CD10, CD15, CD11b, CD56 being additional useful markers could identify 70% of low-risk MDS cases with 94% specificity [120]. In children, for distinction between SAA and RCC, which generally present with hypocellular bone marrow, a cutoff of 2 flow cytometric abnormalities was found to have

60% sensitivity and 88% specificity which changed as 76% and 84% respectively, when combined with other diagnostic parameters [121]. In nonclonal disorders either no or only one flow cytometric abnormality was found. In low-risk MDS, in rare patients no flow-cytometric abnormality was found [58].

However, abnormal flow patterns were encountered in AML, MPN, and natural aging also [58]. Current knowledge on normal and abnormal patterns in the elderly and in normal controls is still inadequate [120].

The flow cytometric analysis of children with RCC (low-risk MDS in childhood) showed no difference in the relative SSC of granulocytes between those in RCC and healthy controls and absence of lineage infidelity markers on myeloid blasts unlike commonly occurring in adult low-risk MDS. The most frequent abnormality in RCC was reported to be heterogeneous expression of CD71 and CD36 on erythrocytes and aberrant expression of CD56 on monocytes (in 58 and 20%). All other abnormalities were observed in RCC in lower frequency than in adulthood low-risk MDS [121].

However, although flow cytometric evaluation is promising in diagnosis of MDS cases which lacked specific diagnostic markers like ring sideroblasts or karyotypic aberrations, it can only be used as a part of a diagnostic work-up consisting of histopathology and cytogenetic analysis [120, 121].

Flow cytometry can be used to rule out PNH; but minor PNH clones are present in 13–23% of adult MDS, and 41% of children with RCC [121].

11. Future recommendations

We recommend that all the aforementioned disorders be considered in the differential diagnosis of MDS. Patients who do not comply with none of a definite diagnosis should be followed-up for a considerable time period in order to assure a spontaneous remission or progression. Spontaneous remission in children and youngsters were reported as 2.2–30 months after the diagnosis [61–68]. In childhood, in the setting of hypocellular bone marrow with absence of cytogenetic abnormality [4] or a bone marrow biopsy with topography and cellularity of the local hematopoiesis [9], two bone marrow biopsies at least two weeks apart are necessary [4]. For cases with refractory cytopenia and cases with less than 15% ring sideroblasts all of which display unilineage dysplasia without excess blasts, repeated bone marrow examination is recommended after a 6 months' observation [5].

Since morphologic dysplasia can be encountered in both clonal and nonclonal disorders, the criteria of dysplasia should be revised in the definition of MDS and attention should be exercised to find out practical laboratory means to detect clonality. Flow cytometry is a promising means to distinguish between clonal and nonclonal cytopenia when used together with other diagnostic tools.

Acknowledgements

The authors thank Hamza Okur PhD, for kindly performing flow cytometric analysis of cell cycle, Prof. Dr Esra Erdemli and Deniz Billur MD, for analyzing the leukocytes for rapid senescence.

Author details

Lale Olcay[1*] and Sevgi Yetgin[2]

*Address all correspondence to: baskent.edu.tr

1 Department of Pediatrics, Başkent University Faculty of Medicine, Unit of Pediatric Hematology, Oncology, Ankara, Turkey

2 Department of Pediatrics, Hacettepe University Faculty of Medicine, Unit of Pediatric Hematology, Oncology, Ankara, Turkey

References

[1] Vardiman JW, Thiele J, Arber DA, Brunning RD, Borowitz MJ, Porwit A, Harris NL, Le Beau MM, Hellström-Lindberg E, Tefferi A, Bloomfield CD: The 2008 revision of the World Health Organization (WHO) classification of myeloid neoplasms and acute leukemia: rationale and important changes. Blood. 2009;114:937–951. DOI: 10.1182/blood-2009-03-209262.

[2] Malcovati L, Hellström-Lindberg E, Bowen D, Adès L, Cermak J, del Cañizo, Porta MGD, Fenaux P, Gattermann N, Germing U, Jansen JH, Mittelman M, Mufti G, Platzbecker U, Sanz GF, Selleslag D, Skov-Holm M, Stauder R, Symeonidis A, van de Loosdrecht AA, de Witte T, Cazzola M: Diagnosis and treatment of primary myelodysplastic syndromes in adults: recommendations from the European LeukemiaNet. Blood. 2013; 122:2943–2964. DOI: 10.1182/blood-2013-03-492884.

[3] Hasle H: Myelodysplastic and myeloproliferative disorders in children. Curr Opin Pediatr. 2007;19:1–8.

[4] Niemeyer CH, Baumann I: Classification of childhood aplastic anemia and myelodysplastic syndrome. Hematol Am Soc Hematol Educ Program. 2011:2011:84–89. DOI: 10.1182/asheducation-2011.1.84.

[5] Invernizzi R, Quaglia F, Porta MGD: Importance of classical morphology in the diagnosis of myelodysplastic syndrome. Mediterr J Hematol Infect Dis. 2015;7:e2015035. DOI: 10.4084/MJHID.2015.035.

[6] Vardiman J: The classification of MDS: from FAB to WHO and beyond. Leuk Res. 2012;36:1453–1458.

[7] Garcia-Manero G. Myelodysplastic syndromes: 2015 update on diagnosis, risk-stratification and management. Am J Hematol. 2015;90:832–841. DOI: 10.1002/ajh.24102.

[8] Bain BJ, Clark DM, Wilkins BS: Bone Marrow Pathology. 4th ed. Singapore: Wiley-Blackwell; 2010. p.166–238.

[9] Hasegawa D: The current perspective of low-grade myelodysplastic syndrome in children. Int J Hematol. 2016. DOI: 10.1007/s12185-016-1965-7.

[10] Steensma DP: Myelodysplastic syndromes: diagnosis and treatment. Mayo Clin Proc. 2015;90:969–983. DOI: 10.1016/j.mayocp.2015.04.001.

[11] Yin CC, Medeiros J, Bueso-Ramos CE: Recent advances in the diagnosis and classification of myeloid neoplasms-comments on the 2008 WHO classification. Int Jnl Lab Hem. 2010;32:461–476. DOI: 10.1111/j.1751-553X.2010.01246.x.

[12] Brunning RD, Hasserjian RP, Porwit A, Bennett JM, Orazi A, Thiele J, Hellstrom-Lindberg E: Refractory cytopenia with unilineage dysplasia. In: Swerdlow SH, Campo E, Harris NL, Jaffe ES, Pileri SA, Stein H, Thiele J, Vardiman JW, editors. WHO Classification of Tumours of Hematopoietic and Lymphoid Tissues. 4th ed, Lyon: IARC Press; 2008. p. 94, 95.

[13] Rajmoldi AC, Fenu S, Kerndrup G, van Weing ER, Niemeyer CM, Baumann I: Evaluation of dysplastic features in myelodysplastic syndromes: experience from the morphology group of the European Working Group of MDS in Childhood (EWOG-MDS). Ann Hematol. 2005; 84:429–433. DOI: 10.1007/s00277-005-1034-4.

[14] Baumann I, Niemeyer CM, Bennett JM, Shannon K: Childhood myelodysplastic syndrome. In: Swerdlow SH, Campo E, Harris NL, Jaffe ES, Pileri SA, Stein H, Thiele J, Vardiman JW, editors. WHO Classification of Tumours of Hematopoietic and Lymphoid Tissues. 4th ed. Lyon: IARC Press; 2008. p. 104–107.

[15] Pagliuca A, Mufti GJ: Clinicomorphological features of myelodysplastic syndromes. In: Mufti GJ, Galton DAG, editors. The Myelodysplastic Syndromes. 1st ed. London: Churchill Livingstone; 1992. p. 1–13.

[16] Bain B: Leukemia Diagnosis. 3rd ed. Oxford: Blackwell Publishing; 2003. P. 144–179.

[17] Olcay L, Yetgin S, Okur H, Erekul S, Tuncer M: Dysplastic changes in idiopathic thrombocytopenic purpura and the effect of corticosteroids to increase dysplasia and cause hyperdiploid macropolycytes. Am J Hematol. 2000;65:99–104.

[18] Bain BJ, Clark DM, Wilkins BS: Bone Marrow Pathology. 4th ed. Singapore: Wiley-Blackwell; 2010. p. 100–165.

[19] Hasle H, Kerndrup G, Jacobsen BB, Heegaard ED, Hornsleth A, Lillevang ST: Chroniv parvovirus infection mimicking myelodysplastic syndrome in a child with subclinical immunodeficiency. Am J Ped Hematol Oncol. 1994;16:329–333.

[20] Baurmann H, Schwarz TF, Oertel J, Serke S, Roggendorf M, Huhn D: Acute parvovirus B19 infection mimicking myelodysplastic syndrome of the bone marrow. Ann Hematol. 1992;64:43–45.

[21] Yarali N, Duru F, Sipahi T, Kara A, Teziç T: Parvovirus B19 infection reminiscent of myelodysplastic syndrome in three children with chronic hemolytic anemia. Pediatr Hematol Oncol. 2000;17:475–482.

[22] Carpenter SL, Zimmerman SA, Ware RE: Acute parvovirus B19 infection mimicking congenital dyserythropoietic anemia. J Pediatr Hematol Oncol. 2004;26:133–135.

[23] Miyahara M, Shimamoto Y, Yamada H Shibata K, Matsuzaki M, Ono K: Cytomegalovirus-associated myelodysplasia and thrombocytopenia in an immunocompetent adult. Ann Hematol. 1997;74:99–101.

[24] Klco JM, Geng B, Brunt EM, Hassan A, Nguyen TD, Kreisel FH, Lisker-Melman M, Frater JL: Bone marrow biopsy in patients with hepatitis C virus infection: spectrum of findings and diagnostic utility. Am J Hematol. 2010;85:106–110.

[25] Yaralı N, Fışkın T, Duru F, Kara A: Myelodysplastic features in visceral leishmaniasis. Am J Hematol. 2002;71:191–195.

[26] Dhingra KK, Gupta P, Saroha V, Setia N, Khurana N, Singh T: Morphological findings in bone marrow biopsy and aspirate smears of visceral kala azar: a review. Ind J Pathol Microbiol. 2010;52:96–100. DOI: 10.4103/0377-4929.59193.

[27] Bain BJ, Clark DM, Wilkins BS. Bone Marrow Pathology. 4th ed. Singapore: Wiley-Blackwell; 2010. p. 500–548.

[28] Yetgin S, Ozen S, Saatci U, Bakkaloglu A, Besbas N, Kirel B: Myelodysplastic features in juvenile rheumatoid arthritis. Am J Hematol. 1997;54:166–169.

[29] Yetgin S, Ozen S, Yenicesu I, Cetin M, Bakkaloğlu A: Myelodysplastic features in polyarteritis nodosa. Pediatr Hematol Oncol. 2001;18:157–160.

[30] Voulgarelis M, Giannouli S, Tasidou A, Anagnostou D, Ziakas PD, Tzioufas AG: Bone marrow histological findings in systemic lupus erythematosus with hematologic abnormalities: a clinicopathological study. Am J Hematol. 2006;81:590–597. DOI: 10.1002/ajh.20593.

[31] Olcay L, Tuncer AM, Okur H, Erdemli E, Uysal Z, Çetin M, Duru F, Uçkan Çetinkaya D: Excessive naked megakaryocyte nuclei in myelodysplastic syndrome mimicking

idiopathic thrombocytopenic purpura: a complicated pre- and post-transplantation course. Pediatr Hematol Oncol. 2009;26:387–397. DOI: 10.3109/08880010902891891.

[32] Fattizzo B, Zaninoni A, Consonni D, Zanella A, Gianelli U, Cortelezzi A, Barcellini W: Is chronic neutropenia always a benign disease? Evidences from a 5-year prospective study. Eur J Intern Med. 2015;26:611–615. DOI: 10.1016/j.ejim.2015.05.019.

[33] Das S, Mishra P, Kar R, Basu D: Gelatinous marrow transformation: a series of 11 cases from a tertiary care centre in South India. Gelatinous marrow transformation: a series of 11 cases from a tertiary care centre in South India. Turk J Hematol. 2014;31:175–179. DOI: 10.4274/Tjh.2012.0151.

[34] Bhasin TS, Sharma S, Chandey M, Bhatia PK, Mannan R: A case of bone marrow necrosis of an idiopathic aetiology: the report of a rare entity with review of the literature. J Clin Diagnostic Res. 2012;7:525–528.

[35] Cotta CV: Gelatinous transformation. Blood. 2012;120:2166.

[36] Yetgin S, Aslan D, Unal S, Tavil B, Kuşkonmaz B, Aytaç Elmas S, Olcay L, Uçkan Çetinkaya D: Dysplasia and disorder of cell membrane entirety in iron-deficiency anemia. Pediatr Hematol Oncol. 2008;25:492–450. DOI: 10.1080/08880010802234804.

[37] Koca E, Buyukasik Y, Cetiner D, Yilmaz R, Sayinalp N, Yasavul U, Uner A: Copper deficiency with increased hematogones mimicking refractory anemia with excess blasts. Leuk Res. 2008;32:495–499. DOI: 10.1016/j.leukres.2007.06.023.

[38] Gregg XT, Reddy V, Prchal JT: Copper deficiency masquerading as myelodysplastic syndrome. Blood. 2002;100:1493–1495. DOI: 10.1182/blood-2002-01-0256.

[39] Lazarchick J: Update on anemia and neutropenia in copper deficiency. Curr Opin Hematol. 2012;19:58–60. DOI: 10.1097/MOH.0b013e32834da9d2.

[40] Sochet AA, Jones A, Riggs CD, Weibley RE: A 3-year-old boy with severe anemia and neutropenia. Pediatric Ann. 2013;42:1.

[41] Cordano A: Clinical manifestations of nutritional copper deficiency in infants and children. Am J Clin Nutr 1998; 67(suppl):1012S–1016S.

[42] Yetgin S, Yalçın SS: The effect of vitamin D3 on CD34 progenitor cells in vitamin D deficiency rickets. Turk J Pediatr. 2004;46:164–166.

[43] Perrotta S, Nobili B, Rossi F, Criscuolo M, Iolascon A, DiPinto D, Passaro I, Cennamo L, Oliva A, Ragione FD: Infant hypervitaminosis A causes severe anemia and thrombocytopenia: evidence of a retinol-dependent bone marrow cell growth inhibition. Blood. 2002;99:2017–2022.

[44] Olcay L, Yetgin S, Erdemli E, Germeshausen M, Aktaş D, Büyükaşık Y, Okur H: Congenital dysgranulopoietic neutropenia. Pediatr Blood Cancer. 2008;50:115–119. DOI: 10.1002/pbc.20877.

[45] Olcay L, Ünal Ş, Öztürk A, Erdemli E, Billur D, Metin A, Okur H, İkincioğulları A, Yıldırmak Y, Büyükaşık Y, Yılmaz-Falay M, Özet G, Yetgin S: Granulocytic and non granulocytic lineages in children with congenital neutropenia and their non neutropenic parents: biochemical, functional, morphological and genetic evaluation. Haematologica. 2012;97 (suppl 3):36–37 (PO 65).

[46] Ozbek N, Derbent M, Olcay L, Yilmaz Z, Tokel K: Dysplastic changes in the peripheral blood of children with microdeletion 22q11.2. Am J Hematol. 2004;77:126–131. DOI: 10.1002/ajh.20139.

[47] Hinson DD, Rogers ZR, Hoffmann GF, Schachtele M, Fingerhut R, Kohlschutter A, Kelley RI, Gibson KM: Hematological abnormalities and cholestatic liver disease in two patients with mevalonate kinase deficiency. Am J Med Genet. 1998;78:408–412.

[48] Jakovleva K, Everaus H: Some aspects of morphological and dysplastic changes of the bone marrow in malignant lymphoma. Acta Haematol. 1998;100:142–146.

[49] Olcay L, Hazırolan T, Yıldırmak Y, Erdemli E, Terzi Y, Arda K: Biochemical, radiologic, ultrastructural, and genetic evaluation of iron overload in acute leukemia and iron-chelation therapy. J Pediatr Hematol Oncol. 2014;36:281–292.

[50] Michot F, Gut J: Alcohol-induced bone marrow damage. A bone marrow study in alcohol-dependent individuals. Acta Haematol. 1987;78:252–257.

[51] Budde R, Schaefer HE: Smokers' dysmyelopoiesis—bone marrow alterations associated with cigarette smoking. Pathol Res Pract. 1989;185:347–350.

[52] Rezuke WN, Anderson C, Pastuszak WT, Conway SR, Firshein SI: Arsenic intoxication presenting as a myelodysplastic syndrome: a case report. Am J Hematol. 1991;36:291–293.

[53] Krajewski W, Kucharska M, Pilacik B, Fobker M, Stetkiewicz J, Nofer JR, Wronska-Nofer T: Impaired vitamin B12 metabolic status in healthcare workers occupationally exposed to nitrous oxide. Br J Anaesth. 2007;99:812–818. DOI: 10.1093/bja/aem280.

[54] Meyerson HJ, Farhi DC, Rosenthal NS: Transient increase in blasts mimicking acute leukemia and progressing myelodysplasia in patients receiving growth factor. Am J Clin Pathol. 1998;109:675–681.

[55] Clatch RJ, Krigman HR, Peters MG, Zutter MM: Dysplastic haemopoiesis following orthotopic liver transplantation: comparison with similar changes in HIV infection and primary myelodysplasia. Br J Haematol. 1994;88:685–692.

[56] Naqvi K, Jabbour E, Bueso-Ramos C, Pierce S, Borthakur G, Estrov Z, Ravandi F, Faderl S, Kantarjian H, Garcia-Manero G: Implications of discrepancy in morphologic diagnosis of myelodysplastic syndrome between referral and tertiary care centers. Blood. 2011;118:4690–4693. DOI: 10.1182/blood-2011-03-342642.

[57] Baumann I, Führer M, Behrendt S, Campr V, Csomor J, Furlan I, de Haas V, Kerndrup G, Leguit R, De Paepe P, Noellke P, Niemeyer C, Schwarz S: Morphological differen-

tiation of severe aplastic anaemia from hypocellular refractory cytopenia of childhood: reproducibility of histopathological diagnostic criteria. Histopathology. 2012;61:10–17. DOI: 10.1111/j.1365-2559.2011.04156.x.

[58] Valent P: Low blood counts: immune mediated, idiopathic, or myelodysplasia. Hematol Am Soc Hematol Educ Program. 2012;2012:485–491. DOI: 10.1182/asheducation-2012.1.485.

[59] Bennett JM, Orazi A: Diagnostic criteria to distinguish hypocellular acute myeloid leukemia from hypocellular myelodysplastic syndromes and aplastic anemia: recommendations for a standardized approach. Haematologica. 2009;94:264–268. DOI: 10.3324/haematol.1375.

[60] Forester CM,Sartain SE, Guo D, Harris MH, Weinberg OK, Fleming MD, London WB, Williams DA, Hofmann I: Pediatric aplastic anemia and refractory cytopenia: a retrospective analysis assessing outcomes and histomorphologic predictors. Am J Hematol. 2015;90:320–326. DOI: 10.1002/ajh.23937.

[61] Mantadakis E, Shannon KM, Singer DA, Finklestein J, Chan KW, Hilden JM, Sandler ES: Transient monosomy 7. A case series in children and review of the literature. Cancer. 1999;85:2655–2661.

[62] Scheurlen W, Borkhardt A, Ritterbach J, Huppertz HI: Spontaneous hematological remission in a boy with myelodysplastic syndrome and monosony 7. Leukemia. 1994;8:1435–1438.

[63] Renneboog B, Hansen V, Heimannn P, De Mulder A, Janssen F, Ferster A: Spontaneous remission in a patient with therapy-related myelodysplastic syndrome (t-MDS) with monosomy 7. Br J Haematol. 1996;92:696–698.

[64] Laver JH, Yusuf U, Cantu ES, Barredo JC, Holt LB, Abboud MR: Transient therapy-related myelodysplastic syndrome associated with monosomy 7 and 11q23 translocation. Leukemia. 1997;11:448–455.

[65] Leung EW, Woodman RC, Roland B, Abdelhaleem M, Freedman MH, Dror Y: Transient myelodysplastic syndrome associated with isochromosome 7q abnormality. Pediatr Hematol Oncol. 2003;20:539–545. DOI: 10.1080/08880010390232754.

[66] Parker TM, Klaassen RJ, Johnston DL: Spontaneous remission of myelodysplastic syndrome with monosomy 7 in a young boy. Cancer Genet Cytogenet. 2008;182:122–125. DOI: 10.1016/j.cancergencyto.2008.01.003.

[67] Wollman MR, Penchansky L, Shekhter-Levin S: Transient 7q- in association with megaloblastic anemia due to dietary folate and vitamin B12 deficiency. J Pediatr Hematol Oncol. 1996;18:162–165.

[68] Bader-Meunier B, Miélot F, Tchernia G, Buisine J, Delsol G, Duchayne E, Allemlerle S, Leverger G, de Lumley L, Manel A-M, Nathanson M, Plantaz D, Robert A, Schaison G, Sommelet D, Vilmer E: Myelodysplastic syndromes in childhood: report of 49 patients

from a French multicentre study. French Society of Paediatric Haematology and Immunology. Br J Haematol. 1996;92:344–350.

[69] Sevilla J, Querol S, Molines A, Gonzalez-Vicent M, Balas A, Carrio A, Estella J, Angel Diaz M, Madero L: Transient donor cell-derived myelodysplastic syndrome with monosomy 7 after unrelated cord blood transplantation. Eur J Haematol. 2006;77:259–263. DOI: 10.1111/j.1600-0609.2006.00716.

[70] Barrios NJ, Kirkpatrick DV, Levin ML, Varela M: Transient expression of trisomy 21 and monosomy 7 following cyclosporin A in a patient with aplastic anemia. Leuk Res. 1991;15:531–533.

[71] Chan GC, Wang WC, Raimondi SC, Behm FG, Krance RA, Chen G, Freiberg A, Ingram L, Butler D, Head DR: Myelodysplastic syndrome in children: differentiation from acute myeloid leukemia with a low blast count. Leukemia.1997;11:206–211.

[72] Frietsch JJ, Dornaus S, Neumann T, Scholl S, Schmidt V, Kunert C, Sayer HG, Hochhaus A, La Rosee P: Paraneoplastic inflammation in myelodysplastic syndrome or bone marrow failure: case series with focus on 5-azacytidine and literature review. Eur J Haematol. 2014;93:247–259. DOI: 10.1111/ejh.12311.

[73] Hiçsönmez G, Çetin M, Yenicesu İ, Olcay L, Koç A, Aktaş D, Tunçbilek E, Tuncer M: Evaluation of children with myelodysplastic syndrome: importance of extramedullary disease as a presenting symptom. Leuk Lymphoma. 2002;42:665–674.

[74] Wu J, Cheng Y, Zhang L: Comparison of immune manifestations between refractory cytopenia of childhood and aplastic anemia in children: a single-center retrospective study. Leuk Res. 2015;39:1347–1352. DOI: 10.1016/j.leukres.2015.09.012.

[75] Dieterich DT, Spivak JL: Hematologic disorders associated with hepatitis C virus infection and their management. CID. 2003;37:533–541.

[76] Zhang W, Nardi MA, Borkowsky W, Li Z, Karpatkin S: Role of molecular mimicry of hepatitis C virus protein with platelet GPIIIa in hepatitis C-related immunologic thrombocytopenia. Blood. 2009;113:4086–4093. DOI: 10.1182/blood-2008-09-181073.

[77] Erlacher M, Strahm B: Missing cells: pathophysiology, diagnosis, and management of (pan)cytopenia in childhood. Front Pediatr. 2015;3:64. DOI: 10.3389/fped.2015.00064.

[78] Krueger GR, Kudlimay D, Ramon A, Klueppelberg U, Schumacker K: Demonstration of active and latent Epstein-Barr virus and human herpesvirus-6 infections in bone marrow cells of patients with myelodysplasia and chronic myeloproliferative diseases. In Vivo (Athens, Greece). 1994;8:533–542.

[79] Olcay L, Billur D, Erdemli E, Baskın SE, Balcı HF, Yetgin S: Myelodysplastic features and cellular senescence in autoimmune disorders: a pilot study on patients with collagen tissue disorders and immune thrombocytopenic purpura. Turk J Med Sci. 2015;45:742–744. DOI: 10.3906/sag-1408-149.

[80] Wang J-D, Chang T-K, Lin H-K, Huang F-L, Wang C-J, Lee H-J: Reduced expression of transforming growth factor-β1 and correlated elevation of interleukin-17 and interferon-γ in pediatric patients with chronic primary immune thrombocytopenia (ITP). Pediatr Blood Cancer. 2011;57:636–640. DOI:10.1002/pbc.22984.

[81] Houwerzijl EJ, Blom NR, van der Want JJL, Louwes H, Esselink MT, Smit JW, Vellenga E, de Wolf JTM: Increased peripheral olatelet destruction ans caspase-3-independent programmed cell death of bone marrow megakaryocytes in myelodysplastic patients. Blood. 2005;105:3472–3479. DOI: 10.1182/blood-2004-06-2108.

[82] Houwerzijl EJ, Blom NR, van der Want JJL, Esselink MT, Koomstra JJ, Smit JW, Louwes H, Vellenga E, de Wolf JT: Ultrastructural study shows morphologic features of apoptosis and para-apoptosis in megakaryocytes from patients with idiopathic thrombocytopenic purpura. Blood. 2004;103:500–506. DOI: 10.1182/blood-2003-01-0275.

[83] Li X, Pu Q. Megakaryocytopoiesis and apoptosis in patients with myelodysplastic syndromes. Leuk Lymphoma. 2005;46:387–391. DOI: 10.1080/10428190400013126.

[84] Shi XD, Hu T, Feng YL, Liu R, Li JH, Chen J, Wang TY: A study on micromegakaryocyte in children with idiopathic thrombocytopenic purpura. Zhonghua Er Ke Za Zhi. 2004;42:192–195.

[85] Uçar C, Ören H, İrken G, Ateş H, Atabay B, Türker M, Vergin C, Yaprak I: Investigation of megakaryocyte apoptosis in children with acute and chronic idiopathic thrombocytopenic purpura. Eur J Haematol. 2003;70: 347–352.

[86] Raza A, Gezer S, Mundle S, Gao X-Z, Alvi S, Borok R, Rifkin S, Iftikhar A, Shetty V, Parcharidou A, Loew J, Marcus B, Khan Z, Chaney C, Showel J, Gregory S, Preisler H: Apoptosis in bone marrow biopsy samples involving stromal and hematopoietic cells in 50 patients with myelodysplastic syndromes. Blood.1995;86:268–276.

[87] Shioi Y, Tamura H, Yokose N, Satoh C, Dan K, Ogata K: Increased apoptosis of circulating T cells in myelodysplastic syndromes. Leuk Res. 2007;31:1641–1648. DOI: 10.1016/j.leukres.2007.03.026.

[88] Olsson B, Andersson P-O, Jacobsson S, Carlsson L, Wadenvik H: Disturbed apoptosis of T-cells in patiemnts with active idiopathic thrombocytopenic purpura. Thromb Haemost. 2005;93:139–144.

[89] Hamada K, Takahashi I, Matsuoka M, Saika T, Mizobuchi N, Yorimitsu S, Takimoto H: Apoptosis of peripheral leukocytes in patients with myelodysplastic syndromes. Rinsho Ketsueki. 1998;39:1079–1084.

[90] Connor DE, Ma DDF, Joseph JE: Flow cytometry demonstrates differences in platelet reactivity and microparticle formation in subjects with thrombocytopenia or thrombocytosis due to primary haematological disorders. Thromb Res. 2013;132:572–577. DOI: 10.1016/j.thromres.2013.09.009.

[91] Bourgeois E, Caulier MT, Rose C, Dupriez B, Bauters F, Fenaux P: Role of splenectomy in the treatment of myelodysplastic syndromes with peripheral thrombocytopenia: a report on six cases. Leukemia. 2001;15:950–953.

[92] Abdul-Wahab J, Naznin M, Suhaimi A, Amir-Hamzah AR: Favourable response to splenectomy in familial myelodysplastic syndrome. Singapore Med J. 2007;48:e206–e208.

[93] Neunert C, Lim W, Crowther M, Cohen A, Solberg L, Crowther MA: The American Society of Hematology 2011 evidence-based practice guideline for immune thrombocytopenia. Blood. 2011;117:4190–4207.DOI: 10.1182/blood-2010-08-302984.

[94] Alcantara O, Kalidas M, Baltathakis I, Boldt DH: Expression of multiple genes regulating cell cycle and apoptosis in differentiating hematopoietic cells is dependent on iron. Exp Hematol 2001;29:1060–1069.

[95] Varkonyi J, Szabo T, Sebestyen P, Tordai A, Andrikovics H, Kollai G, Karadi I: New aspects of copper and iron metabolism in the myelodysplastic syndromes. Chemotherapy. 2006;52:66–68. DOI: 10.1159/000091307.

[96] Lorand-Metze I: The importance of bone marrow histology in MDS. In: Lopes LF, Hasle H, editors. Myelodysplastic and Myeloproliferative Disorders in Children. 1st ed. Brazil: Lemar Livraria; 2003. p. 89–102.

[97] Yetgin S, Ozsoylu S, Ruacan S, Tekinalp G, Sarialioglu F: Vitamin D-deficiency rickets and myelofibrosis. J Pediatr. 1989;114:213–217.

[98] Yetgin S, Ozsoylu S: Myeloid metaplasia in vitamin D deficiency rickets. Scand J Haematol. 1982;28:180–185.

[99] Olcay L,Yetgin S, Okur H, Erdemli E: Rapid cell senescence and apoptosis in lymphocytesand granulocytes and absence of GM-CSF receptor in congenital dysgranulopoietic neutropenia. Leuk Res. 2008;32:235–242. DOI: 10.1016/j.leukres.2007.06.017.

[100] Olcay L, Koç A: Autoimmune hemolytic anemia preceding T-ALL in a five-year-old girl. Ped Hematol Oncol. 2005;22:207–213. DOI: 10.1080/08880010590921478.

[101] Kaymak-Cihan M, Yıldırım ÜM, Paç A, Gül S, Duman R, Tekgündüz E, Terzi YK, Kutlay NY, Dalva K, Yurtçu A, Ünver S, Olcay L. A case with therapy-related myelodysplastic syndrome secondary to acute myelod leukemia. Haematologica. 2012;97(suppl 3):PO-22.

[102] Arana-Yi C, Block AMW, Sait SN, Ford LA, Barcos M, Baer MR: Therapy-related myelodysplastic syndrome and acute myeloid leukemia following treatment of acute myeloid leukemia: possible role of cytarabine. Leuk Res. 2008;32:1043–1048. DOI: 10.1016/j.leukres.2007.11.006.

[103] Colman N, Herbert V: Hematologic complications of alhoholism. Semin Hematol. 1980;17:164–167.

[104] Du Y, Fryzek J, Sekeres MA, Taioli E: Smoking and alcohol intake as risk factors for myelodysplastic syndromes (MDS). Leuk Res. 2010;34:1–5. DOI: 10.1016/j.leukres.2009.08.006.

[105] Chatterjee T, Choudhry VP: Childhood myelodysplastic syndrome. Indian J Pediatr. 2013;80:764–771. DOI: 10.1007/s12098-013-1130-8.

[106] Olcay L, Çetin M: Vitamin B12 deficiency presenting with hemorrhagic diathesis due to thrombocytopenia in childhood. Turk J Haematol. 1998;15:97–99.

[107] Das KC, Mohanty D, Garewal G: Cytogenetics in nutritional megaloblastic anaemia: prolonged persistence of chromosomal abnormalities in lymphocytes after remission. Acta Haematol. 1986;76:146–154.

[108] Chintagumpala MM, Dreyer ZAE, Steuber CP, Cooley LD: Pancytopenia with chromosomal fragility: vitamin B12 deficiency. J Pediatr Hematol Oncol. 1996;18:166–170.

[109] Aitelli C, Wasson L, Page R: Pernicious anemia: presentations mimicking acute leukemia. South Med J. 2004;97:295–297.

[110] Podberezin M, Angeles R, Peace D, Rondelli D, Quigley J, Lindgren V, Gaitonde S: Acute myeloid leukemia with myelodysplasia-related changes. A new entity defined by the WHO 2008 classification of hematopoietic and lymphoid neoplasms. Labmedicine. 2009;40:397–400. DOI: 10.1309/LMHEN4FTDQ3F2MYU.

[111] Akyay A, Olcay L, Kuzu I, Bozdoğan N, Ünal-İnce E, İleri T, Tükün A, Yürür-Kutlay N: A child with myelodysplastic syndrome with hypocellular fibrosis. J Pediatr Hematol Oncol. 2010;32:617–620. DOI: 10.1097/MPH.0b013e3181e6262c.

[112] Steensma DP, Bejar R, Jaiswal S, Lindsley RC, Sekeres MA, Hasserjian RP, Ebert BL: Clonal hematopoiesis of indeterminate potential and its distinction from myelodysplastic syndromes. Blood. 2015;126:9–16. DOI: 10.1182/blood-2015-03-631747.

[113] Valent P, Horny HP: Minimal diagnostic criteria for myelodysplastic syndromes and separation from ICUS and IDUS: update and open questions. Eur J Clin Invest. 2009;39:548–553. DOI: 10.1111/j.1365-2362.2009.02151.x.

[114] Valent P, Bain BJ, Bennett JM, Wimazal F, Sperr WR, Mufti G, Horny H-P: Idiopathic cytopenia of undetermined significance (ICUS) and idiopathic dysplasia of uncertain significance (IDUS), and their distinction from low risk MDS. Leuk Res. 2012;36:1–5. DOI: 10.1016/j.leukres.2011.08.016.

[115] Giagounidis A, Haase D: Morphology, cytogenetics and classification of MDS. Best Practise Res Clin Haematol. 2013;26:337–353. DOI: 10.1016/j.beha.2013.09.004.

[116] Schroeder T, Ruf L, Bernhardt A, Hildebrandt B, Aivado M, Aul C, Gattermann N, Haas R, Germing U: Distinguishing myelodysplastic syndromes (MDS) from idiopathic cytopenia of undetermined significance (ICUS): HUMARA unravels clonality in a subgroup of patients. Annals Oncol. 2010;21:2267–2271. DOI: 10.1093/annonc/mdq233.

[117] Kwok B, Hall JM, Witte JS, Xu Y, Reddy P, Lin K, Flamholz R, Dabbas B, Yung A, Al-Hafidh J, Balmert E, Vaupel C, El Hader C, McGinniss MJ, Nahas SA, Kines J, Bejar R: MDS-associated somatic mutations and clonal hematopoiesis are common in idiopathic cytopenias of undetermined significance. Blood. 2015;126:2355–2361. DOI: 10.1182/blood-2015-08-667063.

[118] Alberts B, Johnson A, Lewis J, Morgan D, Raff M, Roberts K, Walter P, Wilson J, Hunt T: Molecular Biology of The Cell. 6th ed. New York: Taylor & Francis Group; 2015. p. 963–1020.

[119] Andreeff M, Goodrich DW, Pardee AB: Cell proliferation, differentiation, and apoptosis. In: Holland JF, Kufe DW, Pollock RE, Weichselbaum RR, Frei EI, Bast Jr RC, Bast Jr RC, editors. Cancer Medicine. 5th ed. Ontario: BC Decker Inc; 2000. p. 17–32.

[120] Westers TM, Ireland R, Kern W, Alhan C, Balleisen JS, Bettelheim P, Burbury K, Cullen M, Cutler JA, Della Porta MG, Drager AM, Feuillard J, Font P, Germing U, Haase D, Johansson U, Kordasti S, Loken MR, Malcovati L, te Marvelde JG, Matarraz S, Milne T, Moshaver B, Mufti GJ, Ogata K, Orfao A, Porwit A, Psarra K, Richards SJ, Subira D, Tindell V, Vallespi T, Valent P, van der Velden VHJ, de Witte TM, Wells DA, Zetti F, Bene M, van de Loosdrecht AA: Standardation of flow cytometry in myelodysplastic syndromes: a report from an international consortium and the European LeukemiaNet Working Group. Leukemia. 2012;26:1730–1741. DOI: 10.1038/leu.2012.30.

[121] Aalbers AM, van den Heuvel-Elbrink MM, Baumann I, Dworzak M, Hasle H, Locatelli F, De Moerloose B, Schmugge M, Mejstrikova E, Novakova M, Zecca M, Zwaan CM, te Marvelde JG, Langerak AW, van Dongen JJM, Pieters R, Niemeyer CM, van der Velden VHJ: Bone marrow immunophenotyping by flow cytometry in refractory cytopenia of childhood. Haematologica. 2015;100:315–323. DOI: 10.3324/haematol.2014.107706.

[122] Özsoylu Ş: High-dose intravenous methylprednisolone (HIVMP) in hematologi disorders. Hematol Rev. 1990;4:197–207.

Chapter 4

Myelodysplastic Disorders, 5q-Syndrome

Khalid Ahmed Al-Anazi

Additional information is available at the end of the chapter

http://dx.doi.org/10.5772/64202

Abstract

The myelodysplastic syndromes (MDSs) are characterized by ineffective erythropoiesis and progressive cytopenia and ultimately affected patients develop acute myeloid leukemia (AML) or die from advanced bone marrow (BM) failure.

Myelodysplastic syndrome (MDS) with isolated del (5q) is a common type of MDS with specific pathological and clinical manifestations including refractory anemia. It is usually treated by (1) supportive measures including blood transfusions that may cause iron overload that requires iron chelation therapy, (2) targeted therapies such as the immunomodulatory drug lenalidomide, and (3) hematopoietic stem cell transplantation (HSCT) in transplant eligible individuals. The establishment of the various prognostic systems, the discovery of the new genetic mutations, and the identification of new targets, in MDSs in general and in 5q-syndrome in particular, will hopefully translate into more pinpointed targeted therapies that will further improve the outcomes of patients having these disorders.

Keywords: myelodysplastic syndrome, 5q-syndrome, iron overload, lenalidomide, hematopoietic stem cell transplantation

1. Introduction

The MDSs are a group of clonal stem cell disorders that are characterized by ineffective erythropoiesis due to excessive apoptosis and progressive peripheral blood cytopenia culminating into acute myeloid leukemia AML or death from progressive BM failure [1–4]. MDS is primarily a disease of the elderly with a median age of 70 years [3]. The MDSs have been linked to several etiologies, risk factors, and environmental associations such as alcohol intake, tobacco use, Sweet's syndrome, vitamin deficiencies, cytotoxic chemotherapy, various hereditary disorders, and BM failure syndromes [5–12].

2. Pathogenesis of MDSs

The pathogenesis of MDS is poorly understood [5, 12]. However, several pathogenic mechanisms have been described and these include the following: (1) genetic mutations as the cell of origin has acquired multiple mutations that result in dysplasia and ineffective erythropoiesis; (2) MDS clonality: MDS is a clonal process thought to develop from a single-transformed hematopoietic progenitor cell. The inciting mutation is unknown for the majority of cases. However, recurrent genetic mutations involving RNA splicing machinery have been identified; (3) haploinsufficiency of ribosomal proteins particularly ribosomal protein (RPS) 14 in del (5q); (4) telomere dysfunction and aberrant or absent expression of micro-RNA species; (5) epigenetic changes: MDS genomes are characterized by global DNA hypomethylation with concomitant hypermethylation of gene-promoter regions relative to normal controls; (6) factors extrinsic to hematopoietic cells such as stromal abnormalities and T-cell dysregulation that may occur causally or secondary to the primary genetic defects; (7) accelerated apoptosis and ineffective erythropoiesis; (8) altered immune responses such as polyclonal expansion of helper T cells (CD4+) and oligoclonal expansion of cytotoxic T cells (CD8+) in the peripheral blood and BM; (10) leukemic transformation in MDS; the estimated risk of leukemic transformation is more than 50% and is more frequent in patients with high-risk MDS such as refractory anemia with excess of blasts (RAEB) II, monosomy 7, deletion of short arm of chromosome 17, deletion of long arm of chromosome 7, and trisomy 8 [5, 12].

3. Chromosome 5 abnormalities in MDS

Approximately, 15% of patients with MDS have abnormalities of chromosome 5 that include insertional deletion of a segment of the long arm of the chromosome [del (5q) or 5q-syndrome], monosomy 5, and unbalanced translocations [13].

3.1. Del (5q) type of MDS

The insertional deletion of the long arm of chromosome 5, del (5q), is the one of the most common cytogenetic abnormality encountered in patients with MDSs as it has been reported in 10–30% of patients with MDS [14–17]. The long arm of chromosome 5 has two distinct commonly deleted regions (CDRs). The more distal CDR lies in 5q33.1 and contains 40 protein coding genes and genes that code for microRNAs (miR-143 and miR-145) [13]. Many genes related to hematopoiesis are located on the long arm of chromosome 5 [18]. In del (5q), one allele is deleted and this accounts for the genetic haploinsufficiency [13]. The gene cluster at 5q31 includes interleukins (ILs) 3, 4, 5, 9, 13, and 17β in addition to granulocyte monocyte-colony-stimulating factor (CSF). Several cytokine receptor genes are also located on the long arm of chromosome 5 including: CSF-1 receptor and platelet-derived growth factor-β [18].

The world health organization (WHO) recognizes del (5q), which was first described by Van den Berghe et al. in the year 1974, as a distinct form of MDS [15, 18–20]. The 5q-syndrome is the most distinct type of all MDSs as it has clear genotype/phenotype relationship [18, 21]. If del (5q) occurs as the only cytogenetic abnormality, it is associated with favorable prognosis but once it is encountered in association with other single or multiple chromosomal abnormalities, particularly in the setting of complex cytogenetics, the clinical outcome is rendered poor [14, 16, 20, 22, 23].

Patients with del (5q) have specific clinical and pathological features [15, 18, 20]. The 5 q-syndrome is usually characterized by the following: (1) female predominance, (2) refractory macrocytic anemia that is often severe, (3) normal or elevated platelet count, (4) BM findings of erythroid hypoplasia, less than 5% blasts as well as abnormal, dysplastic or hypolobulated megakaryocytes, (5) del (5q) chromosomal abnormality as the sole karyotypic abnormality, and (6) a rather benign clinical course with approximately 10% of patients ultimately progressing to AML [13, 14, 18–20].

Despite the remarkable progress that has been achieved recently, certain unclear issues related to the pathogenesis of del (5q) need further evaluation [18, 20]. Del (5q) MDS is considered a disorder of the hematopoietic stem cells with lympho-myeloid potential. Also, involvement of B cells, rather than T cells, was documented by combining immunophenotyping and fluorescence *in situ* hybridization (FISH) analysis [18]. Cytogenetic and FISH analysis in BM progenitor cells have revealed that, in del (5q) MDS, the deletion was generally present in the pluripotent hematopoietic stem cells (CD34+ and CD38+) with the persistence of the normal progenitor cells in the BM [20]. Genomic stability in 5q-syndrome is related to the infrequency of additional cytogenetic abnormalities [18]. The lack of mutations in the genes mapping the CDR suggests that haploisufficiency is the basis of 5q-syndrome [13, 18, 20]. Candidate genes that show haploinsufficiency in del (5q) include SPARC (secreted protein acidic and cysteine rich), a tumor suppressor gene, and RPS14, which is a component of the 40s ribosomal subunit [13]. Only in advanced forms of the disease, rare mutations involving p53, JAK2, and MPL genes have been described [13, 18, 20].

The erythroid defect or failure in del (5q) appears to be multifactorial as it has been reported to involve in the following: (1) the decreased expression or haploinsufficiency of the ribosomal protein S14 [RPS14] gene, (2) the upregulation of the p53 pathway induced by ribosomal stress, and (3) enhancement of the endogenous erythropoietin production that ultimately leads to red cell transfusion dependence in most patients [13, 15, 18, 21]. On the other hand, loss of the microRNA genes miR-145 and miR-146a has been associated with the thrombocytosis observed in 5q-syndrome patients [21]. Also, the increased expression of Friend leukemia virus integration 1(FLI1), which is one of the target genes of miR-145, maintains effective megakaryopoiesis in del (5q) MDS resulting in normal or elevated platelet (PLT) counts [13].

Isolated del (5q) has been reported in in higher grade MDSs such as RAEB and RAEB-thrombocytosis (RAEB-T), thus contributing to the heterogeneity of the disease [20, 22]. MDS with del (5q) occurs not only in myelodysplastic disorders, but also in AML and it contributes to the pathogenesis of both myeloid diseases by deleting one or more of the tumor suppressor genes [22]. Once associated with additional cytogenetic abnormalities and once new genetic mutations are acquired, such as TP53 mutation, MDS with del (5q) becomes an aggressive disease with rapid evolution into AML [20, 22]. Therefore, isolated del (5q) MDS should be differentiated from other forms of myelodysplasia having del (5q) associated with other cytogenetic abnormalities and an excess of BM blasts [20]. Other specific aspects of 5q- syndrome will be discussed separately in the subsequent sections of the review manuscript.

3.2. Monosomy 5 type of MDS

Loss of the whole chromosome 5 has been described in about 3–8% MDS cases. Recent studies have shown that many suspected monosomies 5 are in fact cryptic translocations or insertions, undetectable by conventional G-banding [24]. The mechanism responsible for the fragmentation of deleted chromosome 5 remains unclear. One of the possible explanations might be the phenomenon called chromothripsis, whereby one or more chromosomes or chromosomal regions shatter into pieces in a single catastrophic event. MDS patients with deleted chromosome 5 involved in complex rearrangements should be considered as a unique entity with extremely poor prognosis [24].

Monosomy 5 does exist but is rarely encountered and the presence of this chromosomal abnormality is usually associated with complex karyotypes, conferring poor prognosis [25]. Studies have shown that, compared to 5q- syndrome, monosomy 5 is more frequently associated with: advanced or higher risk MDS, other chromosomal abnormalities including chromosome 7 abnormalities and inferior overall survival [26]. Monosomy 5 has been reported in therapy-related MDS (t-MDS) with complex cytogenetics and rapid progression to death [27].

4. Clinical manifestations and complications of MDS

MDS has nonspecific signs and symptoms at presentation. However, many patients are asymptomatic at presentation. The main manifestations of MDS are those related to cytopenia. Anemic manifestations include fatigue, weakness, dizziness, exercise intolerance, angina, cognitive impairment, and altered sense of well-being [12, 28]. Patients having thrombocytopenia present with bleeding from various sites such as skin and mucous membranes. Easy bruising, epistaxis, petechiae, ecchymoses, and gum bleeding are the main manifestations [12, 28]. Patients with neutropenia may develop fever and infections may be due to viruses, bacteria, fungi, and mycobacteria [12, 28, 29]. Physical examination in patients with MDS usually reveals: pallor, petechiae or ecchymoses, hepatosplenomegaly, and lymphadenopathy uncommonly, weight loss in advanced cases and skin manifestations in case of associated Sweet’s syndrome [12, 28].

Autoimmune abnormalities may be present in MDS patients and they include cutaneous vasculitis, monoarticular arthritis, pericarditis, pleural effusions, edema formation, skin ulcerations, iritis, myositis, peripheral neuropathy, fever, and pulmonary infiltrates [12]. Other abnormalities that may be encountered in patients with MDS include pure red cell aplasia, acquired HbH disease, myeloid sarcomas, Sweet's syndrome, myocardial ischemia, and thrombocytosis in patients with del (5q) and RARS-T [12, 28].

http://dx.doi.org/10.5772/64202

5. Diagnosis and subtypes of MDS

Minimal morphological diagnostic criteria in MDS include the following: (1) BM findings: ≥ 10% dysplastic cells in ≥ 1 myeloid lineages, (2) highly suggestive features: (a) granulocytic series: agranular neutrophils and Pelger–Huet neutrophils, (b) megakaryocytes, small binucleated megakaryocytes and small round separated nuclei in megakaryocytes, and (c) erythroid series: multinuclear or asymmetrical nuclei, nuclear bridging, and ring sideroblasts [6, 30, 31].

The minimal diagnostic criteria in MDS include the following: (1) prerequisite criteria that include (a) constant cytopenia in ≥ 1 of the following lineages: erythroid: Hb < 11 g/dL, neutrophilic; absolute neutrophil count (ANC) < 1.5 × 10^9/L or megakaryocytic, PLTs < 100 × 10^9/L. (b) exclusion of all other hematopoietic and nonhematopoietic disorders as primary reasons for cytopenia or dysplasia; (2) MDS-related or decisive criteria: (a) dysplasia in at least 10% of all cells in one of the following lineages in the BM smear; erythroid, neutrophilic or megakaryocytic or > 15% ring sideroblasts on iron staining, (b) 5–19% blasts on BM smears, and (c) typical chromosomal abnormality by FISH or conventional karyotype. (3) cocriteria for patients fulfilling (1) but not (2): (a) abnormal phenotype of BM cells clearly indicative of a monoclonal population of erythroid and/ or myeloid cells determined by flow cytometry, (b) clear molecular signs of a monoclonal cell population in human androgen receptor (HUMARA) assay, gene chip profiling or point mutation analysis such as RAS mutation, (c) markedly or persistently reduced colony formation of BM and/or circulating progenitor cells by colony-forming unit assay [6, 30, 31]. The subtypes of MDS according to the WHO classification are illustrated in **Table 1** [6, 30, 31].

Subtype of MDS	Proportion of MDS patients	Peripheral blood findings	Bone marrow findings
RAEB I [refractory anemia with excess of blasts I]	–	Cytopenia (s) <5% blasts No Auer rods Monocytes: <1G/L or <1 × 10^9/L	Unilineage or multilineage dysplasia No Auer rods 5–10% blasts
RAEB II [refractory anemia with excess of blasts II]	40%	Cytopenia(s) 5–19% blasts Possible Auer rods Monocytes: <1 G/L or <1 × 10^9/L	Unilineage or multilineage dysplasia 5–19% blasts Possible Auer rods
RCUD [refractory anemia with unilineage dysplasia, uni	**Refractory:** Anemia: 10–20% Neutropenia: < 1%	Anemia Neutropenia Thrombocytopenia	Only one cytopenia with dysplasia in >10% of cells. > 5% blasts< 15% ring

Subtype of MDS	Proportion of MDS patients	Peripheral blood findings	Bone marrow findings
or bicytopenia]	↓ PLT: < 1%	No or < 1% blasts	sideroblasts
RARS [refractory anemia ring sideroblasts]	3–11%	Anemia No blasts	Unilineage erythroid dysplasia < 5% blasts ≥ 15% ring siderblasts
RCMD [refractory anemia with multi lineage dysplasia with or without ring sideroblasts]	30%	Cytopenia(s) < 1% blasts No Auer rods Monocytes < 1 G/L	Dysplasia in ≥ 10% of cells belonging to at least 2 cell lines < 5% blasts without Auer rods ± 15% ring sideroblasts
MDS with isolated del (5q)	Uncommon	Anemia Normal or high PLT count < 1% blasts	5% blasts without Auer rods Megakaryocytes: normal or ↑; hypolobulated
MDS-U [unclassified MDS]	Unknown percentage	Cytopenia ≤ 1% blasts	Dysplasia in < 10% cells but cytogenetic abnormalities are considered presumptive for MDS < 5% blasts

MDS: myelodysplastic syndrome; PLT: platelet; ↑: increased.

Table 1. WHO classification of MDS.

5.1. Cytogenetics in MDS

Several cytogenetic abnormalities can be encountered in patients with MDSs, some of these are balanced, while others are unbalanced as illustrated in **Table 2** [6]. Cytogenetic abnormalities are major determinants in the pathogenesis of MDS. They are becoming increasingly recognized as the basis of selecting drugs in individual patients with MDS and they play a significant role in monitoring response to treatment [32]. Chromosomal abnormalities are detected in approximately 50% of patients with *de novo* MDS and 80% of patients with t-MDS [32]. Recently, our ability to define the prognosis of the individual patient with MDS has improved significantly [6]. Cytogenetic abnormalities are becoming essential in determining the prognosis of MDS because they constitute the basis of the new cytogenetic scoring system as shown in **Table 3** [31, 33, 34]. The values of the new prognostic systems will certainly become higher as new genetic-based therapy move through trials and into clinical practice [6].

Balanced chromosomal abnormalities		Unbalanced chromosomal abnormalities	
Abnormality	Frequency	Abnormality	Frequency
t (11,16) (q23;p13.3)	–	+8	10%
t (3,21) (q26. 2; q22.1)	–	−7 or del (7q)	10%
t (1,3) (p36.3; q21.2)	–	−5 or del (5q)	5–8%
t(2,11) (p21; q23)	1%	Del (20q)	5%
inv (3) (q21; q26.2)	1%	−Y	3–5%
t (6,9) (p23; q34)	1%	I (17q) or t (17p)	3%
		−13 or del (13q)	3%
		Del (11q)	10%
		Del (12p) or t (12p)	3%
		Del (9q)	1–2%
		Idic (x) (q13)	1–2%

*MDS: myelodysplastic syndrome.

Table 2. Chromosomal abnormalities in MDS.

Prognostic class	Proportion of patients	Karyotype or cytogenetic abnormalities	Median survival in years	Time to 25% AML transformation
Very good	4%	−Y del (11q)	5.4	Not reached
Good	72%	Normal del (5q) del (20q) del (12q) Double including del (5q)	4.8	9.4
Intermediate	13%	del (72) +8 +19 isochromosome (17q) Any other single or double independent clones	2.7	2.5
Poor	4%	−7 inv (3); *t*(3q); del (3q) Double including -7/del (7q) Complex: 3 cytogenetic abnormalities	1.5	1.7
Very poor	4%	Complex > 3 cytogenetic abnormalities	0.7	0.7

MDS: myelodysplastic syndrome; AML: acute myeloid leukemia.

Table 3. New cytogenetic scoring system for MDS.

5.2. Impact of monosomal karyotype on the prognosis of MDS

A monosomal karyotype (MK) is defined by the presence of ≥ 2 distinct autosomal chromosome monosomies or a single autosomal monosomy associated with ≥ 1 structural abnormality [1]. In AML, MK has been associated with a worse prognosis than an otherwise complex karyotype, regardless the specific type of autosome involved [1].

Studies have shown that MK in MDS identifies a prognostically worse subgroup of patients than a complex karyotype regardless of whether monosomy 7 or 5 is part of the MK component [1]. Chromosomal abnormalities are present in 20–70% of patients with MDS, but complex cytogenetics are universally considered unfavorable as they are associated with poor overall survival (OS) and high rates of leukemic transformation [1, 32, 34].

5.3. Genetic mutations described in MDSs and 5q-syndrome

Several classes of genetic mutations have been described in patients with MDS as shown in **Tables 4–6** [34–40]. These mutations are essential in not only determining the prognosis but also constituting a platform for the current and future novel and targeted therapies for various types of myelodysplasia (**Tables 4** and **6**) [34–39].

Class	Mutation	Chromosomal location	Frequency	Prognostic significance	– Associations: phenotypes and MDS types – Application to treatment
(1) RNA- splicing machinery (50%)	**SF3B1** [Splicing factor 3b, subunit 1]	2q33.1	15–60%	Good	**– Phenotype:** ring sideroblasts **– MDS types:** – RARS – RCMD – RS – RARS – T
	SRSF2 [Serine/arginine-rich splicing factor-2]	17q22.3	6–20%	Poor	**– MDS types:** – RCMD – RAEB – CMML
	U2AF1 [U_2 small nuclear RNA auxiliary factor-1]	21q22.3	5–12%	Unclear/poor	**– MDS types:** – RCMD – RAEB – CMML
	ZRSR2 [Zinc finger RNA-binding mofit and serine/arginine rich 2]	Xp22.1	3–10%	Unknown	**– MDS types:** – RCMD – RAEB – CMML

http://dx.doi.org/10.5772/64202

Class	Mutation	Chromosomal location	Frequency	Prognostic significance	– Associations: phenotypes and MDS types – Application to treatment
	ZRSF2	17q25.1	6–12%	Poor	–
	PRPF8	17p13.3	3.3%	Unclear	–
(2) Epigenetic pathways: DNA methylation and chromatin modification (45%)	**DNMT3A** [DNA methyltransferase 3 alpha]	2 p23	8–12%	Adverse/ negative – Decreased survival – Increased risk of sAML	– All MDS types
	TET 2 [tetmethylcytosine deoxygenase-2]	4q 24	15–30% 2%	Unclear / possibly positive – Improved response to azacitidine – Inconsistent impact on survival	**– Phenotype:** myeloid dominancy **– MDS types:** dominancy – all MDS types – Normal karyotype – CMML
	IDH1 [isocitrate dehydrogenase-1] (soluble)	2q 33.3	2%	Unclear – Advanced MDS – AML progression	**– MDS types:** – RCMD – RAEB – CMML
	IDH2 [isocitrate dehydrogenase-2] (mitochondrial)	15q 26.1	2%	Poor prognosis – Decreased survival	**– MDS types:** – RCMD – RAEB – CMML
	EZH2 [enhancer of zeste homolog 2]	-7/7q- 7q35–q36	2–6%	Poor prognosis – Decreased survival	**– MDS types:** – RCMD – RAEB – CMML
	ASXL1 [additional sex combs like 1]	20q 11	10–21%	Poor prognosis – Decreased survival	**– MDS types:** – RCMD – RAEB – CMML
(3) Signal transduction	**NRAS** [neuroblastoma	1 p13.2	10%	Unclear/ adverse	**– MDS types:** – All MDS types

Class	Mutation	Chromosomal location	Frequency	Prognostic significance	– Associations: phenotypes and MDS types – Application to treatment
(kinase signaling)	RAS viral oncogene homolog]			– Increased risk of progression to AML	– CMML – JMML
	KRAS	12 p12.1	2–6%	Unclear/ adverse – Increased risk of progression to AML	– **MDS types**: – All MDS types – CMML – JMML
	CBL [cbl proto-oncogene E3 ubiquitin protein ligase]	11q 23.3	1–5%	Unknown	– **MDS types:** – All MDS types – CMML – JMML
	JAK 2 [Janus kinase 2]	9p24	6.2–8.3%	Unknown – Does not appear to alter prognosis	– **Phenotype:** – Megakaryocytosis – **MDS types:** – all types/RARS-T/RA – JAK2 Inhibitors
	NF1	–	<5%	Poor	– **MDS types:** – all MDS types – JMML
	FLT3 [Fms-related tyrosine -kinase 3]	13 q12	<5%	– Poor prognosis – Progression to AML	– **MDS types:** – All MDS types – FLT 3 Inhibitors
(4) Cohesin family-complex pathway	**RAD 21**	8 p24	2%	– Adverse prognosis	–
	STAG 2	X q25	5–10%	– Adverse prognosis	– **MDS types:** – RCMD – CMML – RAEB
	SMC1 A	Xp 11.22-P11.121	<1%	– Adverse prognosis	–
	SMC 3	10q25	2%	– Adverse prognosis	–

http://dx.doi.org/10.5772/64202

Class	Mutation	Chromosomal location	Frequency	Prognostic significance	– Associations: phenotypes and MDS types – Application to treatment
(5) Transcriptional factors and corepressors	**TP 53** [tumor protein P53]	17q13.1	5–10%	– Very poor – Adverse outcome	– **Phenotype:** – Complex karyotype – Poor prognosis – Rapid progression to AML – **MDS types:** – RAEB – Isolated del (5q) – Therapy related MDS
	RUNX1 [runt-related transcription factor 1]	21q22.3	9–20%	– Adverse outcome – Very poor – Associated with -7/del (7q) – *High risk of progression to AML	– **Phenotype:** thrombocytopenia – **MDS types:** – RCMD – RAEB – CMML
	BCOR1/BCORL1	Xp 11.4/X q25-q26.1	6–9.1%	– Adverse outcome	– **MDS types:** – RCMD – RAEB
	CEBPA [CCAAT/enhancer-binding protein, alpha]	19q13.1	<5%	– Poor prognosis	– **MDS types:** – RCMD – RAEB
	ETV6 Ets variant-6	12 p13	<5%	– Poor outcome	– **MDS types:** – RCMD – RAEB
	SETBP1 SET-binding protein$_1$	18q21.1	2–5%	– Negative/ adverse outcome	
	KMT2A Lysine -K-specific methyltransferase-2A	11q21.1	Approximately 4%	– Negative/ adverse outcome	–
	NPM1 nucleophosmin	5q35.1	Approximately 2%	Unknown	–
	KIT	4q11-q12	Approximately 1%	Unclear	–

Class	Mutation	Chromosomal location	Frequency	Prognostic significance	– Associations: phenotypes and MDS types – Application to treatment
	[V-KitHardy-Zuckerman 4 Feline sarcoma viral oncogene homolog]				
(6) Other genetic mutations	**GNAS** [GNAS complex 10ms]	20q 13.3	Approximately 1%	Unknown	
	PTPN11 Protein tyrosine phosphatase non-receptor type11	12q 24	Approximately 1%	Unknown	
	PTEN	10q 23	<1%	–	
	CDKN2A	9q (12)	<1%	–	
	BRAF	7q 34	<1%	–	
	CSF1R	–	–	– Poor prognosis – Advanced MDS – Progression to AML	– Normal karyotype predominantly
	ATRX	–	Rare		Associated with acquired α-thalassemia, often with severe anemia
	MPL	–	–	– Poor prognosis – Advanced MDS – Progression to AML	5% of RARS – T

MDS: myelodysplastic syndrome; CMML: chronic myelomonocytic leukemia; JMML: juvenile myelomonocytic leukemia; AML: acute myeloid leukemia; RCMD: refractory cytopenia with multilineage dysplasia; RA: refractory anemia; RAEB: refractory anemia with excess of blasts; RARS: refractory anemia with ring sideroblasts; RARS-T: refractory anemia with ring sideroblasts thrombocytosis.

Table 4. Genetic mutations in MDS.

TP53 encodes a cytoplasmic protein p53 that regulates cell growth and death. TP53 mutations have been found mainly in intermediate to high-risk MDS patients [41]. Patients having TP53

http://dx.doi.org/10.5772/64202

mutations often present with severe thrombocytopenia, complex cytogenetic abnormalities, an increased risk of leukemic transformation, and a shorter survival [41, 42]. Patients with mutant p53, compared to patients carrying wild-type p53, have the following features: older age, anemia, and leucopenia at the time of diagnosis and shorter median survival. Molecular identification of mutant p53 contributes to the risk stratification of patients with lower-risk MDS that may alter the treatment approach [41]. TP53 mutations develop at an early disease stage in almost 20% of patients with lower-risk MDS having del (5q) [42].

Biological process	Genetic mutation	
Transcriptional regulators	– SF3 B1 nm	– SRSF2 nm
	– UZ AF1	– CUX1
	– SETBP1	
Epigenetic regulators	– ASXL1	– TET2 nm
	– DNMT3 A	– EZH2
Cell cycle regulators	– TP53	
	– NPM1	
Apoptosis	– BCL2	
Translation	– RPS14 nm	–RPL 23
	– RPS 4x	– RPS 25
	– RPA 19	
Signaling or differentiation	– RUNX1	– N-RAS
	– ETV 6	– FMS
	– FLT 3	– SET BP1

*MDS: myelodysplastic syndrome;

* nm: non-mutated

Table 5. Genetic mutations associated with poor prognosis in MDS.

Mouse models of the 5q-syndrome have indicated that a p53-dependent mechanism underlies the pathophysiology of this disorder. Importantly, activation of p53 has been demonstrated in the human 5q-syndrome [43]. Recurrent TP53 mutations have been associated with an increased risk of AML disease evolution and with decreased response to lenalidomide therapy in del (5q) MDS patients [43].

TP53 mutations are usually present years before disease progression. They are associated with p53 overexpression but are not associated with specific clinical manifestations [42]. The presence of TP53 mutations in low-risk MDS with del (5q) contributes to the heterogeneous disease and may significantly affect clinical decision making [42].

Pathway	Examples of genetic mutations	Frequency in MDS (%)	Application to treatment
DNA splicing machinery	- SF3B1, - UZAF1 - SRSF1, - PRPF8 - SRSR2/SRSF2, - UTx	60–70%	None
DNA methylation	- DNMT3A - TET2 - IDH1/IDH2	40–50%	- DNA methyl transferase inhibitors - IDH1/IDH2 inhibitors
Chromatin modification	- ASXL1 - EZH2	20–30%	- Deacetylyase inhibitors
Signal transduction	- NRAS/KRAS - CBL - JAK2 - NF1 - FLT3	20–30%	- Kinase inhibitors - JAK inhibitors - FLT3 inhibitors
Cohesion complex/family pathway	- STAG2 - RAD21 - SMC1A - SMC3	10%	None
Transcription factors and corepressors	- TP53 - RUNX1 - BCOR1/BCORL1 - CEBPA - ETV6	20–40%	None

MDS: myelodysplastic syndrome.

Table 6. Point mutations in MDS.

In patients with 5q-syndrome, TP53 mutations are present in a small fraction of patients and they cause p53 overexpression subsequently. These aberrant subclones remain quiescent during treatment with lenalidomide and they expand at transformation into acute leukemia [44]. Studies have confirmed that in patient with low-risk MDS having 5q-syndrome, TP53 mutations are associated with strong p53 expression and that p53 positivity is the strongest independent predictor of transformation into AML [45]. Patients with MDS having del (5q) may have mutations other than TP53 such as FOXP1, TP63, JAK2, and MPL mutations [19, 46]. FOXP1 and TP63 mutations may be involved not only in the pathogenesis of the disease, but also they may play a role in the progression into AML [46]. JAK2 and MPL mutations may be found in a small proportion of patients, but their presence does not seem to affect phenotype or progression [19].

Potential new therapeutic agents for del (5q) MDS include the translation enhancer L-leucine, as it may have some efficacy in ribosomopathies. L-leucine has shown increased hemoglobinization and red cell numbers and reduced developmental defects both in humans and in mouse models [43].

6. Prognostic systems in MDSs

In MDS, there are several prognostic scoring systems and these include the following: (1) the international prognostic scoring index (IPSS), (2) the revised IPSS (R-IPSS) (**Table 7**), (3) the WHO prognostic scoring system (WPSS), (4) MD Anderson Cancer Center (MDACC) MDS model that includes the global and the lower-risk scoring systems, and (5) the French prognostic scoring system (FPSS) [30, 31, 33, 47, 48]. The components of the prognostic stratification systems of MDS are as follows: BM blast cells, age, comorbid medical conditions, serum lactic dehydrogenase (LDH), cytogenetics, number of cytopenia, severity of anemia, and high white blood cell (WBC) count [4].

Prognostic variable	**Points**						
	0	**0.5**	**1**	**1.5**	**2**	**3**	**4**
Cytogenetics	Very good	–	Good	–	Intermediate	Poor	Very poor
Bone marrow blasts %	≤2	–	>2–5%	–	5–10%	>10%	–
Hb (g/dL)	≥10	–	8– < 10	<8	–	–	–
PLT count $\times 10^9$/L	≥100	50–100	<50	–	–	–	–
ANC $\times 10^9$/L	≥0.8	<0.8	–	–	–	–	–

MDS: myelodysplastic syndrome; Hb: hemoglobin; ANC: absolute neutrophil count – indicates not applicable; PLT: platelet.

Table 7. (R-IPSS) Revised international prognostic scoring system for MDS.

The IPSS is composed of: blast percentage, karyotype or cytogenetics and the number of cytopenia. The IPSS is classified into low, intemediate-1, intemediate-2, and high-risk score [6, 49]. The R-IPSS model incorporates: BM blasts, cytogenetics, hemoglobin (Hb) level, PLTs, and ANC. The R-IPSS is divided into five risk categories: very low, low, intermediate, high, and very high risks (**Table 7**) [30, 31, 33, 47]. The R-IPSS is an excellent predictor of MDS in the era of disease modifying therapies. The early recognition of patients at high risk of progression to aggressive disease may optimize the timing of treatment before worsening of comorbidities [50]. The precise definition of a prognostic score, such as the R-IPSS, and the probability of leukemia evolution are particularly important in patients with lower-risk MDS in which new approaches including allogeneic HSCT may be addressed in younger patients in a refined manner [50].

The WPSS incorporates the following variables: WHO classification of MDS, cytogenetics, and the need for RBC transfusions [6, 47]. The MD Anderson prognostic model depends on the following factors: age, performance status, prior blood transfusion, WBC and PLT counts, Hb level, BM blasts, and karyotype [47, 49]. The scoring system is divided into four risk categories: low, intermediate-1, intermediate-2, and high [47, 49]. The FPSS includes the following items: the Eastern Cooperative Oncology Group (ECOG) performance status, IPSS cytogenetic risk, the presence of circulating blasts, and packed red blood cell (RBC) transfusion dependency [48]. The prognostic models of MDS are important, as they are used as tools in determining the severity of the illness, the prognosis of MDS, and the best line of management to be considered, that is, supportive care, hypomethylating agents, immunomodulatory drugs or HSCT [49]. The proliferation index (PI) of specific compartments of BM cells is a dynamic parameter that reflects the ongoing rate of production of hematopoietic cells in MDS. It is directly related to the maturation-associated alteration of distinct subgroups of hematopoietic cells in individual patients [4]. Assessment of the PI of nucleated RBCS and other components of BM precursors, such as myeloid CD34+ hematopoietic progenitor cells, could significantly contribute to a better management of MDS. The PI of nucleated RBCS is emerging as an independent prognostic factor for both OS and progression-free survival (PFS) in MDS [4].

7. Anemia and iron overload in MDSs and 5q-syndrome

Anemia is a very common finding in MDS patients [51, 52]. Packed RBC transfusions are the only therapeutic option in 40% of MDS patients [51, 52]. RBC transfusions are considered in MDS patients when Hb level falls below 8 g/dL and may provide temporary relief of anemic symptoms [51, 52]. Anemia contributes to cardiac dysfunction predominantly in elderly individuals [51]. In MDS patients, anemia can be corrected by the following: (1) RBC transfusions, (2) administration of hematopoietic growth factors such as erythropoietin, (3) administration of certain drugs such as lenalidomide, cyclosporine-A, and antithymocyte globulin (ATG), and (4) allogeneic HSCT that is the only curative therapeutic approach [51, 52].

Anemia and blood transfusions have significant impact on the quality of life (QOL) of MDS patients [51]. Transfusion dependency is associated with shortened overall and leukemia-free survival in MDS patients [51]. In these patients, transfusion dependency and iron overload have been retrospectively associated with: (1) inferior survival, (2) worse clinical outcome including cardiac, hepatic, and endocrine dysfunction and in some studies, (3) leukemic transformation, and infectious complications [52].

The most serious side effects of regular blood transfusion are elevation of iron blood levels and iron overload, that is, deposition of iron in body tissues [51–54]. Magnetic resonance imaging (MRI) of the heart and liver is an excellent noninvasive diagnostic tool for (1) the assessment of iron overload and (2) monitoring the response to iron chelation therapy [51, 55, 56]. MRI of the heart and liver is superior to the surrogate markers of iron overload such as serum ferritin, liver iron, ventricular ejection fraction, and tissue-related parameter [51]. The diagnostic parameters used for the evaluation of iron overload in MDS are shown in **Table 8**

[55]. Serum erythropoietin is a predictive factor for response to therapy with subcutaneous erythropoietin [57]. MDS patients with higher values of erythropoietin have poorer response to the administration of erythropoietin therapy even at higher doses [57].

Method	Normal level	Mild to moderate iron overload	Severe iron overload
Serum ferritin (ng/mL)	<400	1000–2500	>2500
Transferrin saturation (%)	20–40	50–70	>70
Labile plasma iron (MM)	<0.4	>0.4	>0.4
Liver T2-MRI (ms)	<6.3	<6.3	<1.4
Cardiac T2-MRI (ms)	>20	8–20	<8

* MDS: myelodysplastic syndrome. * MRI: magnetic resonance imaging.

Table 8. Diagnostic parameters used for evaluation of iron overload in MDS.

7.1. Iron overload in low-risk MDS

In patients with low-risk MDS, packed RBC transfusion are required to correct anemia. Ultimately, these patients become transfusion dependent [55, 58, 59]. Also, more aggressive disease is usually associated with a high transfusion rate and thus significant transfusion dependency becomes a surrogate marker of aggressive disease [59]. On the long-term, transfusion dependence leads to the development of iron overload, which becomes an important clinical problem, that is associated with an increase in morbidity and mortality [59]. However, in some transfusion-independent low-risk MDS patients, an increased erythropoietic activity results in the suppression of hepcidin and contributes to iron loading [55].

In patients with low-risk MDS who are chronically transfused, transfusion-related morbidity is an emerging challenge [58]. Blood transfusion therapy may lead to organ toxicity due to the formation of nontransferrin bound iron and resulting in oxidative stress. Therefore, in low-risk MDS patients with longer life expectancy, preventing organ damage due to iron overload is an important concern [59].

Recently, high serum ferritin level has been identified as a prognostic factor for short time to progression to acute leukemia [59]. Transfusion-dependent patients with an isolated erythroid dysplasia and a low risk of leukemic transformation are more likely to develop parenchymal iron overload and its toxicity and hence benefit from iron chelation therapy [56]. In low-risk MDS patients with relatively lower RBC transfusion requirements, T2-MRI is indicated every 10–20 units of packed RBCS in order to evaluate the need to: (1) initiate iron chelation therapy, (2) assess the effectiveness of treatment, and (3) determine the need for dose adjustment [55].

Currently, the initiation of iron chelation therapy is based on: (1) the total number of RBC transfusions and (2) increased serum ferritin in transfusion-dependent patients [55]. Iron chelation therapy is generally recommended for selected patients with low-risk MDS [52–54]. It is reasonable to offer iron chelation therapy to low-risk MDS patients who are at high risk of developing iron overload [55, 59]. Data from multiple retrospective studies have demonstrated that iron chelation therapy results in marked survival benefit in patients with low-risk MDS [52, 55].

8. Management of MDSs and 5q-syndrome

Most patients with MDS are treated with supportive measures due to their old age and comorbid medical conditions [3]. However, there are various therapeutic options for patients with low or intermediate-1 risk MDS and these include the following: (1) blood product transfusions: packed RBCS and PLTs, (2) iron chelation therapy with: deferasirox, deferoxamine, and deferiprone, (3) erythropoietin with or without granulocyte-CSF, (4) ATG and cyclosporine-A, (5) danazol, (6) pyridoxine, (7) valproic acid, (8) lenalidomide, (9) 5-azacitidine, (10) decitabine, and (11) low-dose cytarabine [60].

8.1. Iron chelation therapy

The role of iron chelation therapy in MDS patients with transfusion dependency and iron overload remains a very controversial issue in the management of MDS, mainly due to lack of solid prospective clinical trials [52, 59, 61]. However, case–control studies, retrospective analyses, and phase-II clinical trials have indicated that iron chelation therapy reduces iron overload as measured by serum ferritin and may even prolong overall survival [54].

Iron chelation therapy is indicated in the following categories of patients: (1) patients with frank iron overload; stable or increasing serum ferritin > 1000 ng/mL without signs of active inflammation or liver disease; who are transfusion-dependent at any frequency and have a life expectancy of >1 year, (2) transfusion-dependent patient who receive > 2 units of packed RBCs per month, at any serum ferritin level, and have a life expectancy of > 2 years, except for patients with frank iron deficiency such as chronic gastrointestinal (GIT) bleeding, and (3) in selected patients, iron chelation therapy is considered when life expectancy < 2 years. Examples include: planned curative treatment such as HSCT, massive iron overload with consecutive organ dysfunction or massive iron overload that is judged to significantly reduce QOL [51, 58]. Additional parameters that may influence decision to treat with iron-chelating agents in selected MDS patients include the following: (1) old age, (2) social and mental circumstances, (3) comorbidity and organ dysfunction, and (4) genetic status such as HFE gene mutations [51, 58]. The guidelines of the National Comprehensive Cancer Network (NCCN) and those of the MDS Foundation for the treatment of iron overload in MDS are illustrated in **Table 9** [52, 55]. The proposed response criteria for iron chelation therapy in MDS are shown in **Table 10** [58].

Source	Transfusion status	Serum ferritin level ng/mL or mg/L	MDS risk category	Patient profile
NCCN	– Received >20 RBC units	>2500 Mg/L	IPSS: low or intermediate	Candidate for allogeneic HSCT
MDS foundation	– Continuing transfusion	>1000 mg/L	– IPSS: low or intermediate – WHO: RA/RARS/5q-	– Candidate for allogeneic HSCT – No erythroid response to primary therapy

MDS: myelodysplastic syndrome; HSCT: hematopoietic stem cell transplantation; IPSS: international prognostic scoring index; WHO: world health organization; RA: refractory anemia; RARS: refractory anemia with ring sideroblasts.

Table 9. Guidelines for the treatment of iron overload in MDS.

Complete response (CR)	Minor response (MR)	Stable iron load	No response
Decrease in serum ferritin to <200 ng/mL or Decrease in serum ferritin by 500 ng/mL	Decrease in serum ferritin to < 200 ng/mL or Decrease in serum ferritin by less than 500 ng/mL	Constantly elevated serum ferritin but <4000 ng/mL	Further increase in serum ferritin by at least 500 ng/mL or serum ferritin level constantly above 400 ng/mL

MDS: myelodysplastic syndrome.

Table 10. Proposed response criteria for iron chelation therapy in MDS.

There are three forms of iron-chelating agents, namely (1) oral deferasirox (exjade), (2) oral deferiprone (feriprox), and (3) parenteral deferoxamine (desferal) [54, 58]. The availability of two effective oral chelating agents, deferasirox and deferiprone, has renewed interest in the evaluation of iron chelation therapy in MDS [52].

The beneficial effects of iron chelation therapy in MDS patients having iron overload include significant reduction of: labile plasma iron, nontransferrin-bound iron and reactive oxygen species (ROS) that mediate tissue damage observed in iron overload [52]. Adverse effects of iron chelation therapy include cost and toxicity. Therefore, MDS patients should be initiated on iron chelation therapy after weighing potential risks and benefits for each patient until more definitive data are available [53]. Application of recent advances in the treatment of MDS can reduce or eliminate the need for blood product transfusions thus minimizing the risk of iron overload [54]. Careful attention to iron parameters with early initiation of iron chelation therapy in patients with evidence of transfusion-related iron overload is an important component of high-quality MDS care [61].

8.2. Lenalidomide

There are 40 genes in the CDR on the long arm of chromosome 5 in MDS with del (5q). Examples of the CDR genes and the effects of lenalidomide on the haplodeficient genes are shown in **Table 11** [13, 62, 63].

Gene	Effect of deletion	phenotype	Effect of lenalidomide	Functional effect of lenalidomide
SPARC	Increased cell adhesion	– Anemia – Thrombocytopenia	Increased expression in MDS CD34+ cells ex vivo	– Inhibition of proliferation and adhesion
RPS 14	Defective ribosomal processing	– Macrocytic anemia	Increased expression in patients with del (5q)	Erythroid response
EGR1	Decrease in tumor suppressors	– Leukocytosis – Anemia – Thrombocytopenia	Increased expression in an MDS-related del (5q) cell line	Reduced proliferation
miR145 miR-146a	Elevated innate immune signaling	– Thrombocytosis – Neutropenia – Megakaryocytic dysplasia	Increased expression in patients with del (5q)	Possible anti-inflammatory
CDC 25C1 PP2A	Defective G2 – M phase regulation	G1 and G2 M arrest and apoptosis	– Direct inhibition of: CDC 25 C – Indirect inhibition of: PP_2 A	G1 and G2 M arrest and apoptosis Restoration of erythropoiesis
DIAPH	Defective cytoskeleton tumor suppression	Clonal dominance	Unknown; to be determined	Unknown Immunomodulatory Antiproliferative

MDS: myelodysplastic syndrome.

Table 11. Genes in the commonly deleted region and effects of lenalidomide on the haplodeficient genes.

Lenalidomide is a novel thalidomide analog that has enhanced immunomodulatory and antiangiogenic effects and diminished thalidomide-related adverse events [60]. The approved indications of lenalidomide treatment in MDS include the following: (1) patients with del (5q) who have symptomatic transfusion-dependent anemia, (2) lower risk, according to IPSS, MDS patients having 5q- syndrome, and (3) other low-risk and intermediate 1 risk types of MDSs [60, 62].

The important clinical trials of lenalidomide in patients with MDS are shown in **Table 12** [60, 62–66]. Lenalidomide has several mechanisms of action that include the following: (1) promotion of erythropoiesis by inhibition of CD45 protein tyrosine phosphatase and activation of EPO-R/STAT5-signaling pathway, (2) the stimulation of production of certain ILs such as

IL-2, IL-10, and interferon (IFN) -δ, (3) inhibition of pro-inflammatory cytokines and chemokines such as tumor necrosis factor (TNF)-α, IL-12, IL-1B, IL-6, monocyte chemotactic protein-1, and macrophage anti-inflammatory protein-1α, (4) anti-angiogenic effects of lenalidomide-mediated through endothelial cell migration inhibition, that is, inhibition of bFGF-, VEGF-, and TNF-α-induced endothelial cell migration, (5) immunomodulatory effects, (6) anti-inflammatory properties, (7) direct antineoplastic activity by the inhibition of malignant clone and upregulation of SPARC gene, (8) direct cytotoxic effect on abnormal del (5q) clones by targeting haploinsufficient genes and their pathways, (9) T-cell activation or stimulation of T-cell proliferation including natural killer (NK) cells number and function and production of multiple cytokines, and (10) inhibition of haplodeficient phosphatases and release of progenitors from p53 arrest [14, 21, 60, 62, 63, 67]. The adverse effects of lenalidomide include the following: (1) myelosuppression: neutropenia, anemia and thrombocytopenia, (2) venous thromboembolism such as deep venous thrombosis in 3.4% of treated patients, (3) infectious complications such as pneumonia, fever and febrile neutropenia, (4) skin rashes, pruritis, and urticaria, (5) GIT upset including nausea and diarrhea, (6) fatigue, muscle cramps, and bone pains, (7) bleeding diathesis, (8) hypokalemia, (9) autoimmune hemolytic anemia, (10) edema formation, and (11) rarely, hypothyroidism and hypogonadism [15, 17, 60, 62, 64, 68]. The mechanisms of resistance to lenalidomide include the following: (1) over expression of PP2A and (2) restoration of p53 expression leading to accumulation of p53 [62].

Cereblon, an E3 ligase protein, was first described to be the molecular target of lenalidomide in a seminal paper, published in the year 2010, that linked its role to the teratogenic effects of thalidomide in zebrafish and chicks [69, 70]. In 2011, cereblon was found to play a key role in mediating the antiproliferative and immunomodulatory activities of lenalidomide and pomalidomide in multiple myeloma (MM) and T cells, respectively [69, 70]. Thalidomide has been shown to bind and inhibit cereblon and cereblon loss had been found to cause birth defects [71]. Studies on MM cell lines have shown lack of correlation between cereblon expression and sensitivity to lenalidomide. However, in MM cell lines, made resistant to lenalidomide and pomalidomide, cereblon protein was greatly reduced [69–71].

The central role of cereblon as a target of lenalidomide and pomalidomide suggests its potential utility as a predictive biomarker of response or resistance to immunomodulatory drug therapy [69]. The currently available commercial assays that are used in measuring cereblon levels have their own limitations. Therefore, standardization and validation of the techniques used are needed to accurately assess the role of cerebron as a predictive biomarker of the response to immunomodulatory drugs [69].

The serine-thionine kinase, casein kinase 1α (CK1α), is encoded by casein kinase 1 A1 (CSNK1A1) gene [72, 73]. CK1α has been implicated in the biology of del (5q) MDS and has been shown to be a therapeutic target in myeloid malignancies and is therefore an attractive candidate for mediating the effects of lenalidomide in del (5q) MDS [73]. CSNK1A1 gene is a putative tumor suppressor gene located in the CDR at 5q 32 for del (5q) MDS and is expressed at haploinsufficiency levels in MDS with del(5q) [72–74]. Haploinsufficiency of CSNK1A1 leads to hematopoietic stem-cell expansion in mice and may play a role in the initial clonal expansion in patients with 5q-syndrome [43]. CSNK1A1 gene plays a central role in the biology or pathogenesis of del (5q) MDS and is a promising therapeutic target [74]. Lenalidomide induces the ubiquitination of CSNK1A1 by the E_3 ubiquitin ligase [CRL4 ^{CRBN}] resulting in CSNK1A1 degradation. Lenalidomide significantly alters the protein abundance of three out of five differentiated ubiquitinated proteins [73].

The development of CK1α inhibitors may provide a new therapeutic opportunity in MDS patients with del (5q) and CSNK1A1 mutations [72]. In MDS patients with del (5q), CSNK1A1 mutations have been found in 7.2% of patients and are associated with older age [72]. CSNK1A1 mutations may coexist with ASKL1 but not with p53 mutations. They are usually responsive to lenalidomide and have no independent prognostic impact on overall survival [72].

In del (5q) MDS, lenalidomide-induced degradation of CSNK1A1 below the haploinsufficiency levels induces p53 activity, that is, CSNK1A1 is a negative regulator of p53 [73]. The deletion of genes on chromosome 5q, such as RPS-14, may further sensitize del (5q) cells to p53 activation. This mechanism of activity is consistent with the acquisition of TP53 mutations in del (5q) MDS patients who develop resistance to lenalidomide [73].

Lenalidomide is a potent therapy for low-risk MDS with del (5q) that causes transfusion independency in 67% of patients and complete cytogenetic remission in 45% of patients [44]. However, 50% of patients responding to lenalidomide relapse within 2 years, and 15% of patients achieving cytogenetic response, and 67% of patients not achieving cytogenetic response are at risk of leukemic transformation within 10 years [44].

8.3. The role of HSCT in MDSs

Allogeneic HSCT is the only known curative therapeutic option for MDS [2, 3, 75–84]. Not only the rates of allogeneic HSCT to treat MDS are continuously increasing, but also survival rates are steadily improving [76, 85]. In patients with MDS, the indications of HSCT are as follows: (1) higher-risk MDS, (2) intermediate-2 MDS, (3) MDS in blast cell crisis, (4) younger patients with MDS having good performance status, and (5) patients with low-risk MDS with poor prognostic features such as: old age, refractory cytopenias and transfusion-dependence [3, 75, 76, 81, 82]. Both blast percentage and percentage of cytogenetically abnormal cells reflect MDS disease burden and predict the outcome of HSCT [86]. Therefore, accurate assessment of MDS disease burden and MDS disease biology based on cytogenetic and molecular profiles is critical to determine the optimal HSCT timing and improve the outcome of HSCT [86]. Incorporation of novel diagnostic techniques such as flow cytometry, molecular cytogenetics and microarray gene expression profiling in the diagnostic algorithms and risk stratification may further optimize therapeutic decisions including the timing of allogeneic HSCT [85].

In patients with MDS undergoing HSCT, predictors of the outcome of HSCT include the following: (1) age, (2) performance status, (3) transfusion dependence, (4) serum erythropoietin level, (5) HSCT-comorbidity index, (6) MK, (7) MDS risk score such as R-IPSS category, and (8) severity of cytopenias [75, 76, 79, 82]. Novel classification schemes for MDS allow for more accurate prognostication and consequently recommendations for HSCT or non-HSCT

http://dx.doi.org/10.5772/64202

therapies [78]. MDS disease classification by IPSS, R-IPSS, and WPSS as well as patient characteristics as assessed by HSCT-comorbidity index provide guidance for optimal patient management [81].

Trial	MDS-001 Open label-single center-phase II	MDS - 003 Single arm-multi center-phase II	MDS - 004 Phase III - randomized - double blind - placebo controlled study
Number of patients	43	148	139
Median Age (years)	72	71	69
IPSS risk category	- Low: 51% - Intermediate I : 27% - Intermediate II : 9% - High : 2%	- Low: 37% - Intermediate I: 44% - Intermediate II: 2-5% - Unclassified: 14%	- Low: 49% - Intermediate I : 51%
FAB subtype	- RA : 47% - RAEB-T 2% - RARS : 30% - CMML : 2% - RAEB : 19%	- RA: 52% - RARS: 12% - RAEB: 20% - CMML: 2%	- RA : 68% - RARS : 15% - RAEB : 10.8% - CMML : 2%
Karyotype	- Del (5q) : 28% - Normal : 53% - Other : 9%	- Isolated del (5q): 74% - Del (5q) + others: 25%	- Isolated Del (5q) : 76% - Del (5q) + others : 24%
Response	**Hematological** **Cytogenetic** - Del(5q): 83% - Del(5q): 75% - Normal cytogenetics 57% - others: 3% - Others: 9%	- Erythroid response: 76% - Transfusion independence: 67% - Cytogenetic response: 73% - Complete response: 45%	- Packed RBC transfusion independence: 49% after 4 cycles (4 weeks)
Time to response	- Median time to response: 9-11.5 weeks - Median duration of response: not reached	- Median time to response: 4.6 weeks - Median duration of response: 115 weeks	- Median duration of response: not reached with either 5mg or 10mg / day of lenalidomide
Adverse effects of lenalidomide encountered	- Neutropenia : 65% - Thrombocytopenia: 53% - Pneumonia: 7% - Fatigue: 5% - Diarrhea: 2%	- Neutropenia: 55% - Thrombocytopenia: 44% - Rash: 6% - Pruritis: 3% - Fatigue: 3% - Nausea: 3% - DVT: 3% - Pneumonia: 3% - Hemorrhage: - Diarrhea: 3%	**5 mg dose** **10 mg dose** - ↓ N1: 74% - ↓ N1: 75% - ↓ PLTS: 33% - ↓ PLT: 41% - ↓ Hb: 5.8% - ↓ Hb: 2.9% - ↓ WBC: 13% - ↓ WBC: 8.7% - DVT: 1.4% - DVT: 5.8%

Trial	Ades et al Phase II trial	Reza et al Phase II trial
Number of patients	47	214
Median age (in years)	69	72
IPSS-risk category	- Intermediate 2 : 60% - High risk : 40%	- Low risk: 43% - Intermediate 1: 36% - Intermediate 2: 4% - Unclassified: 18%
FAB subtype	-	- Normal karyotype: 75% - Clonal (non-5q) cytogenetic abnormalities: 22%
Karyotype	- Isolated del (5q): 9% - Del (5q) + additional abnormalities: 23% - Del (5q) + > 2 additional abnormalities: 58%	- Hematological overall response: 43% - Transfusion independence: 26%
Response	- Over all response: 27% - Complete hematological response: 15% - Transfusion independence: 25%	- Median time to transfusion independence: 4.8 weeks - Median duration of transfusion independence: 41 weeks - Cytogenetic overall response: 19%
Time to response	- Median duration of complete hematological response: 11 months - Median overall response: 9 months	-
Adverse effects encountered	Grade 3/4 cytopenias: 76%	- Neutropenia: 28% - Thrombocytopenia: 26%

- MDS: myelodysplastic syndrome
- CMML: chronic myelomonocytic leukemia
- IPSS: international prognostic scoring index
- FAB: French-American-British
- RBC: red blood cell
- PLT: platelet
- RAEB: refractory anemia with excess of blasts
- RARS: refractory anemia with ring sideroblasts
- RARS-T: refractory anemia with ring sideroblasts thrombocytosis
- RA: refractory anemia
- WBC: white blood cell
- DVT: deep venous thrombosis

Table 12. Clinical trials on lenalidomide in MDS.

The age of MDS patients undergoing HSCT has increased significantly over the last 30 years. While HSCT is being carried out in older patients with MDS, this enthusiasm has been over shadowed by the impact of the procedure and its complications, namely graft versus host disease (GVHD) on the QOL and socioeconomic status [78]. Comorbid medical conditions are the major patient characteristics impacting transplantation success. Validation of comorbidity scoring systems has provided the basis for risk assignment to a given patient [78]. HSCT comorbidity index allows estimation of the probability of non-relapse mortality after HSCT [81].

Pre-HSCT serum ferritin > 100 mg/L has been shown to have an adverse impact on OS following HSCT [75]. Adverse consequences of iron overload on the outcome of HSCT include increased risk of septicemia, invasive fungal infections, and sinusoidal obstruction syndrome [75]. BM blast percentage < 5% at the time of HSCT is the major predictor of improved disease-free survival (DFS) and disease relapse [80]. Prior treatment to decrease blast percentage < 5% prior to allogeneic HSCT is recommended as it has been shown to improve DFS particularly in patients undergoing nonmyeloablative (NMA)-conditioning therapy [80].

The major factors that have a negative effect on relapse-free survival in MDS patients subjected to HSCT are pretransplant karyotype and pre-HSCT BM blast count [76, 81]. Patients with very poor cytogenetics, including MK, have a 10% or less probability of long-term survival [81]. Studies have also shown that a patient with MDS having MK has lower survival rates, higher relapse rates, and higher overall mortality following allogeneic HSCT [76]. The presence of p53, DNMT3A, and TET_2 genetic mutations in the pre-HSCT period decreases the probability of post-transplant survival by a factor of 3–4 [76, 81]. On the other hand, $SF3B_1$ mutations are associated with superior leukemia-free survival and OS in MDS patients subjected to allogeneic HSCT [81].

In MDS patients receiving allogeneic HSCT, the stem cell sources are the following: peripheral blood, BM, and umbilical cord blood (UCB) have yielded similar outcomes [80, 83]. Peripheral blood progenitor cells are currently the preferred source of stem cells due to faster engraftment and higher risk of GVHD giving rise to more potent graft versus tumor (GVT) effect [81, 83]. Cord blood cells are typically associated with slow engraftment and hence higher risk of infections and bleeding complications [81]. UCB-derived hematopoietic grafts provide the advantage of transplanting rather immature cells that allows successful HSCT in some patients even in the presence of HLA mismatches [87]. The following forms of allografts are available for MDS patients who are eligible for transplantation: HLA-matched sibling grafts, matched unrelated donor (MUD) allografts, UCB grafts, and HLA-haploidentical donor allografts [78, 83]. The availability of: HLA matched related and unrelated donors, HLA-haploidentical relatives and UCB helps to identify donors for the vast majority of MDS patients [81]. Traditionally, transplantation of HLA-haploidentical cells carries an increased risk of graft rejection and an increased risk of GVHD. However, the recently introduced conditioning regimens have reduced the risk of graft rejection and the administration of cyclophosphamide in the early post-transplant period has minimized the risk of GVHD to similar or even lower rates than observed following HLA-matched donor cell [81].

An increased use of unrelated donors and the establishment of protocols for cord blood HSCT and HLA-haploidentical HSCT have made HSCT available for a rapidly growing number of patients [78]. Haploidentical HSCT performed using T-cell replete allografts and post-transplant cyclophosphamide can achieve outcomes equivalent to those of conventional HSCT using HLA-matched related or unrelated donors [87]. The preferred donor for MDS patients undergoing allogeneic HSCT is an HLA-matched sibling or alternatively a fully matched unrelated donor as both have comparable survival rates. However, MUD form of HSCT is associated with higher treatment-related mortality (TRM) [82].

Development of a broad range of conditioning regimens has allowed clinicians to offer HSCT taking into consideration: stage of the disease and patient characteristics [78]. Conventional myeloablative conditioning (MAC) protocols include the following: total body irradiation (TBI), cyclophosphamide, busulfan, and fludarabine, while reduced intensity conditioning (RIC) regimens incorporate low-dose TBI, fludarabine, cyclophosphamide, ATG, and alemtuzumab in various doses and schedules [75]. MAC therapy is associated with lower relapse rate particularly in patients in complete remission or with < 5% blasts. MAC therapy is also associated with increased toxicity and nonrelapse mortality [78, 80]. Long-term survival results in remission following allogeneic HSCT from HLA-matched related or unrelated donor and high-intensity conditioning treatment are as follows: lower-risk MDS: 75%, intermediate-1 MDS: 60%, intermediate-2 MDS: 45% and high-risk MDS: 30% [81]. NMA or RIC conditioning regimens may be considered for MDS patients who are not candidates for MAC regimens due to comorbidities or old age, but such regimens should ideally be used within the context of a clinical trial [82]. Since approximately 75% of MDS patients are > 60 years of age at diagnosis, MAC-allogeneic HSCT can only be offered to a subset of individuals [82]. In patients unfit for MAC therapy, NMA conditioning yields equivalent: TRM, DFS, and OS [80]. For patients with *de novo* MDS aged 60–70 years, the favored therapy varies according to the IPSS risk for patients with low risk and intermediate-1 IPSS risk, nontransplantation approaches are preferred and for patients with intermediate-2 and high-IPSS risk, RIC-allogeneic HSCT offers overall and quality-adjusted survival benefit [88]. In patients with MDS, emphasis should be shifted from high-dose chemotherapy aimed at maximum tumor-cell kill to RIC allogeneic HSCT relying on the donor cell-mediated GVT effect that is most prominent in patients having chronic GVHD in particular in order to eradicate the disease [81]. RIC regimens for allogeneic HSCT have the capacity to result in long-term remissions in MDS patients who are ineligible for conventional allogeneic HSCT [89]. The role of RIC-allogeneic HSCT in MDS patients is to induce chronic GVHD which in turn reduces relapse rate and improves DFS and OS [82, 89].

Autologous HSCT is applicable only to a minority of younger patients with MDS because of difficulty in harvesting adequate numbers of CD34+ cells even in low-risk MDS patients and lack of graft versus leukemia or GVT effect thus resulting in high risk of MDS relapse [3].

8.4. HSCT in lower risk MDS patients

In patients with low- or intermediate-1-risk MDS, aged 60–79 years, life expectancy following RIC-allogeneic HSCT is about 38 months compared to 77 months in patients not subjected to HSCT, that is, there is no survival benefit of HSCT in this category of patients [81]. Patients with low or very low-risk MDS should ideally be treated with supportive measures and low intensity therapies, such as lenalidomide, erythropoiesis stimulating agents, hypomethylating agents or immunosuppressive therapies rather than allogeneic HSCT [81, 84].

8.5. Road blocks and other unresolved issues related to HSCT in MDSs

The major road blocks to a universally successful HSCT are relapse of MDS and NRM, often related to GVHD [75, 78, 83]. Allogeneic HSCT in MDS patients can lead to considerable mortality and morbidity mostly as a consequence of toxicity to organs, infectious complications and GVHD [87]. Acute and chronic GVHD are frequent causes of morbidity after HSCT in MDS patients [78]. Additional research is required to prevent GVHD while maintaining the GVT effect [81]. The graft versus dysplasia resulting from allogeneic HSCT and the infusion of donor leukocytes has led to a great understanding of the immunological mechanisms that govern the outcome of HSCT in MDS patients [3]. Post-transplant relapse is a major hurdle to greater success, particularly in patients with high-risk cytogenetics [78]. Pretransplant cytogenetics and BM blasts are the strongest risk factors for post-HSCT relapse [81]. The time interval from allogeneic HSCT until relapse represents a crucial factor to predict response to salvage therapy and survival in patients with high-risk MDS relapsing after allogeneic HSCT [90]. Strategies to reduce relapse and TRM and improve outcome of HSCT include the following: (1) modification of the intensity of conditioning therapy taking into consideration: age, organ function and comorbid medical conditions, (2) pretransplantation strategies that include (A) improvement of remission: (a) hypomethylating agents and/or histone deacetylase inhibitors (HDACs), (b) induction therapy followed by RIC (FLAMSA), and (c) clofarabine and/or cytosine arabinoside. (B) induction of cytogenetic remission by lenalidomide for 5q- syndrome and hypomethylating agents for monosomy 7, and (3) post-transplantation strategies that include (a) boosting GVL effect by immune enhancers such as lenalidomide, CTLA4 (cytotoxic T-lymphocyte-associated protein 4), anti-PDL1 (programmed death-ligand 1) and adoptive transfer of tumor-reactive T cells and natural killer cells, (b) maintenance with HDACs and/or donor lymphocyte infusion (DLI), and (c) maintenance with lenalidomide and/or DLI [83, 91].

The following represent the unresolved issues related to HSCT in MDS: (1) timing of the transplant; standard conditioning for younger patients and RIC for older patient with comorbidities, (2) disease status at transplant, (3) pre-HSCT therapy or pretransplant tumor debulking with traditional chemotherapeutic agents or the novel DNA hypomethylating drugs, (4) the intensity of the conditioning therapies, (5) stem cell source and alternative donors, (6) optimal therapy for intermediate-risk MDS, and (7) the combination of HSCT with novel therapies such as hypomethylating agents and immunomodulatory drugs [3, 79, 80, 84, 92]. As MDS patients are usually on the old side, QOL is a top priority for most patients, so discussion regarding transplantation in older patients must include not only the acute effects of transplantation but also the delayed effects [81]. Incorporation or integration of novel non-HSCT therapeutic modalities in the overall management of MDS patients undergoing allogeneic HSCT is needed [78].

9. Prognosis in low-risk MDS

There are several poor prognostic factors in patients with MDS. The poor prognostic factors in MDS in general are listed in **Table 13** [47]. However, in low-risk disease, the following factors have been found to correlate with poor prognosis: (1) severe anemia, (2) transfusion dependence, (3) poor performance status, (4) older age, (5) number and severity of medical comorbidities, (6) leukocytosis, and (7) elevated level of serum LDH [4].

1. Old age
2. Poor performance status
3. Presence of comorbid medical conditions
4. WBC count > 20 × 10^9/L
5. Severe anemia
6. Severe or refractory thrombocytopenia; PLTs <30 × 10^9/L
7. Eosinophilia: > 350/microliter (μL) and basophilia: > 250/μL
8. Absolute lymphocytic count < 1200/mL
9. Reduced platelet mass
10. Transfusion dependence
11. Presence of bone marrow fibrosis
12. CD34 positivity of nucleated BM cells
13. RBC-MCV (mean corpuscular volume) < 100 FL
14. Increased expression of WT_1 (Wilm's tumor gene)
15. Monsomy 5 or del (5q) associated with other chromosomal abnormalities
16. Specific genetic mutations: TP53/TET2/DNMT3A/FLT3/EZH2/ETV6/BCOR
17. Reduced circulating endothelial cells
18. Increased levels of: TNF-α, single-nucleotide polymorphism in TNF gene
19. Increased serum B2 microglobulin concentration
20. Downregulation of granulopoiesis regulator lymphoid enhancer-binding factor 1 (LEF1)
21. Abnormal localization of immature precursors (ALIP)
22. Increased DNA methylation
23. Failure of decitabine therapy

Table 13. Adverse prognostic factors in MDS.

In patients with del (5q), the following factors have been found to be independent predictors of shortened survival: age, transfusion need at diagnosis and dysgranulopoiesis [18, 19].

10. Conclusions and future perspectives

MDSs including 5q-syndrome are often complicated by BM suppression reflected by cytopenias, infectious complications, iron overload and transformation into AML. Management of these disorders includes the following: (1) supportive care that comprises transfusion of blood products, antimicrobials, growth factors, and iron chelation therapy; (2) targeted therapies, such as lenalidomide, and (3) various forms of HSCT. The role of allogeneic HSCT in MDSs is surging as the recently introduced conditioning therapies have allowed application of this curative therapy to older patients and those with comorbid medical conditions. The recent developments in the science of MDSs will allow more advanced targeted therapies to be integrated into the therapeutic algorithms of these disorders.

The role of cereblon as a molecular target for lenalidomide and pomalidomide and that of CK1α in mediating the effects of lenalidomide will ultimately translate into more refined targeted therapies for patients with del (5q) MDS. Also, early incorporation of more pinpointed targeting of clones harboring TP53 mutations and utilization of the translation enhancer, L-leucine, will further improve not only the management but also the outcome of patients with 5q-syndrome.

Author details

Khalid Ahmed Al-Anazi*

Address all correspondence to: kaa_alanazi@yahoo.com

Department of Adult Hematology and Hematopoietic Stem Cell Transplantation, Oncology Center, King Fahad Specialist Hospital, Dammam, Saudi Arabia

References

[1] Patnaik MM, Hanson CA, Hodnefield JM, Knudson R, Van Dyke DL, Tefferi A. Monosomal karyotype in myelodysplastic syndromes, with or without monosomy 7 or 5, is prognostically worse than an otherwise complex karyotype. Leukemia 2011; 25 (2): 266–270. doi: 10.1038/leu.2010.258. Epub 2010 Nov 12.

[2] Giralt SA, Horowitz M, Weisdorf D, Cutler C. Review of stem-cell transplantation for myelodysplastic syndromes in older patients in the context of the decision memo for allogeneic hematopoietic stem cell transplantation for myelodysplastic syndrome

emanating from the centers for medicare and medicaid services. J Clin Oncol 2011; 29 (5): 566–572. doi: 10.1200/JCO.2010.32.1919. Epub 2011 Jan 10.

[3] Ingram W, Lim ZY, Mufti GJ. Allogeneic transplantation for myelodysplastic syndrome (MDS). Blood Rev 2007; 21 (2): 61–71. Epub 2006 Jun 8.

[4] Matarraz S, Teodosio C, Fernandez C, Albors M, Jara-Acevedo M, López A, et al. The proliferation index of specific bone marrow cell compartments from myelodysplastic syndromes is associated with the diagnostic and patient outcome. PLoS One 2012; 7 (8): e44321. doi: 10.1371/journal.pone.0044321. Epub 2012 Aug 31.

[5] Tefferi A, Vardiman JW. Myelodysplastic syndromes. N Engl J Med 2009; 361: 1872–1885. doi: 10.1056/NEJMra0902908

[6] Invernizzi R, Filocco A. Myelodysplastic syndrome: classification and prognostic systems. Oncol Rev 2010; 4 (1): 25–33. doi: 10.1007/s12156-009-0033-4

[7] Pagano L, Caira M, Fianchi L, Leone G. Environmental risk factors for MDS/AML. Haematol Rep 2006; 2 (15): 42–45.

[8] Ma X. Epidemiology of myelodysplastic syndromes. Am J Med 2012; 125 (7 Suppl): S2–S5. doi: 10.1016/j.amjmed.2012.04.014

[9] Jin J, Yu M, Hu C, Ye L, Xie L, Chen F, et al. Alcohol consumption and risk of myelodysplastic syndromes: a meta-analysis of epidemiological studies. Mol Clin Oncol 2014; 2 (6): 1115–1120. Epub 2014 Aug 7.

[10] Lv L, Lin G, Gao X, Wu C, Dai J, Yang Y, et al. Case–control study of risk factors of myelodysplastic syndromes according to World Health Organization classification in a Chinese population. Am J Hematol 2011; 86 (2): 163–169. doi: 10.1002/ajh.21941

[11] Strom SS, Gu Y, Gruschkus SK, Pierce SA, Estey EH. Risk factors of myelodysplastic syndromes: a case-control study. Leukemia. 2005; 19 (11): 1912–1918.

[12] Aster JC, Stone RM. Clinical manifestations and diagnosis of the myelodysplastic syndromes. Edited by Larson RA, Connor RF. Up To Date 2015. Topic last updated: Dec 1, 2015.

[13] Fuchs O. Important genes in the pathogenesis of 5q- syndrome and their connection with ribosomal stress and the innate immune system pathway. Leuk Res Treat 2012; 2012: 179402. doi: 10.1155/2012/179402. Epub 2012 Feb 13.

[14] Fuchs O, Jonasova A, Neuwirtova R. Lenalidomide therapy of myelodysplastic syndromes. J Leuk (Los Angel) 2013; 1: 104. doi: 10.4172/2329-6917.1000104

[15] List A, Dewald G, Bennett J, Giagounidis A, Raza A, Feldman E, et al. Myelodysplastic Syndrome-003 Study Investigators. Lenalidomide in the myelodysplastic syndrome with chromosome 5q deletion. N Engl J Med 2006; 355 (14): 1456–165.

[16] Musto P, Simeon V, Guariglia R, Bianchino G, Grieco V, Nozza F, et al. Myelodysplastic disorders carrying both isolated del(5q) and JAK2(V617F) mutation: concise review,

with focus on lenalidomide therapy. Onco Targets Ther 2014; 7: 1043–1050. doi: 10.2147/OTT.S59628. e Collection 2014.

[17] Komrokji RS, List AF. Short- and long-term benefits of lenalidomide treatment in patients with lower-risk del (5q) myelodysplastic syndromes. Ann Oncol 2016; 27 (1): 62–68. doi: 10.1093/annonc/mdv488. Epub 2015 Oct 26.

[18] Boultwood J, Pellagatti A, McKenzie AN, Wainscoat JS. Advances in the 5q-syndrome. Blood 2010; 116 (26): 5803–5811. doi: 10.1182/blood-2010-04-273771. Epub 2010 Aug 23.

[19] Patnaik MM, Lasho TL, Finke CM, Gangat N, Caramazza D, Holtan SG, et al. WHO-defined 'myelodysplastic syndrome with isolated del (5q)' in 88 consecutive patients: survival data, leukemic transformation rates and prevalence of JAK2, MPL and IDH mutations. Leukemia 2010; 24 (7): 1283–1289. doi: 10.1038/leu.2010.105. Epub 2010 May 20.

[20] Fenaux P, Kelaidi C. Treatment of the 5q-syndrome. Hematol Am Soc Hematol Educ Program 2006 (1): 192–198.

[21] Pellagatti A, Jädersten M, Forsblom AM, Cattan H, Christensson B, Emanuelsson EK, et al. Lenalidomide inhibits the malignant clone and up-regulates the SPARC gene mapping to the commonly deleted region in 5q-syndrome patients. Proc Natl Acad Sci U S A 2007; 104 (27): 11406–11411. Epub 2007 Jun 18.

[22] Tasaka T, Tohyama K, Kishimoto M, Ohyashiki K, Mitani K, Hotta T, et al.; Japanese Cooperative Study Group for Intractable Bone Marrow Diseases. Myelodysplastic syndrome with chromosome 5 abnormalities: a nationwide survey in Japan. Leukemia 2008; 22 (10): 1874–1881. doi: 10.1038/leu.2008.199. Epub 2008 Jul 31.

[23] Oelschlaegel U, Alexander Röhnert M, Mohr B, Sockel K, Herold S, Ehninger G, et al. Clonal architecture of del (5q) myelodysplastic syndromes: aberrant CD5 or CD7 expression within the myeloid progenitor compartment defines a subset with high clonal burden. Leukemia 2016; 30 (2): 517–520. doi: 10.1038/ leu.2015.158. Epub 2015 Jun 24.

[24] Zemanova Z, Michalova K, Buryova H, Brezinova J, Kostylkova K, Bystricka D, et al. Involvement of deleted chromosome 5 in complex chromosomal aberrations in newly diagnosed myelodysplastic syndromes (MDS) is correlated with extremely adverse prognosis. Leuk Res 2014; 38 (5): 537–544. doi: 10.1016/j.leukres.2014.01.012. Epub 2014 Feb 3.

[25] Galván AB, Mallo M, Arenillas L, Salido M, Espinet B, Pedro C, et al. Does monosomy 5 really exist in myelodysplastic syndromes and acute myeloid leukemia? Leuk Res 2010; 34 (9): 1242–1245. doi: 10.1016/j.leukres.2010.03.022. Epub 2010 Apr 1.

[26] Kantarjian H, O'Brien S, Ravandi F, Borthakur G, Faderl S, Bueso-Ramos C, et al. The heterogeneous prognosis of patients with myelodysplastic syndrome (MDS) and

chromosome 5 abnormalities: how does it relate to the original lenalidomide experience in MDS? Cancer 2009; 115 (22): 5202–5209. doi: 10.1002/cncr.24575

[27] Ogasawara T, Yasuyama M, Kawauchi K. Therapy-related myelodysplastic syndrome with monosomy 5 after successful treatment of acute myeloid leukemia (M2). Am J Hematol 2005; 79 (2): 136–141.

[28] Goldberg SL, Chen E, Corral M, Guo A, Mody-Patel N, Pecora AL, et al. Incidence and clinical complications of myelodysplastic syndromes among United States medicare beneficiaries. J Clin Oncol 2010; 28 (17): 2847–2852. doi: 10.1200/JCO.2009.25.2395

[29] Toma A, Fenaux P, Dreyfus F, Cordonnier C. Infections in myelodysplastic syndromes. Haematologica 2012; 97 (10): 1459–1470. doi: 10.3324/haematol.2012.063420

[30] Fenaux P, Haase D, Sanz GF, Santini V, Buske C; ESMO Guidelines Working Group. Myelodysplastic syndromes: ESMO clinical practice guidelines for diagnosis, treatment and follow-up. Ann Oncol 2014; 25 (Suppl 3): iii57–iii69. doi: 10.1093/annonc/mdu180. Epub 2014 Jul 25.

[31] Eclache V. Classification of myelodysplastic syndromes 2015. Atlas Genet Cytogenet Oncol Haematol. In Press. On line version: http://AtlasGeneticsOncology.org/Anomalies/classifMDS1058.html

[32] Haase D, Germing U, Schanz J, Pfeilstöcker M, Nösslinger T, Hildebrandt B, et al. New insights into the prognostic impact of the karyotype in MDS and correlation with subtypes: evidence from a core dataset of 2124 patients. Blood 2007; 110 (13): 4385–4395. Epub 2007 Aug 28.

[33] Greenberg PL, Tuechler H, Schanz J, Sanz G, Garcia-Manero G, Solé F, et al. Revised international prognostic scoring system for myelodysplastic syndromes. Blood 2012; 120 (12): 2454–2465. Epub 2012 Jun 27.

[34] Otrock ZK, Tiu RV, Maciejewski JP, Sekeres MA. The need for additional genetic markers for myelodysplastic syndrome stratification: what does the future hold for prognostication? Expert Rev Hematol 2013; 6 (1): 59–68. doi: 10.1586/ehm.12.67

[35] Nybakken GE, Bagg A. The genetic basis and expanding role of molecular analysis in the diagnosis, prognosis, and therapeutic design for myelodysplastic syndromes. J Mol Diagn 2014; 16 (2): 145–158. doi: 10.1016/j.jmoldx.2013.11.005. Epub 2014 Jan 21.

[36] Visconte V, Tiu RV, Rogers HJ. Pathogenesis of myelodysplastic syndromes: an overview of molecular and non-molecular aspects of the disease. Blood Res 2014; 49 (4): 216–227. doi: 10.5045/ br.2014.49.4.216. Epub 2014 Dec 23.

[37] Bejar R, Steensma DP. Recent developments in myelodysplastic syndromes. Blood 2014; 124 (18): 2793–2803. doi: 10.1182/blood-2014-04-522136. Epub 2014 Sep 18.

[38] Harada H, Harada Y. Recent advances in myelodysplastic syndromes: molecular pathogenesis and its implications for targeted therapies. Cancer Sci 2015; 106 (4): 329–336. doi: 10.1111/cas.12614. Epub 2015 Feb 25.

[39] Odenike O, Anastasi J, Le Beau MM. Myelodysplastic syndromes. Clin Lab Med 2011; 31 (4): 763–784. doi: 10.1016/j.cll.2011.08.005. Epub 2011 Oct 10.

[40] Greenberg PL, Stone RM, Bejar R, Bennett JM, Bloomfield CD, Borate U, et al.; National Comprehensive Cancer Network. Myelodysplastic syndromes, version 2.2015. J Natl Compr Cancer Netw 2015; 13 (3): 261–272.

[41] Yao DC, de Lima M. Utility of the p53 mutant protein in patients with low-risk myelodysplastic syndrome. Rev Bras Hematol Hemoter 2014; 36 (3): 173–174. doi: 10.1016/j.bjhh.2014.03.014. Epub 2014 Apr 4.

[42] Jädersten M, Saft L, Smith A, Kulasekararaj A, Pomplun S, Göhring G, et al. TP53 mutations in low-risk myelodysplastic syndromes with del (5q) predict disease progression. J Clin Oncol 2011; 29 (15): 1971–1979. doi: 10.1200/JCO.2010.31.8576. Epub 2011 Apr 25.

[43] Pellagatti A, Boultwood J. Recent Advances in the 5q-syndrome. Mediterr J Hematol Infect Dis 2015; 7 (1): e2015037. Published online 2015 May 20. doi: 10.4084/MJHID.2015.037

[44] Jädersten M, Saft L, Pellagatti A, Göhring G, Wainscoat JS, Boultwood J, et al. Clonal heterogeneity in the 5q- syndrome: p53 expressing progenitors prevail during lenalidomide treatment and expand at disease progression. Haematologica 2009; 94 (12): 1762–1766. doi: 10.3324/haematol.2009.011528. Epub 2009 Oct 1.

[45] Saft L, Karimi M, Ghaderi M, Matolcsy A, Mufti GJ, Kulasekararaj A, et al. p53 protein expression independently predicts outcome in patients with lower-risk myelodysplastic syndromes with del(5q). Haematologica 2014; 99 (6): 1041–1049. doi: 10.3324/haematol.2013.098103. Epub 2014 Mar 28.

[46] L'Abbate A, Lo Cunsolo C, Macrì E, Iuzzolino P, Mecucci C, Doglioni C, et al. FOXP1 and TP63 involvement in the progression of myelodysplastic syndrome with 5q- and additional cytogenetic abnormalities. BMC Cancer 2014; 14: 396. doi: 10.1186/1471-2407-14-396

[47] Estey EH, Schrier SL. Prognosis of the myelodysplastic syndromes in adults. Edited by Larson RA, Connor RF. Up To Date 2015. Topic last updated: May 12, 2015.

[48] Jonas BA, Greenberg PL. MDS prognostic scoring systems – past, present, and future. Best Pract Res Clin Haematol 2015; 28 (1): 3–13. doi: 10.1016/j.beha.2014.11.001. Epub 2014 Nov 11.

[49] Santos FP, Kantarjian H, Garcia-Manero G, Ravandi F. The search for better prognostic models in myelodysplastic syndromes. Curr Hematol Malig Rep 2011; 6 (1): 13–21. doi: 10.1007/s11899-010-0070-x

[50] Voso MT, Fenu S, Latagliata R, Buccisano F, Piciocchi A, Aloe-Spiriti MA, et al. Revised International Prognostic Scoring System (IPSS) predicts survival and leukemic evolution of myelodysplastic syndromes significantly better than IPSS and WHO Prognostic Scoring System: validation by the Gruppo Romano Mielodisplasie Italian Regional Database. J Clin Oncol 2013; 31 (21): 2671–2677. doi: 10.1200/JCO.2012.48.0764. Epub 2013 Jun 24.

[51] Petrou E, Mavrogeni S, Karali V, Kolovou G, Kyrtsonis MC, Sfikakis PP, et al. The role of magnetic resonance imaging in the evaluation of transfusional iron overload in myelodysplastic syndromes. Rev Bras Hematol Hemoter 2015; 37 (4): 252–258. doi: 10.1016/j.bjhh.2015.03.014. Epub 2015 May 19.

[52] Mitchell M, Gore SD, Zeidan AM. Iron chelation therapy in myelodysplastic syndromes: where do we stand? Expert Rev Hematol 2013; 6 (4): 397–410. doi: 10.1586/17474086.2013.814456

[53] Leitch HA. Optimizing therapy for iron overload in the myelodysplastic syndromes: recent developments. Drugs 2011; 71 (2): 155–177. doi: 10.2165/11585280-000000000-00000.

[54] List AF. Iron overload in myelodysplastic syndromes: diagnosis and management. Cancer Control 2010; 17(Suppl): 2–8.

[55] Shenoy N, Vallumsetla N, Rachmilewitz E, Verma A, Ginzburg Y. Impact of iron overload and potential benefit from iron chelation in low-risk myelodysplastic syndrome. Blood 2014; 124 (6): 873–881. doi: 10.1182/blood-2014-03-563221. Epub 2014 Jun 12.

[56] Cazzola M, Della Porta MG, Malcovati L. Clinical relevance of anemia and transfusion iron overload in myelodysplastic syndromes. Hematol Am Soc Hematol Educ Program 2008 (1): 166–175. doi: 10.1182/asheducation-2008.1.166

[57] Cortesão E, Tenreiro R, Ramos S, Pereira M, César P, Carda JP, et al. Serum erythropoietin as prognostic marker in myelodysplastic syndromes. Acta Med Port 2015; 28 (6): 720–725. Epub 2015 Dec 31.

[58] Valent P, Krieger O, Stauder R, Wimazal F, Nösslinger T, Sperr WR, et al. Iron overload in myelodysplastic syndromes (MDS) – diagnosis, management, and response criteria: a proposal of the Austrian MDS platform. Eur J Clin Invest 2008; 38 (3): 143–149. doi: 10.1111/j.1365-2362.2007.01915.x. Epub 2008 Jan 24.

[59] Messa E, Cilloni D, Saglio G. Iron chelation therapy in myelodysplastic syndromes. Adv Hematol 2010; 2010: 756289. doi: 10.1155/2010/756289. Epub 2010 Jun 20.

[60] Giagounidis AA, Germing U, Haase S, Aul C. Lenalidomide: a brief review of its therapeutic potential in myelodysplastic syndromes. Ther Clin Risk Manag 2007; 3 (4): 553–562.

[61] Steensma DP. The role of iron chelation therapy for patients with myelodysplastic syndromes. J Natl Compr Cancer Netw 2011; 9 (1): 65–75.

[62] Abou Zahr A, Saad Aldin E, Komrokji RS, Zeidan AM. Clinical utility of lenalidomide in the treatment of myelodysplastic syndromes. J Blood Med 2014; 6: 1–16. doi: 10.2147/JBM.S50482. e Collection 2015.

[63] Giagounidis A, Mufti GJ, Fenaux P, Germing U, List A, MacBeth KJ. Lenalidomide as a disease-modifying agent in patients with del (5q) myelodysplastic syndromes: linking mechanism of action to clinical outcomes. Ann Hematol 2014; 93 (1): 1–11. doi: 10.1007/s00277-013-1863-5. Epub 2013 Sep 10.

[64] Duong VH, Komrokji RS, List AF. Efficacy and safety of lenalidomide in patients with myelodysplastic syndrome with chromosome 5q deletion. Ther Adv Hematol 2012; 3 (2): 105–116. doi: 10.1177/2040620711435659

[65] Adès L, Boehrer S, Prebet T, Beyne-Rauzy O, Legros L, Ravoet C, et al. Efficacy and safety of lenalidomide in intermediate-2 or high-risk myelodysplastic syndromes with 5q deletion: results of a phase 2 study. Blood 2009; 113 (17): 3947–3952. doi: 10.1182/blood-2008-08-175778. Epub 2008 Nov 5.

[66] Raza A, Reeves JA, Feldman EJ, Dewald GW, Bennett JM, Deeg HJ, et al. Phase 2 study of lenalidomide in transfusion-dependent, low-risk, and intermediate-1 risk myelodysplastic syndromes with karyotypes other than deletion 5q. Blood 2008; 111(1): 86–93. Epub 2007 Sep 24.

[67] Rizzieri DA. MDS: unraveling the mystery. Blood 2012; 120 (25): 4906–4908. doi: 10.1182/blood-2012-09-452755

[68] List A, Kurtin S, Roe DJ, Buresh A, Mahadevan D, Fuchs D, et al. Efficacy of lenalidomide in myelodysplastic syndromes. N Engl J Med 2005; 352 (6): 549–557.

[69] Gandhi AK, Mendy D, Waldman M, Chen G, Rychak E, Miller K, et al. Measuring cereblon as a biomarker of response or resistance to lenalidomide and pomalidomide requires use of standardized reagents and understanding of gene complexity. Br J Haematol 2014; 164 (2): 233–244. doi: 10.1111/bjh.12622. Epub 2013 Oct 28.

[70] Lopez-Girona A, Mendy D, Ito T, Miller K, Gandhi AK, Kang J, et al. Cereblon is a direct protein target for immunomodulatory and antiproliferative activities of lenalidomide and pomalidomide. Leukemia 2012; 26 (11): 2326–2335. doi: 10.1038/leu.2012.119. Epub 2012 May 3.

[71] Lu G, Middleton RE, Sun H, Naniong M, Ott CJ, Mitsiades CS, et al. The myeloma drug lenalidomide promotes the cereblon-dependent destruction of Ikaros proteins. Science 2014; 343 (6168): 305–309. doi: 10.1126/science.1244917. Epub 2013 Nov 29.

[72] Heuser M, Meggendorfer M, Cruz MM, Fabisch J, Klesse S, Köhler L, et al. Frequency and prognostic impact of casein kinase 1A1 mutations in MDS patients with deletion

of chromosome 5q. Leukemia 2015; 29 (9): 1942–1945. doi: 10.1038/leu.2015.49. Epub 2015 Feb 24.

[73] Krönke J, Fink EC, Hollenbach PW, MacBeth KJ, Hurst SN, Udeshi ND, et al. Lenalidomide induces ubiquitination and degradation of CK1α in del (5q) MDS. Nature 2015; 523 (7559): 183–188. doi: 10.1038/nature14610. Epub 2015 Jul 1.

[74] Schneider RK, Ademà V, Heckl D, Järås M, Mallo M, Lord AM, et al. Role of casein kinase 1A1 in the biology and targeted therapy of del (5q) MDS. Cancer Cell 2014; 26 (4): 509–520. doi: 10.1016/j.ccr.2014.08.001. Epub 2014 Sep 18.

[75] Parmar S, de Lima M. Hematopoietic stem cell transplantation for myelodysplastic syndrome. Biol Blood Marrow Transplant 2010; 16 (1 Suppl): S37–44. doi: 10.1016/j.bbmt.2009.10.018. Epub 2009 Oct 24.

[76] Odenike O, Onida F, Padron E. Myelodysplastic syndromes and myelodysplastic/myeloproliferative neoplasms: an update on risk stratification, molecular genetics, and therapeutic approaches including allogeneic hematopoietic stem cell transplantation. Am Soc Clin Oncol Educ Book 2015: e398–412. doi: 10.14694/EdBook_AM.2015.35.e398.

[77] Robin M, Porcher R, Adès L, Raffoux E, Michallet M, François S, et al. HLA-matched allogeneic stem cell transplantation improves outcome of higher risk myelodysplastic syndrome A prospective study on behalf of SFGM-TC and GFM. Leukemia 2015; 29 (7): 1496–1501. doi: 10.1038/leu.2015.37. Epub 2015 Feb 13.

[78] Karoopongse E, Deeg HJ. Allogeneic hematopoietic cell transplantation for myelodysplastic syndrome: the past decade. Expert Rev Clin Immunol 2012; 8 (4): 373–381. doi: 10.1586/eci.12.18.

[79] Cutler C. Allogeneic hematopoietic stem-cell transplantation for myelodysplastic syndrome. Hematol Am Soc Hematol Educ Program 2010; 2010: 325–329. doi: 10.1182/asheducation-2010.1.325

[80] Warlick ED, Cioc A, Defor T, Dolan M, Weisdorf D. Allogeneic stem cell transplantation for adults with myelodysplastic syndromes: importance of pretransplant disease burden. Biol Blood Marrow Transplant 2009; 15 (1): 30–38. doi: 10.1016/j.bbmt.2008.10.012

[81] Deeg HJ. Hematopoietic cell transplantation for myelodysplastic syndrome. Am Soc Clin Oncol Educ Book 2015; e375–380. doi: 10.14694/EdBook_AM.2015.35.e375

[82] Negrin RS. Hematopoietic cell transplantation in myelodysplastic syndromes. Up To Date 2015. Topic edited by: Chao NJ, Connor RF. Topic last updated: Oct 27, 2015.

[83] Kröger N. Epigenetic modulation and other options to improve outcome of stem cell transplantation in MDS. Hematol Am Soc Hematol Educ Program 2008; 60–67. doi: 10.1182/asheducation-2008.1.60

[84] Sekeres MA. Bone marrow transplantation (BMT) in myelodysplastic syndromes: to BMT or not to BMT – that is the question. J Clin Oncol 2013; 31 (21): 2643–2644. doi: 10.1200/JCO.2013.48.9146. Epub 2013 Jun 24.

[85] Bacher U, Haferlach C, Kröger N, Schnittger S, Kern W, Wiedemann B, et al. Diagnostic tools in the indications for allogeneic stem cell transplantation in myelodysplastic syndromes. Biol Blood Marrow Transplant 2010; 16 (1): 1–11. doi: 10.1016/j.bbmt.2009.08.007. Epub 2009 Sep 30.

[86] Trottier BJ, Sachs Z, DeFor TE, Shune L, Dolan M, Weisdorf DJ, et al. Novel disease burden assessment predicts allogeneic transplantation outcomes in myelodysplastic syndrome. Bone Marrow Transplant 2016; 51 (2): 199–204. doi: 10.1038/bmt.2015.274. Epub 2015 Nov 23.

[87] Platzbecker U. Who benefits from allogeneic transplantation for myelodysplastic syndromes? New insights. Hematol Am Soc Hematol Educ Program 2013; 2013: 522–528. doi: 10.1182/asheducation-2013.1.522

[88] Koreth J, Pidala J, Perez WS, Deeg HJ, Garcia-Manero G, Malcovati L, et al. Role of reduced-intensity conditioning allogeneic hematopoietic stem-cell transplantation in older patients with de novo myelodysplastic syndromes: an international collaborative decision analysis. J Clin Oncol 2013; 31 (21): 2662–2670. doi: 10.1200/JCO.2012.46.8652. Epub 2013 Jun 24.

[89] Valcárcel D, Martino R, Caballero D, Martin J, Ferra C, Nieto JB, et al. Sustained remissions of high-risk acute myeloid leukemia and myelodysplastic syndrome after reduced-intensity conditioning allogeneic hematopoietic transplantation: chronic graft-versus-host disease is the strongest factor improving survival. J Clin Oncol 2008; 26 (4): 577–584. Epub 2007 Dec 17.

[90] Sauer T, Silling G, Groth C, Rosenow F, Krug U, Görlich D, et al. Treatment strategies in patients with AML or high-risk myelodysplastic syndrome relapsed after Allo-SCT. Bone Marrow Transplant 2015; 50 (4): 485–492. doi: 10.1038/bmt.2014.300. Epub 2015 Jan 19.

[91] Barrett AJ. Stem cell transplants for myelodysplastic syndromes: refining the outcome predictions. Haematologica 2014; 99 (10): 1536–1537. doi: 10.3324/haematol.2014.113555

[92] Oliansky DM, Antin JH, Bennett JM, Deeg HJ, Engelhardt C, Heptinstall KV, et al. The role of cytotoxic therapy with hematopoietic stem cell transplantation in the therapy of myelodysplastic syndromes: an evidence-based review. Biol Blood Marrow Transplant 2009; 15 (2):137–172. doi: 10.1016/j.bbmt.2008.12.003.

Chapter 5

Myelodysplastic Disorders, Monosomy 7

Khalid Ahmed Al-Anazi

Additional information is available at the end of the chapter

http://dx.doi.org/10.5772/64549

Abstract

Myelodysplastic syndromes (MDSs) are heterogeneous hematopoietic disorders associated with various degrees of myelosuppression and transformation into acute leukemia. Chromosome 7 abnormalities occur at any age, have several disease associations, and are generally associated with poor outcome. Treatment of the associated disease conditions may have a positive impact on the outcome of certain types of MDSs. For patients eligible for hematopoietic stem cell transplantation (HSCT), allografts are the standard of care, while supportive measures and the use of hypomethylating agents, such as 5-azacytidine and decitabine, constitute the mainstay of management in individuals who are not fit for allogeneic HSCT. However, the use of hypomethylating agents in conjunction with allogeneic HSCT using nonmyeloablative conditioning therapies may be an appealing therapeutic option for older patients with comorbid medical conditions.

Keywords: myelodysplastic syndrome, monosomy 7, 5-azacytidine, decitabine, hematopoietic stem cell transplantation

1. Introduction

MDSs are a heterogeneous group of clonal hematopoietic stem cell disorders characterized by ineffective hematopoiesis, dysplastic changes in the peripheral blood and bone marrow (BM), and a variable risk of progression into acute myeloid leukemia (AML) [1–4]. Primary MDS has a bimodal age incidence. It is usually a disease of old age as more than 50% of patients are ≥70 years of age [5]. Primary MDS is less common in the pediatric population and it includes specific pediatric syndromes such as juvenile chronic myeloid leukemia (JCML) and infantile monosomy 7 syndrome [5].

The clinical, pathologic, and cytogenetic features of primary MDS in younger patients appear to be different from those in elderly individuals suggesting that this may represent a biologically different disease [5]. In patients with MDS, with or without abnormal chromosomal karyotype, the type and the quantity of the abnormal karyotype have clinical values in predicting transformation to acute leukemia [6]. The use of granulocyte-monocyte colony stimulating factor (GM-CSF) in congenital BM failure syndromes may induce or accelerate the onset of leukemic transformation [7].

2. Pathogenetic mechanisms in MDSs

Several mechanisms are involved in the pathogenesis of MDSs and these include: (1) enhancement of a self-renewal of a hematopoietic stem cell or acquisition of self-renewal in a progenitor cell, (2) enhancement of proliferative capacity in the disease-sustaining clone and/or in its more differentiated progeny, (3) impairment or blockade of differentiation, (4) genetic or epigenetic instability, (5) antiapoptotic mechanisms in the disease-sustaining cells, (6) evasion of the immune system, and (7) suppression of normal hematopoiesis leading ultimately to BM failure [8].

3. Epigenetics in MDSs

Epigenetics is the heritable alteration in gene expression without DNA sequence change. The primary epigenetic modifiers are DNA methylation and histone modifications, both of which are potentially reversible [9]. DNA methylation plays a major role in tissue- and stage-specific gene regulation and it increases with age. Aberrant methylation of certain promoter regions can occur in diseases particularly cancers and correlates with gene silencing [9]. Epigenetic changes in the form of modification of the transcriptional capacity of the cell via processes such as DNA methylation and histone deacetylation can also alter gene expression impacting disease biology [10].

Advances in the science of epigenetics have led to better understanding of the specific pathogenetic mechanisms underlying MDSs. DNA methylation provides a major epigenetic code of lineage and development-specific genes that control expression of normal cells [8]. The most relevant molecular mediators of the epigenetic state in MDS are gene expression patterns maintained by methylation of cytosine residues in DNA and covalent modification of histones. TET2 status may be a genetic predictor of response to azacytidine, independently of karyotype and holds promise as one of the tools available to help in better selection of patients for treatment [8].

Cancer is characterized by global DNA hypomethylation and regional promoter hypermethylation of genes [9, 10]. Promoter methylation of CDKN2B [encoding $p15^{INK4b}$] has been shown to be restricted to the malignant hematological disorders [9, 10]. Several tumor suppressor genes (TSGs) are inactivated by promoter hypermethylation. Potentially reversible

http://dx.doi.org/10.5772/64549

silencing of genes, such as CDKN2B, by promoter methylation has been shown to occur in MDS and it increases with disease progression [9, 10].

1. Unknown etiology.		
2. Old age; more than 50 years		
3. Obesity		
4. Alcohol intake		
5. Tobacco use		
6. Sweet's syndrome		
7. Vitamin deficiency: B_{12} and folate		
8. Infections:	- Human immunodeficiency virus	- Epstein-barr virus
	- Tuberculosis	- Brucellosis
9. Autoimmune disorders:		
	- Behcet syndrome	
	- Fibrosing alveolitis	
	- Systemic lupus erythromatosis	
10. Exposure to:	- Solvents	- Lead
	- Benzene	- Arsenic
	- Herbicides	- Hair dyes
	- Pesticides	- Agricultural chemicals
11. Cytotoxic chemotherapy:	- Alkylating agents	- Topoisomerase Π inhibitors
12. Radiotherapy		
13. Bone marrow failure syndromes:	- Aplastic anemia	- Fanconi anemia
	- Dyskeratosis congenita	- Diamond Blackfan syndrome
	- Paroxysmal nocturnal hemoglobinuria	
	- Congenital neutropenia (Kostmann's syndrome)	
14. Genetic, familial and hereditary disorders:	- Ataxia telangiectasia	- Trisomy 8 mosaicism
	- Xeroderma pigmentosa	- Down syndrome
	- Bloom's syndrome	- Neurofibromatosis
15. Miscellaneous:		
	- Polycythemia rubra vera	
	- Familial myelodysplastic syndromes; monosomy 7	
	- Germ cell tumors (embryonal dysgenesis)	
	- Mutagen detoxification [$GSTq_1$ - null]	
	- Family history of hematopoietic cancer	

Table 1. .Etiology, risk factors and epidemiological associations of myelodysplastic syndromes.

4. Etiology and associations of MDSs

MDSs have several etiologies, risk factors, and epidemiological associations as shown in **Table 1** [11–43]. Also, several hereditary diseases predispose to familial forms of MDS/AML as shown in **Table 2** [11, 16, 18, 23, 25, 27, 44–48].

4.1. Familial MDSs

Familial MDSs are rare diseases. The most common form of familial MDSs is familial platelet disorder, caused by heterozygous germline RUNX1 mutations, which has the propensity to evolve into myeloid malignancy. Many patients lack history of bleeding or thrombocytopenia [44, 46, 47]. Several cases of T-acute lymphoblastic leukemia (ALL) have been reported in patients with inherited RUNX1 mutations [44]. Novel causative mechanisms such as RUNX1 deficiency result in constitutional microdeletions of 21q22 and myelodysplasia associated with telomerase deficiency [44]. Treatment of familial MDS is allogeneic hematopoietic stem cell transplantation (HSCT) but donors have to be screened for deficiency of RUNX1 and deficiency of telomerase [44].

The following genetic mutations have been described in familial MDS/AML: TERC, TERT, CEBPA, GATA2, and RUNX1 [16, 44, 46–48].

4.2. MonoMac syndrome

MonoMac syndrome is a familial disorder associated with GATA2 deficiency, inherited as autosomal dominant and causes early onset of MDS/AML [47, 48]. Additional acquisitions include: monosomy 7 and ASXL1 mutations. Genetic mutations are detected in dendritic cells, monocytes, natural killer (NK) cells and B-lymphocytes. Many carriers are asymptomatic. The syndrome is associated with severe infectious complications and familial predisposition to cancer. Aggressive therapeutic strategies are needed as the disease has poor outcome [47, 48]. GATA2 mutations have also been described in familial MDS/AML and Emberger syndrome [46–48].

5. Cytogenetic abnormalities in MDSs

Chromosomal abnormalities are detectable in 40–60% of patients with *de novo* MDS and approximately 90% of patients with secondary therapy-related MDSs (t-MDSs) [1]. The most frequent cytogenetic abnormalities are del(5q), monosomy 7, del(7q), trisomy 8, complex karyotype, and -Y [1]. Chromosome 5 and 7 abnormalities are considered to be the most frequent recurrent genetic abnormalities in myeloid malignancies (MDS and AML) as they occur in 10–20% of myeloid neoplasms [49].

http://dx.doi.org/10.5772/64549

Pure familial MDS	Familial MDS/AML
1. Familial monosomy 7	- Bone marrow failure syndromes:
2. Chromosome 21q22 deletions	1. Diamond-Blackfan syndrome
3. Telomere deficiency-associated familial MDS	2. Severe congenital neutropenia
[occult dyskeratosis congenita]	3. Congenital amegakaryocytic thrombocytopenia
4. Familial platelet disorder with propensity to myeloid	4. Dyskeratosis congenita
malignancy	5. Schwachman-Diamond syndrome
	- DNA repair deficiency syndrome:
	1. Fanconi anemia
	2. Bloom syndrome
	3. Li-Fraumeni syndrome
	- Signal transductions:
	1. Noonan syndrome
	2. Neuorofibromatosis-1
	- Numerical chromosomal abnormalities:
	1. Trisomy 21

Abbreviations: MDS, myelodysplastic syndrome; AML, acute myeloid leukemia.

Table 2. Familial MDS/AML.

6. Chromosome 7 abnormalities

Abnormalities involving chromosome 7 occur in approximately 20% of patients with MDS having clonal cytogenetic abnormalities. Abnormalities of chromosome 7 include: (1) total loss of chromosome 7 [monosomy 7], (2) deletion of a segment of the long arm of chromosome 7 [del(7q)], and (3) translocations involving chromosome 7 [2]. However, these cytogenetic anomalies have different prognostic significance [1, 2, 50, 51]. MDS with monosomy 7 has poor prognosis, while isolated del (7q) has a better outcome compared to isolated monosomy 7 [2]. Del(7q) which has distinct clinical and pathological characteristics should no longer be considered in the same prognostic category as monosomy 7 [2]. Also, the prognostic impact of der(7) t(1,7) (q10 or p10) is less adverse once compared to monosomy 7 or del (7q) [1]. In a series of 246 patients with myeloid disorders: monosomy 7 or -7 was the most frequent chromosomal abnormality as it was reported in 51% of patients with secondary myeloid disorders, del(7q) was found in 7% of cases, and partial monosomy was found in 8% of secondary myeloid diseases, while in *de novo* myeloid disorders, monosomy 7 and del(7q) were reported in only 10% of patients [52].

6.1. Disease associations

Chromosome 7 abnormalities are associated with: (1) de novo and t-MDS, (2) de novo and therapy related AML (t-AML), (3) JCML, (4) juvenile myelomonocytic leukemia [JMML], (5) familial monosomy 7, (6) primary myelofibrosis, (7) Down's syndrome, (8) Fanconi anemia, and (9) lymphoma [50, 51, 53]. Monosomy 7 is the commonest chromosomal abnormality in all of the above conditions except in primary myelofibrosis, where del(7q) is the commonest chromosome 7 anomaly [53]. In adults, chromosome 7 abnormalities are associated with: (1) advanced age, (2) antecedent MDS, and (3) resistance to current therapies [54]. In patients with MDS and AML, chromosome 7 abnormalities usually carry poor prognosis [54].

6.2. Genes on chromosome 7 and their detection

Genes that have been reported to have microdeletions involving chromosome 7q21.2-q21.3 include: SAMD9, SAMD9L, and HEPACAM2 [55]. The following acquired somatic deletions have also been reported at chromosome 7q36.1: EZH2, CUL1, and TET2 [56, 57]. Examples of additional genetic mutations that have been reported in monosomy 7 and del(7q) include: ASXL1, RUNX1, CBL, ETV6, FAM40B, FAM115A, SEMA3A, LUC7L2, SSPO, NRCAM, GRM8, HYAL4, RABL5, TRIM24, FISI, and CUX1 [51, 57, 58]. Chromosome 7 abnormalities can be detected by conventional cytogenetics or interphase fluorescence *in situ* hybridization (FISH) [59]. Interphase FISH is a very useful method in detecting -7/7q- in patients with MDS. Also, it is more sensitive in detecting chromosome 7 abnormalities than conventional cytogenetics [59]. Refined chromosomal analysis has emerged as a tool that has considerable impact on decision making and development of treatment protocols in patients with MDS and AML [60].

6.3. The commonly deleted segments (CDSs)

Several studies on MDS and AML specimens with interstitial deletions on chromosome 7 have implicated three putative CDSs at the following chromosome bands: 7q22, 7q34, and 7q35-36. However, 7q22 is the most frequently deleted band in patients with MDS/AML having del(7q) [3]. The following genes in monosomy 7/del(7q) MDS/AML have been reported to be inactivated or to harbor recurrent genetic mutations such as EZH2, LUC7L2, and CUX1 [3].

The CDS on the long arm of chromosome 7 between 7q22 and 7q36 has been identified to harbor a number of haploinsufficient myeloid TSGs [49, 50, 54]. Loss of function of at least one TSG contributes to disease progression and leukemogenesis or leukemic transformation [50, 54]. It is feasible to somatically delete a large chromosomal segment that is implicated in tumor suppression in hematopoietic cell population *in vitro* [54]. The CDSs that occur at chromosomal bands7q22, 7q34, and 7q35-q36 contain the following genes: TRIM24, SVOPL, ATP6V0A4, TMEM213, KIAA1549, LUC7L2, KLRG2, CLEK2L, HIPK2, TBXAS1, ZC34AV1L, ZC3HAV1, TTC26, UBN2, C7orf55, TPK1, CNTNAP2, MIR548F3, C7orf33, CUL1, and EZH2 [49].

Loss of TP53 is more frequently associated with del5q rather than del7q, while loss of ETV6 is particularly associated with concurrent del(5q) and del(7q) [49]. CUX1, a gene encoding a homeodomain-containing transcription factor, has been identified within the CDS on chromosome 7 (7q22.1) [61]. CUX1 is expressed at haploinsufficient levels in leukemias with chromosome 7 abnormalities. Haploinsufficiency of CUX1 gave human hematopoietic cells a significant engraftment advantage on transplantation in immunodeficient mice [61].

Monosomy 7 and del(7q) are highly recurrent chromosomal abnormalities in myeloid malignancies including: AML, *de novo* MDS, and t-MDS/AML [51, 54, 61]. Also, monosomy 7 and del(7q) are common findings in children and adults who develop MDS as a second malignant neoplasm [27]. In t-MDS/AML with chromosome 7 abnormalities, the peak incidence is between 3 and 7 years after cessation of cytotoxic chemotherapy such as alkylating agents [27]. Under such circumstances, monosomy 7 and del(7q) are not equivalent in prognosis and spectrum of disease phenotype [51].

Monosomy 7 and del(7q) are highly prevalent in acquired cytogenetic abnormalities in *de novo* MDS/AML and t-MDS/AML [3]. The proportion of -7/del (7q) cells is markedly increased in hematopoietic stem cell (HSC) and progenitor cell compartments of MDS patients relative to T and B lymphocytes [3]. Recent studies demonstrating quantitative changes in the frequencies of phenotypic primitive long-term HSCs, common myeloid progenitors, and granulocyte-monocyte progenitors in MDS patients with -7/del(7q) further support the diverse effects on hematopoiesis [3].

After many attempts, mice with 5A3 deletions in the CDS of chromosome band 7q22 have been successfully generated [54]. The 5A3 deleted mice have shown normal hematologic parameters but have not developed myeloid malignancies spontaneously [54]. Animal studies have also shown that heterozygous 5A3 deletion does not accelerate the evolution of leukemia or modulate the responsiveness to antileukemic drugs, while homozygous 5A3 deletions are embryonically lethal [54].

The following 7q genes have been implicated in contributing to leukemogenesis by haploinsufficiency or epigenetic transcriptional repression: SAMD9L, RASA4, dedicator of cytokinesis 4 (DOCK4), and MLL3 [3]. Animal studies have shown that the long-term HSC compartment is expanded in $5A3^{+/del}$ mice and that the 5A3 deletion partially rescues defective repopulation in GATA2 mutant mice [3]. Studies have also shown that 7q22 deletions are implicated in playing a strong haploinsufficiency role in leukemogenesis [3]. Mutations in DOCK4 gene which is a putative 7q gene have been identified in prostate and ovarian cancers and studies have demonstrated that DOCK4 gene acts as a tumor suppressor [62]. Depletion of DOCK4 levels in MDS stem and progenitor cells leads to erythroid dysplasia by disrupting the action of cytoskeleton in developing red blood cells (RBCs) ultimately leading to dysplastic morphology of erythroid cells both *in vivo* and *in vitro* [62].

7. Monosomy 7 MDS

Monosomy 7 is characterized by (1) lower median age of affected patients than that of 5q- syndrome, (2) severe refractory cytopenias, (3) rapid disease progression, (4) resistance to therapy, and (5) increased susceptibility to infectious complications [52, 63]. Infections encountered in monosomy 7 may be life-threatening and they include (1) bacterial infections: these are the most common types of infections and may be complicated by sepsis, and (2) invasive aspergillosis [63, 64]. Infectious complications in monosomy 7 are caused by neutropenia, dysfunctional neutrophils, and chemotherapy or targeted therapy given to control the disease [64].

In patients having monosomy 7, isolated monosomy 7 occurs in 36% of the cases, monosomy 7 and one additional chromosomal abnormality are encountered in 14% of patients, and monosomy 7 associated with complex cytogenetics in seen in approximately 50% of the cases [63]. Monosomy 7 can be associated with the following chromosomal abnormalities: trisomy 8, chromosome 5 abnormalities, and t(1,7) [63]. Chromosomal microarray analysis is a clinically useful tool in the diagnosis and follow-up of MDS patients with monosomy 7 [65]. In monosomy 7, there is an association between DNA loss and functional impairment or defect of granulocytes [66]. Monosomy 7 is not rare in acute lymphoblastic leukemia as it has been reported in 3–6% of the cases of ALL and in 16% of Philadelphia chromosome positive ALL as it occurs as a secondary anomaly to t(9,22) [52]. Monosomy 7 carries poor prognosis as studies have shown that (1) relapse rate of monosomy 7 at 1 year to be 81%, and (2) event-free survival at 7 years to be 6% [52]. Monosomy 7 does not usually affect lymphoid subpopulations but it is restricted to committed progenitor cells with the capacity to differentiate into mature myeloid cells [67].

Analysis of expression profiles in CD34+ cells from MDS patients with monosomy 7 has shown a malignant phenotype with highly proliferative potential expressing HOX9A, PRAME, BMI-1, PLAB, and BRCA2 (DNA repair gene) [63]. Gene therapy for chronic granulomatous disease has been reported to cause activation of ectopic viral integration site 1 (EVI1) which in turn induces development of genomic instability that ultimately results in clonal progression toward myelodysplasia and monosomy 7 [68].

Conventional chemotherapy in monosomy 7 carries a high risk of early death and poor response. Even if complete remissions are obtained, they are usually short-lived [63]. Targeted therapies such as 5-azacytidine and lenalidomide are more effective than cytotoxic chemotherapy in patients with monosomy 7 MDS. However, lenalidomide is more effective in patients having monosomy 7 and 5q- syndrome. Complete hematological and even cytogenetic responses have been documented in patients with monosomy 7 MDS treated with lenalidomide [63].

In transplant-eligible patients, allogeneic HSCT is the treatment of choice in patients with monosomy 7 [25, 63, 69]. Following allogeneic HSCT, presence of monosomy 7 is a predictor of unfavorable outcome [52].

Masked monosomy 7 refers to monosomy 7 that is detected by FISH but not by conventional cytogenetics. It has been reported in varying frequencies in patients with MDS [70]. Masked monosomy 7 is less common than has been thought and does not seem to carry the same prognostic weight as monosomy 7 diagnosed by metaphase cytogenetics [70].

7.1. Monosomy 7 in children

MDS is uncommon in children as it accounts for less than 5% of all hematopoietic neoplasms [33, 71]. Viral infections including Epstein-Barr virus (EBV) may contribute to the pathogenesis of MDS by stimulating a preexisting clone and may induce certain genetic mutations [33]. Chromosome 7 abnormalities, monosomy 7 and del (7q), are common cytogenetic abnormalities in MDS and they are found in 31% of children with myeloid neoplasms [22, 71]. They are

http://dx.doi.org/10.5772/64549

characterized by ineffective erythropoiesis, BM dysplasia, and increased risk of leukemic transformation [22]. Monosomy 7 is the most common chromosomal abnormality in children with MDS [33, 71]. In children, monosomy 7 implies poor prognosis because it is associated with high risk of transformation into acute leukemia including ALL [33, 71].

Treatment of children with MDS/AML associated with monosomy 7 with allogeneic HSCT, using a variety of donor types such as sibling donor, unrelated donor, and umbilical cord blood, as well as different sources such as BM and peripheral blood, is an effective therapeutic modality [69]. In patients with more advanced disease, optimization of conditioning therapies may further improve disease-free survival [69]. Graft versus leukemia effect appears to play a major role in leukemia control for some patients and quality of life (QOL) in patients surviving allogeneic HSCT is usually very good [69].

7.2. Familial monosomy 7 syndrome

Familial monosomy 7 syndrome is a rare familial disorder [44, 45]. It is inherited as autosomal dominant with incomplete penetrance [45]. Familial monosomy 7 can be partial or complete monosomy and it is associated with the following chromosomal abnormalities: trisomy 8, 5q-, and t(1;7) [45]. It has even sex distribution and often presents before the age of 18 years and the median age at diagnosis in 8 years [45]. Allogeneic HSCT in this category of MDS is problematic due to familial predisposition to cancer, hence the prognosis is usually poor [44, 45]. Familial monosomy 7 has several associations including: (1) inherited BM failure syndromes, (2) secondary MDS/AML, (3) occupational exposure to chemical toxins, (4) exposure to cytotoxic chemotherapy, particularly alkylating agents, (5) Noonan syndrome, (6) Fanconi anemia, and (7) cerebellar ataxia [44, 45]. The cell origin or phenotype is multipotential progenitor cell [45]. The clinical manifestations of familial monosomy 7 syndrome include complications of cytopenias, dysplasia, and acute leukemic transformation in addition to features of the associated disease conditions [44, 45].

7.3. JMML

JMML is a rare clonal MDS/myeloproliferative neoplasm (MPN) of young children [44, 45, 72, 73]. It has also been described as juvenile CML and was formerly grouped in the French-American-British (FAB) classification of MDS [74]. Without treatment, the 10-year overall survival (OS) of patients with JMML is 6% [74]. Allogeneic HSCT is the only curative therapy for children with JMML [72, 74]. Studies have also shown that event-free survival is 52% at 5 years post-HSCT [72]. Also, relapse is expected to occur in 50% of transplanted patients [72, 73]. Treatment options of relapsed JMML after the first HSCT include: (1) withdrawal of immunosuppressive therapy and/or donor lymphocyte infusion, and (2) second allogeneic HSCT, which may be the treatment of choice in such situations [72]. The major causes of HSCT failure in patients with JMML are treatment-related mortality and relapse [74].

8. Anemia in MDS

Severe anemia should be considered a major criterion for deciding not only the type but also the timing of therapeutic interventions in patients with MDS [75]. Once anemia is symptomatic, transfusion of packed RBCs is the mainstay of therapy in MDS [76]. The redistribution of transfusion iron from reticuloendothelial cells to parenchymal cells is modulated by hepcidin. Ineffective erythropoiesis has a suppressive effect on hepcidin production and hence increases iron redistribution [76].

9. Iron overload in high-risk MDS

Transfusion history should be considered in transplantation decision making in patients with MDS because pre-HSCT transfusion history and serum ferritin levels have been shown to have significant prognostic value in patients with MDS undergoing allogeneic HSCT [77]. Elevated serum ferritin and elevated liver iron content in patients with MDS and acute leukemia prior to HSCT are associated with inferior post-HSCT survival [78]. Studies have shown that transfusion dependency is independently associated with (1) reduced overall survival, (2) increased nonrelapse mortality (NRM), and (3) increased risk of acute graft versus host disease (GVHD) in patients with MDS undergoing allogeneic HSCT [77].

In patients with high-risk MDS, iron overload has adverse consequences on the outcome of HSCT as it has been associated with (1) increased transfusion-related mortality, (2) infectious complications, and (3) AML progression [79]. Iron chelation therapy in patients with higher risk MDS should be considered to possibly (1) reduce infectious complications, (2) delay leukemic transformation, and (3) improve the outcome of HSCT [80].

Nuclear factor-kappaB (NF-kB) is key regulator of many cellular processes and its impaired activity has been described in different myeloid malignancies including MDS [81]. NF-kB inhibition by deferasirox could prove to be an important therapeutic option in higher risk MDS patients by targeting blast cells in which increased NF-kB activity has been extensively demonstrated thus acting as a possible enhancer of chemosensitivity of the malignant clone [81].

10. Management of MDS

The following therapeutic modalities are available for patients with MDS: (1) supportive measures: packed RBCs and platelet (PLT) transfusions, antimicrobial therapy, and hematopoietic growth factors, (2) drug therapies including novel agents such as lenalidomide, azacytidine, and decitabine, and (3) various forms of HSCT [82].

10.1. Epigenetic therapies of MDS

Epigenetic therapies cause potentially reversible epigenetic changes that can alter gene expression patterns [83]. Epigenetic therapies in MDS include (1) histone deacetylase inhibitors, and (2) hypomethylating agents, such as azacytidine and decitabine, that inhibit the DNA methyltransferase enzymes (DNMT) [83].

Epigenetic silencing is a universal mechanism of gene inactivation in malignant cells, probably exceeding mutational events. Recent therapeutic approaches targeting the aberrant epigenome of cancer has been developed [84]. The hypomethylating agents, azacytidine and decitabine, have shown remarkable activity in older individuals with higher risk MDSs including patients with poor-risk cytogenetic profiles. Translational studies performed on BM biopsies obtained from MDS patients with both azanucleoside demethylating agents have indicated that both azanucleosides can revert the aberrant hypermethylation state *in vivo* [84].

10.2. Hypomethylating agents

The azanucleosides, 5-azacytidine and decitabine, were originally synthesized more than 50 years ago in order to be used as classical cytotoxic agents [85–88]. Azacytidine was first described by Sorm in 1964 as a cancerostatic agent [89]. Both hypomethylating agents, 5-azacytidine and decitabine, had demonstrated activity against lymphoid leukemic cells as well as hemopoietic tissues in experimental leukemia mice models [90–93].

10.2.1. 5-Azacytidine

Azacytidine is a pyrimidine nucleoside analog that differs from cytosine by the presence of nitrogen, rather than ring carbon, at position 5 [8, 9]. It was first manufactured in Europe in the 1960s [8, 9]. Azacytidine is a DNA methyltransferase inhibitor (DMTI) that has *in vitro* and *in vivo* demethylating effects [9]. The hypomethylating effects of azacytidine appear to primarily depend on the structural alternations at position 5 [8]. Azacytidine was the first hypomethylating agent to be approved by the Food and Drug Administration (FDA) in United States of America for the treatment of all subtypes of MDS in May 2009 [8, 10, 94]. In patients with high-risk MDS, the benefits of azacytidine therapy on survival compared to conventional chemotherapy have not been established outside clinical trials [95, 96]. Despite the wide spread use of azacytidine in the treatment of high-risk MDSs, there is lack of improvement in long-term survival. Therefore, identification of predicting factors of response and survival is mandatory [95, 96].

Hypomethylating agents or azanucleosides are becoming the standard therapy for patients with higher-risk MDSs [97]. Patients with high-risk MDSs treated with azanucleosides have a median overall survival of 11–16 months, so they should be strongly considered for upfront allogeneic HSCT or experimental therapies [97]. In patients with high-risk MDSs planned for allogeneic HSCT, azacytidine treatment may be valuable in stabilizing the disease and preventing relapse [98]. Additionally, pretransplant administration of azacytidine does not adversely affect transplant outcome [98]. Preemptive azacytidine therapy has an acceptable safety profile and can substantially prevent or at least delay relapse in patients with MDS or AML with minimal residual disease after allogeneic HSCT [99].

Name of trial	CALG-B/8421 trial	CALG-B/8921 trial
Phase	Phase I	Phase II
Azacytidine therapy	IV administration Initial dose: 75 mg/m^2 continuous IV infusion over 7 days every 28 daysdose escalated to 150 mg/m^2	SC administration 100 mg/m^2
Number of patients evaluated	43	68
Complete response	5 patients (12%)	8 patients (12%)
Partial response	11 patients (25%)	10 patients (15%)
Improvement	5 patients (12%)	18 patients (27%)
Total response	21 Patients (49%)	36 patients (53%)

Abbreviations: MDS, myelodysplastic syndrome; IV, intravenous; CALG-B, cancer and leukemia group B; SC, subcutaneous.

Table 3. Phase I and phase II CALG-B clinical trials on azacytidine in MDS.

The outcome of patients with high-risk MDSs after failure of azacytidine treatment is generally poor [100]. After failure of azacytidine treatment, the options are rather limited to (1) best supportive care in patients unfit for allogeneic HSCT, and (2) allogeneic HSCT and investigational agents in patients who are eligible for such therapies [100]. Mechanisms of action of 5-azacytidine are multifactorial and they include (1) demethylation of several key genes, that is, reduction of DNA methylation by inhibition of methyltransferase enzymes, (2) cytotoxic action by inhibition of protein translation, and (3) enhancement of apoptosis [8–10]. In patients with MDSs, 5-azacytodine is indicated in (1) high-risk MDSs, and (2) intermediate 2 risk MDSs [8, 10, 95, 97, 100–102]. The side effects of azacytidine therapy include myelosuppression (leucopenia, anemia, and thrombocytopenia); gastrointestinal (GIT) upset (nausea, vomiting, diarrhea, and constipation); injection site reactions and erythema; serum sickness-like illness; abnormal liver function tests; fatigue; weakness; lethargy; anorexia; headache; arthralgias; febrile neutropenia; cytomegalovirus infection; and pneumonia [9, 10, 99, 101, 103].

The effects of azacytidine in patients with MDSs include (1) prolongation of survival, (2) improvement in QOL, and (3) delayed leukemic transformation [8, 10, 95, 101, 102]. Responses to azacytidine according to karyotypes are as follows: (1) excellent responses are expected in patients with normal cytogenetics, (2) durable remission and 80% response rate are expected in patients having chromosome 7 abnormalities as the sole karyotypic abnormalities, and (3) good early responses but early relapses in patients with trisomy 8 [9]. Predictors of positive responses to DMTIs is include (1) doubling of PLT count, (2) mutated TET2, (3) mutated EZH2, (4) Phosphoinositide-phospholipase C beta hypomethylation, and (5) low serum level of micro-RNA-21 [96, 104, 105]. Predictors of poor response to DMTIs include (1) BM blasts >15%,

(2) previous therapy, (3) transfusion dependency, (4) grade 3 marrow fibrosis, (5) mutated p53, (6) abnormal karyotype of complex cytogenetics, (7) high serum level of micro-RNA-21, and (8) increased cytidine deaminase expression of activity in males [96, 104, 106].

Trial	AZA-001 trial			CALG-B 9221 trial		
Phase	Phase III randomized controlled multicenter international study			Phase III randomized controlled study		
Study design	Azacytidine	Conventional care	*P*-value	Azacytidine	Best supportive care	*P*-value
Number of patients	179	179	–	99	92	–
IPSS class intermediate 2 and high risk	158 patients (89%)	155 patients (87%)	–	20%	26%	–
Median survival (months)	24.5 months	15 months	≤0.0001	18 months	11 months	0.03
2 year overall survival	50.8%	26.2%	<0.0001	–	–	–
Transformation to AML				15%	38%	0.001
Median time to AML transformation	17.8 months	11.5 months	≤0.0001	21 months	13 months	0.007
Complete response	30 patients (17%)	14 patients (4%)	0.015	7%	0%	0.01
Partial response	21 patients (12%)	7 patients (4%)	0.0094	16%	0%	<0.0001
Improvement	Stable disease 75 patients (42%)	Stable disease 65 patients (36%)	0.33	37%	5%	<0.0001
Overall response	HI in 87 patients (49%)	HI in 51 patients (29%)		60%	5%	-

Abbreviations: MDS, myelodysplastic syndrome; AML, acute myeloid leukemia; IPSS, International Prognostic Scoring System; CALG-B, cancer and leukemia group B; AZA, azacytidine HI: hematological improvement.

Table 4. Phase III randomized controlled clinical trials on azacytidine.

In patients with high-risk MDSs and AML, the combination of 5-azacytidine, valproic acid, and all-trans retinoic acid (ATRA) are safe and they are active and associated with induction of global DNA hypomethylation and histone acetylation [107, 108]. Lessons learned from clinical experience with hypomethylating agents include (1) in the majority of treated patients, the beneficial effects are only noted after approximately four cycles of therapy, (2) the achievement of hematological improvement is sufficient to ensure prolonged OS, (3) in almost all patients, interruption of treatment induces relapse, (4) patients who relapse after treatment or who are refractory to therapy have extremely limited survival, and (5) patients with complex karyotype involving monosomy 7 or monosomy 5 have negligible survival advantage from hypomethylating agents despite achievement of response [96]. Clinical phase I, II, and III trials on the use of azacytidine in patients with MDSs are shown in **Tables 3** and **4** [9, 10, 101, 103, 109]. Investigational agents that can be used in the treatment of MDSs in case of failure of hypomethylating agents include (1) rigosertib, (2) sapacitabine, (3) clofarabine, and (4) BCL2 inhibitors (proapoptotic drug therapy) including ABT-737 and ABT-199 [96, 110].

Conclusion that can be drawn from phase III trials on azacytidine include: (1) in CALG-B 9221 trial: compared to best supportive care (BSC), azacytidine therapy resulted in (a) significantly higher response rates, (b) improved QOL, (c) improved survival, and (d) reduced risk of leukemic transformation; and (2) in AZA-001 trial: compared to conventional therapy, that Included BSC, low dose cytarabine ± intensive chemotherapy, azacytidine increased OS in patients with high-risk MDS [101, 109]. In patients with chromosome 7 abnormalities [monosomy 7 and del(7q)], the median survival was 13.1 months in patients treated with azacytidine compared to 4.6 months in patients who received conventional therapies [101].

10.2.2. Decitabine

Decitabine (5-aza-2-deoxycytidine) inhibits DNMT. It was approved by the FDA in the United States for the treatment of MDS in the year 2006 [83, 111, 112]. It is postulated that initially the drug and the DNMT enzymes become attached, then the outcome will be: (1) enzyme degradation resulting in low DNMT levels, and (2) ultimately achievement of hypomethylation [83]. Although decitabine antitumor activity is not fully understood, there are several possible mechanisms of action that include (1) induction of hypomethylation or reversal of cancer-associated hypermethylation effects, (2) reactivation of genes responsible for cellular differentiation, (3) stimulation or induction of immune responses, (4) induction of DNA damage pathways or apoptotic response pathways, that is, induction of changes in the rates of apoptosis, and (5) augmentation of stem cell renewal [83, 105]. Various doses, schedules, and even routes of administration have been used: 10, 15, or 20 mg/m^2 intravenously (IV) or subcutaneously (SC) for 3–5 days, each cycle for at least four cycles that are given at 4- to 6-week intervals [83, 111, 112].

Although it has been used in the treatment of all FAB subtypes of MDS, the specific indications are as follows: (1) intermediate 1, intermediate 2, and high-risk MDS, (2) *de novo* and secondary MDS, including t-MDS, (3) MDS transforming into AML, in individuals unfit for intensive cytotoxic chemotherapy, as upfront therapy, (4) treatment of MDS refractory to lenalidomide, (5) debulking treatment prior to HSCT in high-risk patients, and (6) patients with chronic myelomonocytic leukemia (CMML) [83, 105, 111]. The adverse effects of decitabine therapy include (1) myelosuppression leading to febrile neutropenia, sepsis, pneumonia, and fungal infections, (2) gastrointestinal effects including nausea, vomiting, diarrhea, and mucositis, (3) hair loss, skin rashes, fatigue, and bleeding, (4) renal failure, (5) cardiovascular complications are uncommon, and (6) pleural effusions and acute lung injury [83, 112, 113]. Encountering myelosuppression that requires decitabine dose modification may truly indicate response to therapy [112].

Despite the efficacy of dectiabine therapy, there are no known definitive predictors of response. However, in patients with high-risk MDS treated with decitabine, high expression of human equilibrative nucleoside transporter-1 (hENT-1) gene appears to predict a good response to decitabine therapy and is associated with prolonged survival [114]. Patients with chromosome 7 abnormalities usually respond more favorably to continuous IV infusion of low-dose decitabine than to conventional chemotherapy with low-dose cytarabine [115]. Results of clinical trials on decitabine are shown in **Table 5** [83, 84, 111, 113]. Unfortunately, there is no head-to-head comparison with 5-azacytidine. Also, decitabine has not shown a statistically significant evidence of prolonged survival benefit in prospective studies. In addition, the role of decitabine after HSCT needs further evaluation [83].

10.2.3. Rigosertib (ON01910.Na)

Rigosertib is a multikinase inhibitor that inhibits both the phosphoinositide 3 kinase and the polo-like kinase pathways [116–120]. It inhibits the cell-cycle progression by selectively inducing a mitotic arrest and apoptosis in cancer cells [116, 118–120]. Recently, it has been highlighted as a novel anticancer agent for the treatment of MDS. Rigosertib has shown activity in the following malignancies: (1) mantle cell lymphoma, (2) chronic lymphocytic leukemia, and (3) MDS [118]. In MDS, rigosertib has several mechanisms of action that include: (a) upregulation of genes related to microtubule kinetics, (b) downregulation of the mRNA degradation system, that is, suppression of nonsense mRNA decay (NMD) gene, (c) suppression of cyclin-D1 in BM CD34+ cells in MDS patients with trisomy 8 and monosomy 7, and (d) induction of cell death by inhibition of PI3kinase/Akt pathway and DNA damage-induced G2/M arrest, that is, induction of mitotic arrest and apoptosis in myeloblasts while sparing normal cells [118–120].

Rigosetib has shown efficacy in all morphologic, prognostic risk and cytogenetic subgroups of MDS and has produced complete responses in some patients [121]. It has shown activity in high-risk MDS patients and in those having monosomy 7 and trisomy 8. It has produced the following beneficial effects: (1) decrease in BM blasts, (2) improvement in hematopoiesis, (3) inhibition of cyclin D1 accumulation, and (4) decrease in trisomy 8 and monosomy 7 aneuploidy [116, 119, 121]. However, a randomized controlled, phase 3, clinical trial that had been performed in 74 institutions in Europe and the United States on the use of rigosertib in patients with high-risk MDS after failure of hypomethylating agents did not show significant OS compared to best supportive care [117]. The drug is available in oral and injectable formulations [120, 121]. Although rigosertib has exhibited a favorable safety profile, the following adverse effects have been reported: syncope, fatigue, nausea, vomiting, abdominal pain, hypotension, anemia, thrombocytopenia, neutropenia, febrile neuropenia, pneumonia, dysuria, and hematuria [116, 117, 120].

Trial	Number of patients	Phase and design of trial	Study focus	Results	Total dose per course/ interval between cycles	Median number of courses	Time to AML progress	Median survival
Kantarjian et al. Cancer 2006	170	Phase II randomized multicenter	Decitabine vs. BSC	OR: 17% CR: 9% PR: 8% HI: 13%	135 mg/m² 6 weekly	3	12.1 months vs. 7.8 months	14 months vs. 14.9 months
Ruter et al. Cancer 2006	22	Phase II pooled analysis of 3 trials	Low dose decitabine as salvage therapy at relapse	OR: 45% CR: 4.5% PR: 9.1% HI: 31.8%	135 mg/m² 6 weekly	3	-	37.5 months
Kantarjian et al. Cancer 2007	115	Phase II 1 single center	Prognostic factors associated with outcome	OR: 70% CR: 35% PR: 2% HI: 10–23%	100 mg/m² 4 weekly	≥7	Not reached	22 months
Kantarjian et al. Blood 2007	95	Phase II randomized single center	Optimal dosage of decitabine	OR: 73% CR: 34–39% PR: 1% HI: 14–24%	100 mg/m² -	≥6	27% over 18 months	19 months
Kantarjian et al. Cancer 2007	491	Phase II historical comparison of 2 groups of patients at single center	Decitabine vs. AML type of intensive chemotherapy	CR: decit: 43% vs. intensive chemotherapy: 34%	100 mg/m² –	–	–	22 months vs. 12 months
Borthakur et al. Leuk Lymphoma 2008	14	Phase II early results	Efficacy of decitabine after failure of vidaza	OR: 28% CR: 21% HI: 7%	100 mg/m² 4 weekly	3	4 months	6 months
Steensma et al. JCO 2009	99	Phase II multicenter non randomized	Efficacy & safety of decitabine as outpatient regimen	OR: 32% CR: 17% HI: 18%	100 mg/m² 4 weekly	5	–	19.4 months
Lubbert et al. JCO 2011	233	Phase III- 2 arms multicenter	Decitabine vs. BSC	CR: 13% PR: 6% HI: 15%	95 mg/m² 6 weekly	4	8.8 months vs. 6.1 months	PFS: 6.6 months vs. 3 months

Trial	Number of patients	Phase and design of trial	Study focus	Results	Total dose per course/ interval between cycles	Median number of courses	Time to AML progress	Median survival
Jabbour et al. Clin Lymphoma Myeloma Leuk 2013	183	Phase III pooled analysis of 2 multicenter trials	Decitabine vs. BSC in *de novo* MDS vs. 2^0 MDS	OR: 28% *de novo* MDS vs. 15.4% in 2^0 MDS	135 mg/m² 4–6 weekly	3 and 5 courses	33 months for 2^0 MDS not reached for *de novo* MDS	OS: 16.6 months vs. 9 months

Abbreviations: MDS, myelodysplastic syndrome; AML, acute myeloid leukemia; OR, overall response; CR, complete response; PR, partial response; HI, hematological improvement; BSC, best supportive care; vs., versus; 2^0, secondary; OS, overall survival.

Table 5. Decitabine trials in MDS patients.

11. The role of HSCT in high-risk MDSs including monosomy 7

11.1. HSCT in adults with MDSs

Allogeneic HSCT is the only potentially curative therapy for MDS patients [4, 82, 122–124]. Recently, HSCT is being used with increasing frequency in patients with MDS, partly due to the development of novel conditioning therapies, such as nonmyeloablative conditioning, that allow HSCT to be offered to older patients [4, 122]. Also, the use of immunomodulatory drugs and hypomethylating agents prior to HSCT has shown efficacy in (1) controlling disease, that is, a bridging approach to HSCT, and (2) tumor debulking before HSCT [4, 122]. The indications of allogeneic HSCT in adults with MDS are shown in **Table 6** [4, 82, 122–125].

MDS patients with monosomy 7 or complex cytogenetics and preserved BM are considered indications for immediate rather than delayed HSCT. Secondary MDS is another special indication for HSCT [82, 125]. Currently, patients with therapy-related MDS (t-MDS) are being treated using the same paradigm as in *de novo* MDS [82]. Despite its curative potential, the role of allogeneic HSCT in the treatment of elderly patients with MDS is less well defined than in younger individuals [4]. The following issues related to HSCT remain an area of intense investigations: (1) pretransplant disease burden, (2) optimal conditioning therapies, (3) optimal donor selection, (4) optimal stem cell source, (5) GVHD prophylaxis, and (6) post-transplant relapse [122]. The following complications of allogeneic HSCT: GVHD, infections, and non-relapse mortality may offset the benefits of allogeneic HSCT over medical therapies [82]. Despite the remarkable improvement in both efficacy and safety of HSCT over the past two decades, therapy-related morbidity and mortality as well as disease relapse still pose significant risks to transplanted patients [82, 122, 123]. Methods employed to prevent and treat relapse of MDS following HSCT include (1) donor lymphocyte infusion (DLI), (2) hypomethylating agents, (3) novel cellular therapies including vaccination, and (4) use of alloreactive natural killer cells [4, 122].

In children	In adults
1- Refractory anemia with excess of blasts	(A) Definite indications:
(RAEB)	1- Intermediate 2 IPSS
2- Refractory anemia with excess of blasts in	2- High-risk IPSS
transformation (RAEB-t)	(B) Probable indications:
3- Chemotherapy or radiotherapy related MDS	1- t-MDS or secondary MDS
(t-MDS)	2- Packed Red blood cell transfusions refractory to:
4- Juvenile myelomonocytic leukemia	- Hematopoietic growth factors
5- Refractory cytopenias associated with:	- Immunomodulatory drugs
a- transfusion dependence	- Hypomethylating agents
b- cytogenetic abnormalities	3- Severe neutropenia or thrombocytopenia
	4- At least one line of cytopenia with multilineage dysplasia
	5- High risk chromosomal abnormalities: monosomy 7 and complex
	cytogenetics
	6- High percentage of blasts [≥10%]

Abbreviations: MDS, myelodysplastic syndrome; t-MDS, therapy-related myelodysplastic syndrome; RAEB, refractory anemia with excess of blasts; RAEB-t, refractory anemia with excess of blasts in transformation; SCT, hematopoietic stem cell transplantation.

Table 6. Indications for allogeneic HSCT in patients with MDS.

Predictors of outcome of allogeneic HSCT in MDS patients include: (1) disease stage including blast count, (2) transfusion dependence, and (3) karyotype, cytogenetic abnormalities and molecular aberrations or genetic mutations such as: monosomal karyotype, complex cytogenetic and TP53 mutation [82, 122, 125].

11.2. HSCT in children with MDSs

Allogeneic HSCT is the only potentially curative therapy for children with MDSs, particularly those having JMML [73, 126]. The indications of allogeneic HSCT in children with MDSs are shown in **Table 6** [73, 126–128]. Relapse rate following allogeneic HSCT performed for JMML may reach 50% or more [73]. Children with MDS and JMML should be referred for allogeneic HSCT soon after making the diagnosis in order to prevent disease progression as pretransplant chemotherapy does not appear to improve outcome [127, 128]. Predictors of poor outcome of allogeneic HSCT in children with MDS include (1) monosomy 7, (2) age more than 4 years at transplant, (3) relapse after HSCT, (4) female gender, and (5) human leukocyte antigen (HLA)-mismatched allografts [73].

11.3. HSCT in higher risk MDS patients

Patients with higher risk MDS who have an HLA-matched donor should be transplanted early before progression of their disease or acquisition of a nonhematological contraindication to HSCT [129]. In patients with intermediate-2 or high-risk MDS, aged 60–79 years, subjected to reduced intensity conditioning allogeneic HSCT, life expectancy is about 36 months compared to 28 months in patients not subjected to HSCT, that is, HSCT in this group of patients has a survival advantage [130]. Patients with higher risk MDS should be treated with either hypomethylating agents or HSCT [131]. It is justified to offer patients with higher risk MDS who have an HLA identical donor an allograft [129]. Retrospective studies have concluded that patients with higher risk MDS have a survival advantage over demethylating agents if they can be offered an early allogeneic HSCT [129]. Transplant-related mortality remains high in HSCT, it ranges between 10% and 40% particularly after myeloablative conditioning therapy in elderly individuals [129]. Long-term survival ranges between 30% and 60% depending on patient characteristics, disease risk, type of donor, source of stem cells, and complications that evolve following HSCT [129].

12. Conclusions and future directions

In children and adults, high-risk MDSs including monosomy 7 are often complicated by various degrees of BM suppression, infectious complications, severe iron overload, and transformation into AML. Management of these disorders includes (1) supportive care that comprises transfusion of blood products, antimicrobials, and iron chelation therapy, (2) epigenetic therapies including histone deacetylase inhibitors and hypomethylating agents such as azacytidine and decitabine, and (3) various types of allogeneic HSCT. Recently, the role of allogeneic HSCT in high-risk MDSs is increasing due to the introduction of the new conditioning therapies that have allowed the application of this curative modality of therapy not only to older patients, but also to individuals with medical comorbidities. However, in patients with familial causes of their MDSs of BM failure planned for allogeneic HSCT using a sibling donor, great caution should be exercised and enough investigations should be performed before clearing the sibling for donation. The role of certain growth factors in the management of patients with high-risk MDS is controversial as G-CSF has been reported to accelerate the progression into acute leukemia.

The recent developments in the diagnostics of MDSs and the recently introduced therapeutic agents such as rigosertib, clofarabine, sapacitabine, and BCL2 inhibitors as well as the evolving modalities of HSCT are likely to improve the outcome of patients with higher risk MDSs significantly.

Author details

Khalid Ahmed Al-Anazi

Address all correspondence to: kaa_alanazi@yahoo.com

Department of Adult Hematology and Hematopoietic Stem Cell Transplantation, Oncology Center, King Fahad Specialist Hospital, Dammam, Saudi Arabia

References

[1] Bacher U, Schanz J, Braulke F, Haase D. Rare cytogenetic abnormalities in myelodysplastic syndromes. Mediterr J Hematol Infect Dis 2015; 7 (1): e2015034. doi: 10.4084/MJHID.2015.034. eCollection 2015.

[2] Cordoba I, González-Porras JR, Nomdedeu B, Luño E, de Paz R, Such E, et al. Spanish Myelodysplastic Syndrome Registry. Better prognosis for patients with del(7q) than for patients with monosomy 7 in myelodysplastic syndrome. Cancer 2012; 118 (1): 127–133. doi: 10.1002/cncr.26279. Epub 2011 Jun 29.

[3] Wong JC, Weinfurtner KM, Alzamora Mdel P, Kogan SC, Burgess MR, Zhang Y, et al. Functional evidence implicating chromosome 7q22 haploinsufficiency in myelodysplastic syndrome pathogenesis. eLife 2015; 4: e07839. doi: 10.7554/eLife.07839

[4] Kröger N. Allogeneic stem cell transplantation for elderly patients with myelodysplastic syndrome. Blood 2012; 119 (24): 5632–5639. doi: 10.1182/blood-2011-12-380162. Epub 2012 Apr 13.

[5] Chang KL, O'Donnell MR, Slovak ML, Dagis AC, Arber DA, Niland JC, et al. Primary myelodysplasia occurring in adults under 50 years old: a clinicopathologic study of 52 patients. Leukemia 2002; 16 (4): 623–631. doi: 10.1038/sj.leu.2402392

[6] Li Y, Li WW, Wang XM, An L, Liu H, Wang ZS, et al. The relevance between quantitative and type of chromosomal abnormality and leukemia transformation in myelodysplastic syndrome. Zhonghua Xue Ye Xue Za Zhi 2013; 34 (3): 221–224. doi: 10.3760/cma.j.issn.0253-2727. 2013. 03.009.

[7] Weinblatt ME, Scimeca P, James-Herry A, Sahdev I, Kochen J. Transformation of congenital neutropenia into monosomy 7 and acute nonlymphoblastic leukemia in a child treated with granulocyte colony-stimulating factor. J Pediatr 1995; 126 (2): 263–265.

[8] Khan C, Pathe N, Fazal S, Lister J, Rossetti JM. Azacitidine in the management of patients with myelodysplastic syndromes. Ther Adv Hematol 2012; 3 (6): 355–373. doi: 10.1177/2040620712464882.

[9] Raj K, Mufti GJ. Azacytidine (Vidaza(R)) in the treatment of myelodysplastic syndromes. Ther Clin Risk Manag 2006; 2 (4): 377–388.

[10] McCormack SE, Warlick ED. Epigenetic approaches in the treatment of myelodysplastic syndromes: clinical utility of azacitidine. Onco Targets Ther 2010; 3: 157–165.

[11] Tefferi A, Vardiman JW. Myelodysplastic syndromes. N Engl J Med 2009; 361: 1872–1885. doi: 10.1056/NEJMra0902908

[12] Strom SS, Gu Y, Gruschkus SK, Pierce SA, Estey EH. Risk factors of myelodysplastic syndromes: a case-control study. Leukemia 2005; 19 (11): 1912–1918. doi: 10.1038/sj.leu.2403945

[13] Pagano L, Caira M, Fianchi L, Leone G. Environmental risk factors for MDS/AML. Haematologica Rep 2006; 2 (15): 42–45.

[14] Lv L, Lin G, Gao X, Wu C, Dai J, Yang Y, et al. Case–control study of risk factors of myelodysplastic syndromes according to World Health Organization classification in a Chinese population. Am J Hematol 2011; 86 (2): 163–169. doi: 10.1002/ajh.21941

[15] Jin J, Yu M, Hu C, Ye L, Xie L, Chen F, et al. Alcohol consumption and risk of myelodysplastic syndromes: a meta-analysis of epidemiological studies. Mol Clin Oncol 2014; 2 (6): 1115–1120. Epub 2014 Aug 7. doi: 10.3892/mco.2014.376

[16] Aster JC, Stone RM. Clinical manifestations and diagnosis of the myelodysplastic syndromes. Topic 4492, version 33.0 Edited by Larson RA, Connor RF. UpToDate 2016. Topic last updated: Dec 1, 2015.

[17] Invernizzi R, Filocco A. Myelodysplastic syndrome: classification and prognostic systems. Oncol Rev 2010; 4 (1): 25–33. doi: 10.1007/s12156-009-0033-4

[18] Shekhter-Levin S, Penchansky L, Wollman MR, Sherer ME, Wald N, Gollin SM. An abnormal clone with monosomy 7 and trisomy 21 in the bone marrow of a child with congenital agranulocytosis (Kostmann disease) treated with granulocyte colony-stimulating factor. Evolution towards myelodysplastic syndrome and acute basophilic leukemia. Cancer Genet Cytogenet 1995; 84 (2): 99–104.

[19] Bakanay SM, Topcuoglu P, Bilgin AU, Yararbas K, Karauzum SB, Ozcan M, et al. Clonal evolution of monosomy 7 in acquired severe aplastic anemia: two cases treated with allogeneic hematopoietic stem cell transplantation. Turk J Hematol 2008; 25: 94–97.

[20] Tsuzuki M, Okamoto M, Yamaguchi T, Ino T, Ezaki K, Hirano M. Myelodysplastic syndrome with monosomy 7 following combination therapy with granulocyte colony-stimulating factor, cyclosporin A and danazole in an adult patient with severe aplastic anemia. Rinsho Ketsueki 1997; 38 (9): 745–751.

[21] Nishimura M, Yamada T, Andoh T, Tao T, Emoto M, Ohji T, et al. Granulocyte colony-stimulating factor (G-CSF) dependent hematopoiesis with monosomy 7 in a patient

with severe aplastic anemia after ATG/CsA/G-CSF combined therapy. Int J Hematol 1998; 68 (2): 203–211.

[22] McDonald S, Wilson DB, Pumbo E, Kulkarni S, Mason PJ, Else T, et al. Acquired monosomy 7 myelodysplastic syndrome in a child with clinical features suggestive of dyskeratosis congenita and IMAGe association. Pediatr Blood Cancer 2010; 54 (1): 154–157. doi: 10.1002/pbc.22283.

[23] Dror Y, Squire J, Durie P, Freedman MH. Malignant myeloid transformation with isochromosome 7q in Shwachman-Diamond syndrome. Leukemia 1998; 12 (10): 1591–1595.

[24] Mellink CH, Alders M, van der Lelie H, Hennekam RH, Kuijpers TW. SBDS mutations and isochromosome 7q in a patient with Shwachman-Diamond syndrome: no predisposition to malignant transformation? Cancer Genet Cytogenet 2004; 154 (2): 144–149.

[25] Cunningham J, Sales M, Pearce A, Howard J, Stallings R, Telford N, et al. Does isochromosome 7q mandate bone marrow transplant in children with Shwachman-Diamond syndrome? Br J Haematol 2002; 119 (4): 1062–1069.

[26] Nifosì G, Sbolli G, Ferrari B, Berte' R, Vallisa D, Civardi G, et al. Sweet's syndrome associated with monosomy 7 myelodysplastic syndrome. Eur J Intern Med 2001; 12 (4): 380–383. doi: http://dx.doi.org/10.1016/S0953-6205(01)00137-6

[27] Maris JM, Wiersma SR, Mahgoub N, Thompson P, Geyer RJ, Hurwitz CG, et al. Monosomy 7 myelodysplastic syndrome and other second malignant neoplasms in children with neurofibromatosis type 1. Cancer 1997; 79 (7): 1438–1446.

[28] Karimata K, Masuko M, Ushiki T, Kozakai T, Shibasaki Y, Yano T, et al. Myelodysplastic syndrome with Ph negative monosomy 7 chromosome following transient bone marrow dysplasia during imatinib treatment for chronic myeloid leukemia. Internal Med 2011; 50 (5): 481–485. doi: 10.2169/internalmedicine.50.4481

[29] [29] Marques-Salles TJ, Soares-Ventura EM, de Oliveira NL, Silva M, Assis R, de Morais VLL, et al. Myeloproliferative syndrome of monosomy 7: a brief report. Gene Mol Biol 2008; 31, 1, 36–38.

[30] Endo M, Sekikawa A, Tsumura T, Maruo T, Osaki Y. A case of myelodysplastic syndrome with intestinal Behçet's disease-like symptoms treated by prednisolone and azacitidine. Am J Case Rep. 2015; 16: 827–831. doi: 10.12659/AJCR.895431

[31] Özbek N, Yazal Erdem A, Arman Bilir Ö, Karaca Kara F, Yüksek M, Yaralı N, et al. A child with psoriasis, hypogammaglobulinemia and monosomy 7-positive myelodysplastic syndrome. Turk J Haematol 2015; 32 (1): 87–88. doi: 10.4274/tjh.2014.0308.

[32] Neas K, Peters G, Jackson J, Tembe M, Wu ZH, Brohede J, et al. Chromosome 7 aberrations in a young girl with myelodysplasia and hepatoblastoma: an unusual association. Clin Dysmorphol 2006; 15 (1): 1–8.

[33] Manor E, Shemer-Avni Y, Boriakovski S, Kafka M, Bodner L, Kapelushnik J. Myelodysplastic syndrome (MDS) associated with EBV infection in a pediatric patient. Open J Pediatr 2013; 3 (1): 28–34. doi: http://dx.doi.org/10.4236/ojped.2013.31006

[34] Maserati E, Minelli A, Olivieri C, Bonvini L, Marchi A, Bozzola M, et al. Isochromosome (7) (q10) in Shwachman syndrome without MDS/AML and role of chromosome 7 anomalies in myeloproliferative disorders. Cancer Genet Cytogenet 2000; 121 (2): 167–171.

[35] Kalra R, Dale D, Freedman M, Bonilla MA, Weinblatt M, Ganser A, et al. Monosomy 7 and activating RAS mutations accompany malignant transformation in patients with congenital neutropenia. Blood 1995; 86 (12): 4579–4586.

[36] Hu J, Shekhter-Levin S, Shaw PH, Bay C, Kochmar S, Surti U. A case of myelodysplastic syndrome with acquired monosomy 7 in a child with a constitutional t(1;19) and a mosaicism for trisomy 21. Cancer Genet Cytogenet 2005; 156 (1): 62–67.

[37] Williamson BT, Leitch HA. Higher risk myelodysplastic syndromes in patients with well-controlled HIV infection: clinical features, treatment, and outcome. Case Rep Hematol 2016; 2016: 8502641. doi: 10.1155/2016/8502641. Epub 2016 Jan 20.

[38] Arathi CA, Puttaraj KR, Shobha SN. An association between hypoplastic myelodysplastic syndrome and T-prolymphocytic leukaemia. J Lab Physicians 2011; 3(1): 49–51. doi: 10.4103/0974-2727.78568.

[39] Al-Anazi KA, Al-Jasser AM. *Brucella* bacteremia in patients with acute leukemia: a case series. J Med Case Rep 2007; 1: 144. doi: 10.1186/1752-1947-1-144

[40] Li JJ, Sheng ZK, Tu S, Bi S, Shen XM, Sheng JF. Acute brucellosis with myelodysplastic syndrome presenting as pancytopenia and fever of unknown origin. Med Princ Pract 2012; 21 (2): 183–185. doi: 10.1159/000333698. Epub 2011 Dec 1.

[41] Shaharir SS, Tumian NR, Yu Lin AB, Abdul Wahid SF. Disseminated tuberculosis masquerading primary myelodysplastic syndrome. J Infect Dev Ctries 2013; 7 (3): 286–288. doi: 10.3855/jidc.2691.

[42] Neonakis IK, Alexandrakis MG, Gitti Z, Tsirakis G, Krambovitis E, Spandidos DA. Miliary tuberculosis with no pulmonary involvement in myelodysplastic syndromes: a curable, yet rarely diagnosed, disease: case report and review of the literature. Ann Clin Microbiol Antimicrob 2008; 7: 8. doi: 10.1186/1476-0711-7-8.

[43] Sultana T, Chowdhury AA, Yunus ABM, Ahmed ANN. Myelodysplastic syndrome with tuberculosis which developed to AML—a case report. Bangladesh J Pathol 2009; 24 (1): 25–27.

[44] Liew E, Owen C. Familial myelodysplastic syndromes: a review of the literature. Haematologica 2011; 96 (10): 1536–1542. doi: 10.3324/haematol.2011.043422. Epub 2011 May 23.

[45] Hess JL. Familial monosomy 7 syndrome. Atlas Genet Cytogenet Oncol Hematol. 2001; 5(3): 220–221. doi: 10.4267/2024/37769.

[46] West AH, Godley LA, Churpek JE. Familial myelodysplastic syndrome/acute leukemia syndromes: a review and utility for translational investigations. Ann N Y Acad Sci 2014; 1310: 111–118. doi: 10.1111/nyas.12346. Epub 2014 Jan 27.

[47] Bödör C, Renneville A, Smith M, Charazac A, Iqbal S, Etancelin P, et al. Germ-line GATA2 p.THR354MET mutation in familial myelodysplastic syndrome with acquired monosomy 7 and ASXL1 mutation demonstrating rapid onset and poor survival. Haematologica 2012; 97 (6): 890–894. doi: 10.3324/haematol.2011.054361. Epub 2012 Jan 22.

[48] Hahn CN, Chong CE, Carmichael CL, Wilkins EJ, Brautigan PJ, Li XC, Babic M, et al. Heritable GATA2 mutations associated with familial myelodysplastic syndrome and acute myeloid leukemia. Nat Genet 2011; 43 (10): 1012–1017. doi: 10.1038/ng.913.

[49] Zhang R, Kim YM, Wang X, Li Y, Lu X, Sternenberger AR, et al. Genomic copy number variations in the myelodysplastic syndrome and acute myeloid leukemia patients with del(5q) and/or -7/del(7q). Int J Mol Sci 2015; 12 (9): 719–726. doi: 10.7150/ijms.12612

[50] Abdelrazik HN, Farawila HM, Sherif MA, AlAnsary M. Molecular characterization of chromosome 7 in AML and MDs patients. Afr J Health Sci 2006; 13: 33–42.

[51] Jerez A, Sugimoto Y, Makishima H, Verma A, Jankowska AM, Przychondzen B, et al. Loss of heterozygosity in 7q myeloid disorders: clinical associations and genomic pathogenesis. Blood 2012; 119: 6109–6117. doi: 10.1182/blood-2011-12-397620

[52] Desangles F. -7/del(7q) in adults. Atlas Genet Cytogenet Oncol Hematol 1999; 3 (3): 139–140. doi: 10.4267/2042/37535

[53] Hussain FTN, Nguyen EP, Raza S, Knudson R, Pardanani A, Hanson CA, et al. Sole abnormalities of chromosome 7 in myeloid malignancies: spectrum, histopathologic correlates and prognostic implications. Am J Hematol 2012; 87: 684–686. doi: 10.1002/ajh.23230

[54] Wong JC, Zhang Y, Lieuw KH, Tran MT, Forgo E, Weinfurtner K, et al. Use of chromosome engineering to model a segmental deletion of chromosome band 7q22 found in myeloid malignancies. Blood 2010; 115 (22): 4524–4532. doi: 10.1182/blood-2009-07-232504. Epub 2010 Mar 16.

[55] Asou H, Matsu H, Ozaki Y, Nagamachi A, Nakamura M, Aki D, et al. Identification of a common microdeletion cluster in7q21.3 subband among patients with myeloid leukemia and myelodysplastic syndrome. Biochem Biophys Res Commun 2009; 383: 245–251. doi: 10.1016/j.bbrc.2009.04.004. Epub 2009 Apr 7.

[56] Nikoloski G, Langemeijer SMC, Kuiper RP, Knops R, Massop M, Tonnissen ERLTM, et al. Somatic mutations of the histone methyltransferase gene EZH2 in myelodysplastic syndromes. Nat Genet 2010; 42: 665–667.

[57] Makishima H, Traina F, Jankowska AM, Sugimoto Y, Guinta KM, Sakaguchi H, et al. Pathogenesis of monosomy 7 in bone marrow failure syndromes. Poster 11, 53rd ASH Annual Meeting and Exposition 2011.

[58] Wall M, Rayeroux KC, Mackinnon RN, Zordan A, Campbell LJ. ETV6 deletion is a common additional abnormality in patients with myelodysplastic syndromes or acute myeloid leukemia. Haematologica 2012; 97 (12): 1933–1936. doi: 10.3324/haematol. 2012.069716

[59] Shen Y, Xue Y, Li J, Guo Y, Pan J, Wu Y. Detection of monosomy 7 or 7q- in cases of myelodysplastic syndrome. Zhonghua Yi Xue Yi Chuan Xue Za Zhi 2001; 18 (4): 255–258.

[60] Yunis JJ, Lobell M, Arnesen MA, Oken MM, Mayer MG, Rydell RE, et al. Refined chromosome study helps define prognostic subgroups in most patients with primary myelodysplastic syndrome and acute myelogenous leukaemia. Br J Haematol 1988; 68 (2): 189–194. doi: 10.1111/j.1365-2141.1988.tb06188.x

[61] McNerney ME, Brown CD, Wang X, Bartom ET, Karmakar S, Bandlamudi C, et al. CUX1 is a haploinsufficient tumor suppressor gene on chromosome 7 frequently inactivated in acute myeloid leukemia. Blood 2013; 121 (6): 975–983. doi:10.1182/ blood-2012-04-426965. Epub 2012 Dec 3.

[62] Sundaravel S, Duggan R, Bhagat T, Ebenezer DL, Liu H, Yu Y, et al. Reduced DOCK4 expression leads to erythroid dysplasia in myelodysplastic syndromes. Proc Natl Acad Sci USA 2015; 112 (46): E6359-E6368. doi: 10.1073/pnas.1516394112. Epub 2015 Nov 2.

[63] Geelani S, Manzoor F, Bashir N, Bhat S, Rasool J, Qadri SM, et al. Myelodysplastic syndrome with monosomy 7—a rare case of morphological and cytogenetic remission with lenalidomide. Case Study Case Rep 2015; 5 (1): 1–4.

[64] Tan NC, Lee KH, Liu TC. Myelodysplastic syndrome with monosomy 7 and pulmonary aspergillosis. Singapore Med J 2000; 41(6): 290–291.

[65] Dwivedi AC, Lyons MJ, Kwiatkowski K, Bartel FO, Friez MJ, Holden KR, et al. Clinical utility of chromosomal microarray analysis in the diagnosis and management of monosomy 7 mosaicism. Mol Cytogenet 2014; 7 (1): 93. doi: 10.1186/s13039-014-0093-4. eCollection 2014.

[66] Kere J, Ruutu T, de La Chapelle A. Monosomy 7 in granulocytes and monocytes in myelodysplastic syndrome. New Engl J Med 1987; 316: 499–503.

[67] Gerritsen WR, Donohue J, Bauman J, Jhanwar SC, Kernan NA, Castro-Malaspina H, et al. Clonal analysis of myelodysplastic syndrome: monosomy 7 is expressed in the myeloid lineage, but not in the lymphoid lineage as detected by fluorescent in situ hybridization. Blood 1992; 80: 217–224.

[68] Stein S, Ott MG, Schultze-Strasser S, Jauch A, Burwinkel B, Kinner A, et al. Genomic instability and myelodysplasia with monosomy 7 consequent to EVI1 activation after

gene therapy for chronic granulomatous disease. Nat Med 2010; 16 (2):198–204. doi: 10.1038/nm.2088. Epub 2010 Jan 24.

[69] Trobaugh-Lotrario AD, Kletzel M, Quinones RR, McGavran L, Proytcheva MA, Hunger SP, et al. Monosomy 7 associated with pediatric acute myeloid leukemia (AML) and myelodysplastic syndrome (MDS): successful management by allogeneic hematopoietic stem cell transplant (HSCT). Bone Marrow Transplant 2005; 35 (2): 143–149. doi: 10.1038/sj.bmt.1704753

[70] Jakovleva K, Ogard I, Arvidsson I, Jacobsson B, Swolin B, Hast R. Masked monosomy 7 in myelodysplastic syndromes is uncommon and of undetermined clinical significance. Leuk Res 2001; 25 (3): 197–203.

[71] Aktas D, Tuncbilek E. Myelodysplastic syndrome associated with monosomy 7 in childhood: a retrospective study. Cancer Genet Cytogenet 2006; 171 (1): 72–75.

[72] Yoshimi A, Mohamed M, Bierings M, Urban C, Korthof E, Zecca M, et al. Second allogeneic hematopoietic stem cell transplantation (HSCT) results in outcome similar to that of first HSCT for patients with juvenile myelomonocytic leukemia. Leukemia 2007; 21 (3): 556–560. doi: 10.1038/sj.leu.2404537. Epub 2007 Feb 1.

[73] Locatelli F, Nöllke P, Zecca M, Korthof E, Lanino E, Peters C, et al; European Working Group on Childhood MDS; European Blood and Marrow Transplantation Group. Hematopoietic stem cell transplantation (HSCT) in children with juvenile myelomonocytic leukemia (JMML): results of the EWOG–MDS/EBMT trial. Blood 2005; 105 (1): 410–419. Epub 2004 Sep 7. doi:10.1182/blood-2004-05-1944

[74] Korthof ET, Snijder PP, de Graaff AA, Lankester AC, Bredius RG, Ball LM, et al. Allogeneic bone marrow transplantation for juvenile myelomonocytic leukemia: a single center experience of 23 patients. Bone Marrow Transplant 2005; 35 (5): 455–461. doi: 10.1038/sj.bmt.1704778

[75] Malcovati L. Red blood cell transfusion therapy and iron chelation in patients with myelodysplastic syndromes. Clin Lymphoma Myeloma 2009; 9 (Suppl 3): S305–S311. doi: 10.3816/CLM.2009.s.029

[76] Cazzola M, Della Porta MG, Malcovati L. Clinical relevance of anemia and transfusion iron overload in myelodysplastic syndromes. Hematology Am Soc Hematol Educ Program 2008; 1: 166–175 doi: 10.1182/asheducation-2008.1.166

[77] Alessandrino EP, Angelucci E, Cazzola M, Della Porta MG, Di Bartolomeo P, Gozzini A, et al. Iron overload and iron chelation therapy in patients with myelodysplastic syndrome treated by allogeneic stem-cell transplantation: report from the working conference on iron chelation of the Gruppo Italiano Trapianto di Midollo Osseo. Am J Hematol 2011; 86: 897–902. doi: 10.1002/ajh.22104

[78] Armand P, Kim HT, Cutler CS, Ho VT, Koreth J, Alyea EP, et al. Prognostic impact of elevated pre-transplant serum ferritin in patients undergoing myeloablative stem cell

transplantation. Blood. 2007; 109(10): 4586–4588. doi: 10.1182/blood-2006-10-054924. Prepublished online January 18, 2007.

[79] Leitch HA. Optimizing therapy for iron overload in the myelodysplastic syndromes: recent developments. Drugs 2011; 71 (2): 155–177. doi: 10.2165/11585280-000000000-00000.

[80] Mitchell M, Gore SD, Zeidan AM. Iron chelation therapy in myelodysplastic syndromes: where do we stand? Expert Rev Hematol 2013; 6 (4): 397–410. doi: 10.1586/17474086.2013.814456

[81] Messa E, Cilloni D, Saglio G. Iron chelation therapy in myelodysplastic syndromes. Adv Hematol 2010; 2010: 756289. doi: 10.1155/2010/756289. Epub 2010 Jun 20.

[82] Kindwall-Keller T, Isola LM. The evolution of hematopoietic SCT in myelodysplastic syndrome. Bone Marrow Transplant 2009; 43 (8): 597–609. doi: 10.1038/bmt.2009.28. Epub 2009 Mar 2.

[83] Garcia JS, Jain N, Godley LA. An update on the safety and efficacy of decitabine in the treatment of myelodysplastic syndromes. OncoTarget Ther 2010; 3: 1–13.

[84] Lubbert M, Suciu S, Baila L, Rüter BH, Platzbecker U, Giagonidis A, et al. Low-dose decitabine versus best supportive care in elderly patients with intermediate-or high-risk myelodysplastic syndrome (MDS) ineligible for intensive chemotherapy: final results of the randomized phase III study of the European Organization for Research and Treatment of Cancer Leukemia Group and the German MDS Study Group. J Clin Oncol 2011; 29 (15): 1987–1996. doi: 10.1200/JCO.2010.30.9245.

[85] Cheng JC, Yoo CB, Weisenberger DJ, Chuang J, Wozniak C, Liang G, et al. Preferential response of cancer cells to zebularine. Cancer Cell 2004; 6(2):151–158.

[86] Amatori S, Bagaloni I, Donati B, Fanelli M. DNA demethylating antineoplastic strategies: a comparative point of view. Genes Cancer 2010; 1 (3): 197–209. doi: 10.1177/1947601910365081.

[87] Saunthararajah Y, Triozzi P, Rini B, Singh A, Radivoyevitch T, Sekeres M, et al. p53-independent, normal stem cell sparing epigenetic differentiation therapy for myeloid and other malignancies. Semin Oncol 2012; 39 (1): 97–108. doi: 10.1053/j.seminoncol.2011.11.011.

[88] Ng KP, Ebrahem Q, Negrotto S, Mahfouz RZ, Link KA, Hu Z, et al. p53 independent epigenetic-differentiation treatment in xenotransplant models of acute myeloid leukemia. Leukemia 2011; 25 (11): 1739–1750. doi: 10.1038/leu.2011.159. Epub 2011 Jun 24.

[89] Šorm F, Piskala A, Čihák A, Veselý J. 5-Azacytidine, a new, highly effective cancerostatic. Experientia 1964; 20 (4): 202–203.

[90] Šorm F, Veselý J. The activity of the new antimetabolite, 5-azacytidine, against lymphoid leukemia in AK mice. Neoplasma 1964; 11: 123–130.

[91] Šorm F, Veselý J. The effect of 5-aza-2-deoxycytidine against leukemic and hemopoietic tissues in AKR mice. Neoplasma 1968; 15: 339–343.

[92] Veselý J, Čihák A, Šorm F. Association of decreased uridine and deoxycytidine kinase with enhanced RNA and DNA polymerase in mouse leukemic cells resistant to 5-azacytidine and 5-aza-2′-deoxycytidine. Cancer Res 1970; 30; 2180–2186.

[93] Karahoca M, Momparler RL. Pharmacokinetic and pharmacodynamic analysis of 5-aza-2′-deoxycytidine (decitabine) in the design of its dose-schedule for cancer therapy. Clin Epigenetics 2013; 5 (1): 3. doi: 10.1186/1868-7083-5-3.

[94] Kaminskas E, Farrell AT, Wang YC, Sridhara R, Pazdur R. FDA drug approval summary: azacitidine (5-azacytidine, Vidaza) for injectable suspension. Oncologist 2005; 10 (3): 176–182.

[95] Bernal T, Martínez-Camblor P, Sánchez-García J, de Paz R, Luño E, Nomdedeu B, et al. Spanish Group on Myelodysplastic Syndromes; PETHEMA Foundation; Spanish Society of Hematology. Effectiveness of azacitidine in unselected high-risk myelodysplastic syndromes: results from the Spanish registry. Leukemia 2015; 29 (9): 1875–1881. doi: 10.1038/leu.2015.115. Epub 2015 May 6.

[96] Santini V. Novel therapeutic strategies: hypomethylating agents and beyond. Hematology Am Soc Hematol Educ Program. 2012; 2012: 65–73.

[97] Zeidan AM, Sekeres MA, Garcia-Manero G, Steensma DP, Zell K, Barnard J, et al. Comparison of risk stratification tools in predicting outcomes of patients with higher-risk myelodysplastic syndromes treated with azanucleosides. Leukemia 2016; 30 (3): 649–657. doi: 10.1038/leu.2015.283. Epub 2015 Oct 14.

[98] Field T, Perkins J, Huang Y, Kharfan-Dabaja MA, Alsina M, Ayala E, et al. 5-Azacitidine for myelodysplasia before allogeneic hematopoietic cell transplantation. Bone Marrow Transplant 2010; 45 (2): 255–260. doi: 10.1038/bmt.2009.134. Epub 2009 Jun 22.

[99] Platzbecker U, Wermke M, Radke J, Oelschlaegel U, Seltmann F, Kiani A, et al. Azacitidine for treatment of imminent relapse in MDS or AML patients after allogeneic HSCT: results of the RELAZA trial. Leukemia 2012; 26 (3): 381–389. doi: 10.1038/leu.2011.234. Epub 2011 Sep 2.

[100] Prébet T, Gore SD, Esterni B, Gardin C, Itzykson R, Thepot S, et al. Outcome of high-risk myelodysplastic syndrome after azacitidine treatment failure. J Clin Oncol 2011; 29 (24): 3322–3327. doi: 10.1200/JCO.2011.35.8135. Epub 2011 Jul 25.

[101] Fenaux P, Mufti GJ, Hellstrom-Lindberg E, Santini V, Finelli C, Giagounidis A, et al. International Vidaza High-Risk MDS Survival Study Group. Efficacy of azacitidine compared with that of conventional care regimens in the treatment of higher-risk

myelodysplastic syndromes: a randomised, open-label, phase III study. Lancet Oncol 2009; 10 (3): 223–232. doi: 10.1016/S1470-2045(09) 70003-8. Epub 2009 Feb 21.

[102] Gurion R, Vidal L, Gafter-Gvili A, Belnik Y, Yeshurun M, Raanani P, et al. 5-azacitidine prolongs overall survival in patients with myelodysplastic syndrome--a systematic review and meta-analysis. Haematologica 2010; 95 (2): 303–310. doi: 10.3324/haematol. 2009.010611. Epub 2009 Sep 22.

[103] Vigil CE, Martin-Santos T, Garcia-Manero G. Safety and efficacy of azacitidine in myelodysplastic syndromes. Drug Des Devel Ther 2010; 4: 221–229.

[104] Kim Y, Cheong JW, Kim YK, Eom JI, Jeung HK, Kim SJ, et al. Serum microRNA-21 as a potential biomarker for response to hypomethylating agents in myelodysplastic syndromes. PLoS ONE 2014; 9 (2): e86933. doi: 10.1371/journal.pone.0086933

[105] Pleyer L, Greil R. Digging deep into dirty drugs-modulation of the methylation machinery. Drug Metab Rev 2015; 47 (2): 252–279. doi: 10.3109/03602532.2014.995379

[106] Mahfouz RZ, Jankowska A, Ebrahem Q, Gu X, Visconte V, Tabarroki A, et al. Increased CDA expression/activity in males contribute to decreased cytidine analogue half-life and likely contributes to worse outcomes with 5-azacytidine or decitabine therapy. Clin Cancer Res 2013; 19 (4): 938–948. doi: 10.1158/1078-0432.CCR-12-1722

[107] Soriano AO, Yang H, Faderl S, Estrov Z, Giles F, Ravandi F, et al. Safety and clinical activity of the combination of 5-azacytidine, valproic acid and all-trans retinoic acid in acute myeloid leukemia and myelodysplastic syndrome. Blood 2007; 110: 2302–2308. doi: 10.1182/blood-2007-03-078576

[108] Raffoux E, Cras A, Recher C, Boëlle PY, de Labathe A, Turlure P, et al. Phase 2 clinical trial of 5-azacytidine, valproic acid and all-trans retinoic acid in patients with high-risk acute myeloid leukemia or myelodysplastic syndrome. OncoTarget 2010; 1(1): 34–42.

[109] Silverman LR, Demakos EP, Peterson BL, Kornblith AB, Holland JC, Odchimar-Reissig R, et al. Randomized controlled trial of azacitidine in patients with the myelodysplastic syndrome: a study of the cancer and leukemia group B. J Clin Oncol 2002; 20 (10): 2429–2440. doi: 10.1200/JCO.2002.04.117

[110] Jilg S, Reidel V, Müller-Thomas C, König J, Schauwecker J, Höckendorf U, et al. Blockade of BCL-2 proteins efficiently induces apoptosis in progenitor cells of high-risk myelodysplastic syndromes patients. Leukemia 2016; 30: 112–123. doi: 10.1038/leu. 2015.179

[111] Jabbour E, Kantarjian H, O'Brien S, Kadia T, Malik A, Welch MA, et al. Retrospective analysis of prognostic factors associated with response and overall survival by baseline marrow blast oercentage in patients with myelodysplastic syndromes treated with decitabine. Clin Lymphoma Myeloma Leuk 2013; 13 (5): 592–596. doi: 10.1016/j.clml. 2013.05.004

[112] Jabbour E, Garcia-Manero G, Cornelison AM, Cortes JE, Ravandi F, Daver N, et al. The effect of decitabine doser modification and myelosuppression on response and survival

in patients with myelodysplastic syndromes. Leuk Lymphoma 2015; 56 (2): 390–394. doi: 10.3109/10428194.2014.914192

[113] Kantarjian H, Oki Y, Garcia-Manero G, Huang X, O'Brien S, cortes J, et al. Results of a randomized study of 3 schedules of low-dose decitabine in higher-risk myelodysplastic syndrome and chronic myelomonocytic leukemia. Blood 2007; 109: 52–57. doi: 10.1182/blood-2006-05-021162

[114] Wu L, Shi W, Li X, Chang C, Xu F, He Q, et al. High expression of the human equilibrative nucleoside transporter 1 gene predicts a good response to decitabine in patients with myelodysplastic syndrome. J Transl Med 2016; 14: 66. doi: 10.1186/s12967-016-0817-9

[115] Rüter B, Wijermans P, claus R, Kunzmann R, Lübbert M. Preferential cytogenetic response to continuous intravenous low-dose decitabine administration in myelodysplastic syndrome with monosomy 7. Blood 2007; 110: 1080–1082. doi: 10.1182/blood-2007-03-080630

[116] Silverman LR, Greenberg P, Raza A, Olnes MJ, Holland JF, Reddy P, et al. Clinical activity and safety of the dual pathway inhibitor rigosertib for higher risk myelodysplastic syndromes following DNA methyltransferase inhibitor therapy. Hematol Oncol 2015; 33 (2): 57–66. doi: 10.1002/hon.2137. Epub 2014 Apr 29.

[117] Garcia-Manero G, Fenaux P, Al-Kali A, Baer MR, Sekeres MA, Roboz GJ, et al. ONTIME Study Investigators. Rigosertib versus best supportive care for patients with high-risk myelodysplastic syndromes after failure of hypomethylating drugs (ONTIME): a randomised, controlled, phase 3 trial. Lancet Oncol 2016 Mar 8. pii: S1470-2045(16)00009-7. doi: 10.1016/S1470-2045(16)00009-7. [Epub ahead of print]

[118] Hyoda T, Tsujioka T, Nakahara T, Suemori Si, Okamoto S, Kataoka M, et al. Rigosertib induces cell death of a myelodsplastic syndrome-derived cell line by DNA damage-induced G2/M arrest. Cancer Sci 2015; 106 (3): 287–293. doi: 10.1111/cas.12605

[119] Olnes MJ, Shenoy A, Weinstein B, Pfannes L, Loeliger K, Tucker Z, et al. Directed therapy for patients with myelodysplastic syndromes (MDS) by suppression of cyclin D1 with ON01910.Na. Leuk Res 2012; 36 (8): 982–989. doi: 10.1016/j.leukres.2012.04.002

[120] Komrokji RS, Raza A, Lancet JE, Ren C, Taft D, Maniar M, et al. Phase I clinical trial of oral rigosertib in patients with myelodysplastic syndromes. Br J Haematol 2013; 162 (4): 517–524. doi: 10.1111/bjh. 12436

[121] Seetharam M, Fan AC, Tran M, Xu L, Renschler JP, Felsher DW, et al. Treatment of higher risk myelodysplastic syndrome patients unresponsive to hypomethylating agents withON01910.Na. Leuk Res 2012; 36 (1): 98–103. doi: 10.1016/j.leukres.2011.08.022

[122] Vaughn JE, Scott BL, Deeg HJ. Transplantation for myelodysplastic syndromes 2013. Curr Opin Hematol 2013; 20 (6): 494–500. doi:10.1097/MOH.0b013e328364f547.

[123] Mori T, Aisa Y, Yokoyama A, Nakazato T, Yamazaki R, Shimizu T, et al. Total body irradiation and granulocyte colony-stimulating factor-combined high-dose cytarabine as a conditioning regimen in allogeneic hematopoietic stem cell transplantation for advanced myelodysplastic syndrome: a single-institute experience. Bone Marrow Transplant 2007; 39 (4): 217–221. doi:10.1038/sj.bmt.1705578. Epub 2007 Jan 15.

[124] Nakamura R, Rodriguez R, Palmer J, Stein A, Naing A, Tsai N, et al. Reduced-intensity conditioning for allogeneic hematopoietic stem cell transplantation with fludarabine and melphalan is associated with durable disease control in myelodysplastic syndrome. Bone Marrow Transplant 2007; 40 (9): 843–850. doi:10.1038/sj.bmt.1705801. Epub 2007 Aug 27.

[125] Armand P, Deeg HJ, Kim HT, Lee H, Armistead P, de Lima M, et al. Multicenter validation study of a transplantation-specific cytogenetics grouping scheme for patients with myelodysplastic syndromes. Bone Marrow Transplant 2010; 45 (5): 877–885. doi: 10.1038/bmt.2009.253. Epub 2009 Sep 28.

[126] Jan S. Stem cell transplantation for a myelodysplastic syndrome in children. Rep Pract Oncol Radiother 2000; 5 (2): 43–47.

[127] Smith AR, Christiansen EC, Wagner JE, Cao Q, MacMillan ML, Stefanski HE, et al. Early hematopoietic stem cell transplant is associated with favorable outcomes in children with MDS. Pediatr Blood Cancer 2013; 60 (4): 705–710. doi: 10.1002/pbc.24390. Epub 2012 Nov 14.

[128] Yusuf U, Frangoul HA, Gooley TA, Woolfrey AE, Carpenter PA, Andrews RG, et al. Allogeneic bone marrow transplantation in children with myelodysplastic syndrome or juvenile myelomonocytic leukemia: the Seattle experience. Bone Marrow Transplant 2004; 33 (8): 805–814. doi:10.1038/sj.bmt.1704438. Epub 2004 Feb 2.

[129] Robin M, Porcher R, Adès L, Raffoux E, Michallet M, François S, et al. HLA-matched allogeneic stem cell transplantation improves outcome of higher risk myelodysplastic syndrome A prospective study on behalf of SFGM-TC and GFM. Leukemia 2015; 29 (7):1496–1501. doi: 10.1038/leu.2015.37. Epub 2015 Feb 13.

[130] Deeg HJ. Hematopoietic cell transplantation for myelodysplastic syndrome. Am Soc Clin Oncol Educ Book 2015; asco.org/edbook: e375-e380. doi: 10.14694/EdBook_AM.2015.35.e375

[131] Sekeres MA. Bone marrow transplantation (BMT) in myelodysplastic syndromes. To BMT or not to BMT—that is the question. J Clin Oncol 2013; 31 (21): 2643–2644. doi: 10.1200/JCO.2013.48.9146. Epub 2013 Jun 24.

Chapter 6

Chronic Myelomonocytic Leukaemia

Andreas Himmelmann

Additional information is available at the end of the chapter

http://dx.doi.org/10.5772/63193

Abstract

The classification, pathobiology and clinical management of chronic myelomonocytic leukaemia (CMML) are reviewed. Three important issues are identified: (1) CMML should be recognised as a unique clinical entity and as distinct from myelodysplastic syndromes (MDSs). Somatic mutations of a restricted set of genes are frequent in CMML. (2) Risk stratification for CMML patients should utilise new CMML-specific prognostic scoring systems. (3) Until randomised clinical trials have defined the role of new drugs (especially of the hypomethylating agents), treatment must focus on the main symptoms and aim at quality-of-life improvement.

Keywords: chronic myelomonocytic leukaemia, myelodysplastic/myeloproliferative syndrome, somatic mutations, prognosis, therapy

1. Introduction

Chronic myelomonocytic leukaemia (CMML) is a rare haematological neoplasm characterised by a persistent peripheral blood monocytosis and both myelodysplastic and myeloproliferative features. Our understanding of this disease has undergone profound changes in recent years. Initially it was classified as a subtype of myelodysplastic syndromes (MDSs), and it is now recognised as a unique disease. This reclassification has been substantiated by recent advances in the genetic and molecular pathogenesis of CMML, which have confirmed that CMML is biologically distinct from MDS with a different pattern of somatic mutations and a different molecular ontogeny [1]. In addition, CMML-specific prognostic scoring systems (CPSSs) have been established by various groups. These differ from those commonly used in MDS and, for the first time, also include molecular markers. Hopefully, these efforts will culminate in CMML-specific treatments in the near future. The following chapter will summarise these developments starting with a discussion of CMML classification and ending with an outlook on new treatment approaches.

2. Diagnosis and classification

The first reports comprising significant numbers of patients with CMML were published around 40 years ago [2, 3]. These early series already noted a considerable clinical diversity, describing myelodysplasia and cytopenia accompanied by leukocytosis and other myeloproliferative symptoms such as splenomegaly. Nevertheless, the first French–American–British (FAB) Cooperative Group classification of MDS in 1982 included CMML as a MDS subtype, emphasising its dysplastic features but not its diversity [4]. The diagnostic criteria proposed included more than 1×10^9/L blood monocytes, bone marrow blasts of 20% or less, peripheral blasts <5%, and bone marrow dysplastic features in at least one haematopoietic lineage (**Table 1**). To account for the clinical diversity mentioned earlier, the FAB group later introduced a subclassification by dividing patients into two groups based on the leukocyte count at diagnosis [5]. Patients with a leukocyte count above 13×10^9/L were considered to have a myeloproliferative form (MPD-CMML), those with a leukocyte count below 13×10^9/L a myelodysplastic form (MDS-CMML). This arbitrary threshold has been controversial, and its clinical relevance was tested in several cohorts of patients with CMML. In a retrospective analysis of 158 patients (81 patients with MDS-CMML and 77 patients with MPD-CMML), Germing et al. found no significant difference in 2-year overall survival (OS) between these subgroups. The likelihood of transformation to AML was higher in the MDS-CMML group, but this difference was not statistically significant [6]. Voglova et al. [7] described the frequent transition of MDS-CMML to MPD-CMML, suggesting that the two subgroups might represent different stages of the same disease rather than two different entities. Onida et al. analysed a cohort of 213 patients with CMML (35% with MDS-CMML and 65% with MPD-CMML) and could also not find a statistically significant difference in survival after 12 months. There was, however, a trend for a better survival of patients with MPD-CMML after 16 months [8]. To resolve these diagnostic inconsistencies, the WHO (2001) classification of myeloid neoplasms defined a new group of overlap syndromes called myelodysplastic/myeloproliferative diseases (MDS/MPS). Besides CMML, atypical (bcr-abl negative) CML (aCML), juvenile myelomonocytic leukaemia (JMML) and myelodysplastic/myeloproliferative disease, unclassifiable (MDS/MPS-U) were placed in this group [9]. The details of the diagnostic criteria for CMML are listed in **Table 1**. Further, two CMML subtypes were recognised: CMML-1 with PB blast <5% and <10% BM blasts and CMML-2 with 5–19% PB blasts and 10–19% BM blasts. The prognostic significance of these subgroups was confirmed in a reanalysis of the Düsseldorf registry of 300 CMML patients. The 5-year risk of transformation to AML was 63% for patients with CMML-2 compared to only 18% for patients with CMML-1 [10]. More recently, the same group found that further subclassification of CMML based on medullary blast count could provide additional prognostic information [11]. Patients with the new subtype of CMML-0 (defined as <5% medullary blasts) had a better prognosis than those with CMML-1 (OS 31 vs. 19 months). These results have not yet been reproduced in an independent cohort.

The 2008 revision of the WHO classification has maintained the main diagnostic criteria for CMML, with one additional feature [12]. In particular, the recognition of an associated eosinophilia is an important clue to an underlying rearrangement of the platelet-derived growth factor receptor, alpha or beta polypeptide (*PDGFRA/B*) gene. If this molecular lesion is found, the case should be classified as a myeloid neoplasm with eosinophilia associated with *PDGFRA/B* rearrangement. These patients often respond exquisitely to imatinib [13].

Diagnostic difficulties most commonly arise in the distinction between CMML and aCML, because a monocytosis can be present in the latter. In difficult cases, the pattern of somatic mutations might be exploited in the future [14, 15]. For example, the co-existence of a serine/arginine-rich splicing factor 2 (*SRSF2*) and a ten–eleven translocation-2 (*TET2*) mutation suggests CMML, a SET nuclear proto-oncogene binding protein1 (*SETBP1*) mutation points towards aCML.

The presence of a peripheral blood monocytosis is a diagnostic prerequisite for the diagnosis of CMML but can also be caused by a number of reactive conditions. In patients with clinical or laboratory signs of inflammation, such as fever, arthritis, increased C-reactive protein or elevated erythrocyte sedimentation rate, the diagnosis of CMML should be made with caution. Often, re-evaluation is necessary once the signs of inflammation have subsided. A recent study suggests that the distinction between reactive monocytosis and CMML might be possible by immunophenotyping, but this finding needs further confirmation in independent studies [16].

FAB classification	WHO classification
Myelodysplastic syndrome	MDS/MPD overlap syndrome
PB Monocytosis >1 × 10^9/L	PB Monocytosis >1 × 10^9/L
Myeloblasts <5% in PB, <20% in BM	Myeloblasts <20% in BM
Dysplasia in one or more haematopoietic lineage	No BCR-ABL1 fusion gene
	No PDGFRA/PDGFRB rearrangement
	Dysplasia in one or more myeloid lineage
	If lacking: acquired clonal cytogenetic abnormality
Subclassification	*Subclassification*
MDS-CMML: WBC < 13 × 10^9/L	CMML-1: Blasts PB < 5%, BM < 10%
MPD-CMML: WBC > 13 × 10^9/L	CMML-2: Blasts PB 5–19%, BM 10–19%

FAB, French-American-British; PB, peripheral blood; BM, bone marrow.

Table 1. Comparison of the FAB and WHO classifications of CMML.

3. Epidemiology and clinical features

CMML is a rare disease of the elderly. Two recent population-based studies found a similar age standardised annual incidence rate of approximately 0.3–0.4/100,000/year [17, 18]. Median age was 70–75 years, and there was a slight male predominance. The study from the Netherlands found that the diagnosis was made in a non-university setting in 78%, indicating that many patients are managed by practising haematologists. This observation emphasises the need to perform clinical studies also in a community-based setting to include as many patients as possible. The 5-year relative survival was poor (16–20%) in this study and did not improve over time. Therapy-related CMML (t-CMML), defined as occurring after chemotherapy, radiotherapy or both, is considered rare but was found in 10% in a recent MD Anderson Cancer Centre (MDACC) series. Patients with t-CMML had a significantly worse median OS compared to patients with de novo disease (13 vs. 20 months), most likely due to a higher rate of intermediate- or high-risk cytogenetic abnormalities [19]. Similar results were reported in a series from the Mayo Clinic (median OS 11 vs. 20 months) [20].

3.1. Clinical features

Monocytosis can be an incidental finding in an otherwise asymptomatic patient. In other cases, it is accompanied by anaemia (in about 50% of patients at diagnosis) and/or thrombocytopenia. Frequently, a haematological prodrome, for example an unclear thrombocytopenia, can be observed. In about 30–60% of patients, leukocyte counts $>13 \times 10^9$/L are found, often with clinical signs of myeloproliferation such as splenomegaly in around 30% [8]. Hepatosplenomegaly is more frequent (25–50% of patients) in the myeloproliferative variant [21]. Many patients experience constitutional symptoms, fatigue, night sweats and occasionally bone pain.

In contrast to MDS, involvement of various organ systems has been described in CMML patients. Skin lesions can be an indicator of leukemic transformation [22]. Serosal infiltration causing pleural or pericardial effusion is quite frequent and can be difficult to treat [23]. Local instillation of mitoxantrone, in combination with systemic chemotherapy, has been used with some success in such cases. A case of widespread gastric involvement mimicking metastatic gastric carcinoma was recently seen in our practice (own unpublished observation). Cases of uncontrollable haematuria caused by CMML involvement of the urogenital tract have also been described [24, 25].

An association with autoimmune-mediated disorders is frequently seen in CMML. For example, in a study of 123 CMML patients, 20% had at least one associated disorder, most commonly immune thrombocytopenia (ITP), gout or psoriasis [26]. Importantly, ITP seems to respond well to standard treatment used in primary ITP, such as steroids and splenectomy [27].

Over time transformation into acute myeloid leukaemia occurs in approximately 30% of patients. The rate of transformation varies according to the risk profile at diagnosis. A sudden rise in the leukocyte count does not necessarily indicate leukemic transformation but can be an expression of increased myeloproliferation. A careful evaluation of the blast count is important in this situation.

3.2. Laboratory and pathologic findings

In the peripheral blood, monocytes can be normal or display atypical features such as fine nuclear chromatin or abnormal nuclear lobulations. In the myeloproliferative variant, median absolute monocyte counts ranging from 4.2×10^9 to 7.7×10^9/L have been reported [21]; in general, the median monocyte count is around 2×10^9–3×10^9/L. Morphologic evidence of dysgranulopoesis is often seen in CMML, while dysmegakaryopoiesis and dyserythropoiesis are less frequent. The bone marrow is usually hypercellular with an elevated myelopoiesis-to-erythropoiesis ratio. By definition, the blast count is <20%. When enumerating blasts, monoblasts and promonocytes should be included. A helpful morphological classification of monocytic precursors, particularly defining promonocytes in CMML, is available [28]. Monocytic precursors including monoblasts are frequently CD34 negative. Therefore, there is a risk of underestimating the blast number by relying only on CD34 staining in bone marrow biopsies or flow cytometry. The medullary blast count should be determined in good quality bone marrow aspirates that have also been stained for esterase.

4. Cytogenetics

Clonal chromosomal abnormalities occur in approximately 30% of patients with CMML [29, 30]. The most frequent abnormalities are +8 (20–25%), -Y (20%), monosomy 7 and deletion 7q (14%), deletion 20q (8%). A complex karyotype was found in 11%. In contrast to MDS, del5q is very rare. Patients with an abnormal karyotype tended to be older, more anaemic and had a higher peripheral blood and bone marrow blast count [30]. Additional sex combs like 1 (*ASXL1*) mutations were associated with an abnormal karyotype, *SRSF2* mutations with a normal karyotype [31]. Cytogenetic abnormalities were also found to be of prognostic relevance (see Section 6).

5. Molecular findings

Large-scale sequencing studies in myeloid malignancies have lead to important insights into disease biology. These studies have shown one of the highest rates of acquired somatic mutations in CMML patients. For example, in a study by Meggendorfer et al. [31], at least one mutation in 9 recurrently mutated genes was found in 93% of 275 CMML patients. This study and several others also identified clear differences in frequency of mutations in key cellular pathways between CMML and MDS. In addition, the genomic landscape in CMML demonstrates a much smaller molecular heterogeneity compared to a more diffuse mutation profile in MDS [32].

Table 2 summarises the frequency of mutations sorted by the cellular pathway affected [33]. In contrast to MDS, genes serving in different signalling pathways are frequently mutated in CMML. As a biological correlate, an increased sensitivity to GM-CSF has been found in vitro. It appears to be mediated by the STAT pathway, since inhibition of proliferation was observed by the JAK2 inhibitor ruxolitinib [34], indicating the therapeutic potential of these agents or anti GM-CSF monoclonal antibodies.

Cellular pathway	Gene	Frequency (%)
Signalling	*KRAS*	8%
	NRAS	11%
	CBL	10%
	JAK2	10%
	SETBP1	10%
RNA splicing	*SRSF2*	46%
	ZRR2	10%
	U2AF35	10%
Epigenetic regulation	*TET2*	58%
	ASXL1	50%
	EZH2	8%
Transcription	RUNX1	15%

Numbers based on Refs. [1, 33].

Table 2. Frequency of somatic mutations in CMML.

Significant differences were also found in the frequency of mutations affecting RNA splicing. While mutations in *SRSF2* are very common in CMML (40–45%), they are found in <10% of MDS patients, with an enrichment in subtypes with blast excess [31, 32]. Similarly, mutations in epigenetic regulators, among them *TET2* and *ASXL1*, occur much more frequently in CMML than in MDS. For example, using next generation sequencing, *TET2* mutations were found in only 39 of 320 patients with MDS (12%) but in 16 of 35 patients with CMML (46%) [35].

TET2 belongs to the ten–eleven translocations family of proteins and participates in the conversion of 5-methylcytosine to 5-hydroxymethylcytosine. TET2 function depends on the presence of alpha-ketoglutarate, which is produced by isocitrate dehydrogenase 1 and 2 (IDH1/2). *TET2* and *IDH1/2* mutations are mutually exclusive and lead to promoter *hyper*methylation [36], providing a potential explanation for the mode of action of the hypomethylating agents (HMAs). *TET2* mutations appear to be particularly important for CMML pathophysiology and development of its characteristic phenotype. In a series of elegant experiments with samples from CMML patients, Itzykson et al. [37] have shown that early clonal dominance, particularly in a *TET2*-mutated clone, promotes granulomonocytic differentiation. Knockdown experiments of *TET2* in human cord blood CD34+ cells have also found perturbation of myeloid development with promotion of the granulomonocytic lineage [38]. Furthermore, the early occurrence of *TET2* mutations could predetermine the acquisition of secondary mutations, for example in *SRSF2*, leading to characteristic mutational combinations. Besides its role in understanding disease biology and classification, mutational analysis is likely to impact on various clinical aspects, for example prognostication (discussed below) and prediction of treatment response.

6. Prognosis

6.1. Individual parameters

The importance of the medullary blast count as a prognostic variable was discussed before and forms the basis of the subclassification of CMML into CMML-1 and CMML-2. The prognostic significance of cytogenetic abnormalities was first described by the Spanish MDS group in a cohort of 414 CMML patients. Three risk cytogenetic categories were identified in that study: low risk (normal karyotype and loss of chromosome Y as single abnormality), intermediate (all other single or double abnormalities) and high risk (trisomy 8, abnormalities of chromosome 7 and complex karyotype). The OS at 5 years for these risk groups was 35, 24 and 4%, respectively [29]. In a recent large collaborative analysis of 409 patients with CMML, slightly different cytogenetic risk groups were defined: low risk [normal, sole -Y, sole der(3q)], intermediate (all karyotypes not belonging to high or low risk group) and high risk (complex and monosomal karyotype). In contrast to the Spanish study, trisomy 8 was placed in the intermediate risk group. The median OS was 41, 20 and 3 months, respectively [30]. The mutational status of several genes has also shown to be of prognostic relevance, although conflicting results were found in different cohorts. For example, mutations in *TET2* were associated with no effect on outcome in one study [35] and with an adverse outcome in another study [39]. In a large series of 312 patients tested for a number of genes, only *ASXL1* mutations had a negative prognostic value in multivariate analysis [40]. This finding was confirmed in a larger cohort of 466 patients (including the 312 patients from the original series) [41]. In another large study of 275 CMML patients, no effect of *SRSF2* mutations on survival was observed [31]. In summary, *ASXL1* mutational status has emerged as a robust prognostic variable and has thus been incorporated into CPSSs, as discussed below.

6.2. Prognostic scoring systems

A number of prognostic scoring systems for CMML patients have been developed in the past, none of which however was universally used [42]. This is in contrast to MDS where the International Prognostic Scoring System (IPSS) and its recently revised version (IPSS-R) form the basis of treatment decisions in studies as well as in clinical practice. More recently, novel CMML-specific scoring systems have been described that incorporate cytogenetic or molecular information. These scores appear to be more precise and will be discussed further. First, the CPSS has been developed by the Spanish MDS group in a cohort of 558 patients [43]. It uses WHO/FAB subtype, a CMML-specific cytogenetic risk categorisation and transfusion dependence to divide patients into four risk groups (low, intermediate-1 or intermediate-2, and high) with a median OS of 72, 31, 13 and 5 months, respectively). This model demonstrated for the first time that cytogenetic abnormalities are of prognostic relevance in CMML. Notably, it highlights that the significance of individual cytogenetic abnormalities can vary between

CMML and MDS. For example, trisomy 8 carries an adverse prognosis in CMML but not in MDS. The CPPS has been externally validated in a cohort of 274 patients. Second, the French cooperative MDS group (GFM) developed a prognostic model that included the presence of *ASXL1* mutations, age (>65 years being an adverse prognostic factor), and haematological parameters (WBC > 15 × 10^9/L, platelet count <100 × 10^9/L and haemoglobin <11 g/dl being adverse factors). It stratifies patients into 3 risk categories with a median OS of not reached, 38.5 and 14.4 months, respectively, and has also been externally validated [40]. Lastly, the group from the Mayo Clinic has improved on their original prognostic model by incorporating *ASXL1* mutational status. This new score has been termed Mayo Molecular Model (MMM) and was developed in corporation with the GFM [41]. Five risk factors affected median survival in multivariate analysis: *ASXL1* mutation status, absolute monocyte count >10 × 10^9/L, haemoglobin levels <10 g/dl, platelet count <100 × 10^9/L, and circulating immature myeloid cells. It divides patients into four risk categories with median survival of 97, 59, 37 and 16 months, respectively. Importantly, this new score can identify low risk patients (by the original Mayo Clinic score) with a high risk of progression (without or with *ASXL1* mutation: median survival 99 vs. 44 months).

Particularly when considering allogeneic stem cell transplantation, prognostication in younger CMML patients, defined as younger than 65 years, is crucial. A retrospective analysis of 261 such patients has identified several adverse prognostic factors that differ from those in the general CMML population. In addition to anaemia and *ASXL1* mutations, an increased circulating blast count, *SRSF2* mutations and the cytogenetic risk classification of the Mayo-French consortium were independently prognostic. In this study, *ASXL1* and *SRSF2* mutation status did not influence response to HMAs or transplantation outcome [44].

In summary, it is evident that CPSSs that include cytogenetic and/or molecular parameters should be employed in the future.

7. Therapy

7.1. General considerations

Although providing little prognostic information, the concept of a myelodysplastic and a myeloproliferative variant of CMML is helpful in guiding treatment. In particular, patients suffering mainly from uncontrolled myeloproliferation may require rapidly acting cytoreductive treatment. On the other hand, patients with symptoms due to marrow failure require treatment aiming at restoring adequate peripheral blood counts. No treatment so far has been shown to prolong survival or to alter the natural history of the disease. However, randomised studies in CMML patients have not yet been performed, with one exception [45]. Typically, CMML patients (excluding those with MPD-CMML) were included in MDS trials, albeit in small numbers precluding a meaningful statistical analysis. For example, in the AZA-001 trial that led to the registration of azacitidine in higher risk MDS only 16 of the 358 enrolled patients had CMML [46].

For the treatment of lower risk patients with symptomatic anaemia, erythropoiesis-stimulating agents (ESA) might be helpful. A 64% erythroid response rate and transfusion independence in 33% of patients was recently reported in a retrospective analysis of 94 CMML patients. Low/intermediate-1 CPSS and low endogenous erythropoietin levels were predictors of response [47]. ESA's should be used with caution in patients with myeloproliferative CMML because of the risk of splenic enlargement or rupture.

Younger patients with high-risk features (for example intermediate-2 or high risk in the MMM) should be evaluated for eligibility for allogeneic stem cell transplantation. Whether high-risk patients benefit from early treatment with HMAs, as in high-risk MDS, must be tested in prospective randomised trials.

7.2. Stem cell transplantation

Allogeneic stem cell transplant (allo-SCT) still remains the only curative option for patients with CMML and should be considered in younger patients with high-risk disease. So far all reports on allo-SCT in CMML have been retrospective and many included patients with CMML as well as MDS. CMML-specific patient series have only been recently reported, with the EBMT series comprising 513 patients being by far the largest [48]. The median age was 53 years, clearly younger than the median age of CMML patients in general. The non-relapse mortality at 1 and 4 years was 31 and 41%, respectively. The incidence of relapse at 4 years was 32%, resulting in an estimated 4-year relapse free survival of 27% and OS of 33%, respectively. Of note, no influence of procedure-related parameters such as stem cell source, type of donor or T-cell depletion on outcome was found. Importantly, the only significant parameter associated with an improved outcome was the presence of a complete remission at the time of transplantation. A similar trend was also found in a smaller study [49]. Thus, allo-SCT can provide long-term remissions in about 30% of younger patients. The procedure should be performed after achievement of the best possible remission status, either with combination chemotherapy or with HMAs. Although the best preparatory regimen is not known, a recent retrospective study of 83 patients from the MDACC supports the use of HMA before allo-SCT. The study found a significantly lower incidence of relapse at 3 years post transplant in patients treated with HMA, compared to patients treated with other agents (22 vs. 35%, $p = 0.03$), resulting in a better 3-year progression-free survival [50]. A selection bias might confound these interesting results, since patients who do not progress while treated with HMA (median of 6 cycles in the study) are likely to have a less aggressive disease.

7.3. Cytoreductive treatment

In patients with symptoms mainly caused by myeloproliferation, cytoreductive treatment is indicated. Several studies have demonstrated the effect of the topoisomerase-I inhibitor topotecan in patients with CMML. As a single-agent, complete response rates of up to 28% have been described [51]. Similarly, clinically meaningful responses, including improvement of life threatening pericardial and pleural effusions, as well as cytopenias were reported for the topoisomerase-II inhibitor etoposide [52]. However, in a randomised study of 105 patients from 43 European centres, hydroxyurea was found to be superior to etoposide in terms of the response rate (60 vs. 36%) and OS (20 vs. 9 months) and has thus remained the treatment of choice for palliative cytoreduction in CMML patients [45]. The experience with intensive chemotherapy in CMML has been disappointing [53]. AML-like induction therapy is only rarely used, usually as a preparatory regimen before allogeneic stem cell transplantation in patients with an aggressive disease.

7.4. Hypomethylating agents

The introduction of the HMAs azacitidine and decitabine is likely to transform clinical management of CMML. A growing number of studies have shown considerable single agent activity with very low toxicity. In the largest study so far (76 patients from France, Cleveland Clinic and Lee Moffitt Cancer Center), a response rate of 43%, with 17% complete remissions, was found [54]. Of note, 46% had a proliferative form of CMML, as defined by a leukocyte count of $>13 \times 10^9$/L. In that study, the presence of more than 10% bone marrow blasts and palpable splenomegaly had a negative impact on survival. A smaller Italian retrospective study analysed the response in 31 patients with CMML (42% with CMML-1, 58% with CMML-2) who were treated with azacitidine at a dose of 75 or 50 mg/m^2 for 7 days. The overall response rate was 51%, including 45% achieving complete remission [55]. A study from the Austrian Azacitidine registry reported on the outcome of 48 patients treated with azacitidine at 11 different centres [56]. Mean age was 71 years; 40% had CMML-1; 60% had CMML-2; and splenomegaly was found in 48%. Even in this unselected cohort with several high-risk features, there was a surprising response rate of 70%, including 22% complete responses. Matched paired analysis suggested a better 2-year-survival when compared to best supportive care (62 vs. 41%, $p = 0.067$).

Other studies have examined the activity of the related HMA decitabine in CMML. One of the first reports was published by the MDACC group on 19 patients with CMML, and a complete response rate of 58% was found. The dose of decitabine was 100 mg/m^2 per course, given in three different treatment schedules [57]. In a phase 2 trial from the GFM, 39 patients with advanced CMML were treated with decitabine at a dose of 20 mg/m^2 for 5 days. The median number of treatment cycles was 10 and the overall response rate 38%, OS at 2 years was 48%. Interestingly, the presence of *ASXL1* mutations had no significant impact on response or survival in that study [58]. A review of CMML patients that were included in several phase 2 and one phase 3 trials of decitabine in MDS was done by Wijermans et al. [59]. Among a total of 271 patients, 31 CMML patients were identified. The overall response rate was 25% with 14% CR, and 39% had stable disease. The treatment schedule was different than in the GFM study, and many patients received only a few cycles of therapy (median of four cycles).

Reliable and easily available predictors of response to treatment with HMA have not yet been identified. Although a correlation of response with *TET2* mutational status would seem plausible, this was not found in two different studies [58, 60]. Likewise, no other somatic mutation frequent in CMML proved to be predictive of response.

A small retrospective analysis has shown activity of decatibine and azacitidine in reducing spleen size in CMML patients. Spleen size was measured by physical examination, and complete or partial spleen response was found in 5 of 11 patients (45%) [61].

http://dx.doi.org/10.5772/63193

Although these data are promising and have led to the registration of both drugs for the treatment of CMML, data from phase 3 trials demonstrating a survival benefit are not yet available. Also, the optimal treatment schedule and treatment duration need to be defined. The results of an ongoing randomised trial (DACOTA trial) comparing hydroxyurea to decitabine in patients with advanced proliferative CMML are, therefore, eagerly awaited. This trial is conducted in three countries (France, Italy and Germany) and will include about 160 patients. The primary endpoint is progression-free survival.

7.5. Investigational agents

A large number of investigational agents have been tested in CMML, among them tyrosine kinase inhibitors, farnesyltransferase inhibitors, immunomodulators and most recently JAK2 inhibitors. The experience with many of these approaches is limited to small phase 1 or phase 2 studies that have not been further developed, either because of limited activity or because of significant toxicity.

Imatinib has shown no effect in CMML patients without a *PDGFRB* rearrangement. Because CMML cells often have *RAS* activating mutations, drugs targeting this pathway have been tested. In a phase 2 trial, 35 patients with CMML were treated with lonafarnib (200–300 mg twice daily), one CR and 7 haematological improvements were reported. Major toxicities were gastrointestinal, fatigue, fever and hypokalemia [62]. Similar results were observed for tipifanib in a study of 10 CMML patients [63]. In several patients treated with lonafarnib, a significant increase in the white blood cell count was noted, sometimes accompanied by oedema and respiratory symptoms. This complication resolved quickly after discontinuation of lonafarnib and treatment with dexamethasone [64]. Disappointingly, translational studies have shown no correlation between responses and inhibition of farnesyl transferase.

Interesting results have been found in a study targeting angiogenesis in MDS and CMML patients with a combination consisting of melphalan (2 mg/day) and lenalidomide (10 mg/day). Changes in circulating endothelial cells and plasma VEGF levels served as biomarkers of angiogenesis. The response rate was 33% in CMML patients (3/9), all of which had a proliferative form of the disease. Interestingly, there was a correlation between response and angiogenesis inhibition in these patients. Dose reductions were frequently necessary, but many patients were cytopenic already at baseline [65].

Most recently, a multicentre phase 1 trial (only published in abstract form) tested the JAK2 inhibitor ruxolitinib in 19 CMML patients. All patients had CMML-1 and those with significant cytopenias were excluded. No dose limiting toxicity was noted. Although there were few haematologic responses, a frequent improvement of splenomegaly and B symptoms was found. A phase 2 trial testing ruxolitinib at a dose of 20 mg BID is planned [66].

8. Summary and outlook

CMML is a rare myeloid neoplasm with an overall poor prognosis. Important progress has been made in recent years in several aspects. First, the recognition of CMML as a unique disease entity, separated from the myelodysplastic syndromes, is an important step towards optimising clinical management. Second, the introduction of CPSSs will improve patient selection in clinical trials. Phase 3 clinical trials in CMML patients will soon define the role of HMA in treatment. The elucidation of the mutational landscape in CMML has not provided disease-specific mutations but highly characteristic mutational combinations, particularly of *TET2* and *SRSF2*. These insights into molecular pathology are very likely to provide the basis for the development of novel therapeutic agents. Individualised therapies based on the predominant gene mutations could be envisaged. For example, while patients with *TET2* mutations are treated with HMA, in patients with mutations affecting signalling, specific pathway inhibitors might be more potent. Clearly, novel strategies and agents are needed for this still difficult to treat disease.

Author details

Andreas Himmelmann*

Address all correspondence to: andreas.himmelmann@hirslanden.ch

Haematology Practice Lucerne, Clinic St. Anna, Lucerne, Switzerland

References

[1] Benton CB, Nazha A, Pemmaraju N, Garcia-Manero G. Chronic myelomonocytic leukemia: forefront of the field in 2015. Crit Rev Oncol Hematol 2015;95:222–42.

[2] Geary CG, Catovsky D, Wiltshaw E, Milner GR, Scholes MC, Van Noorden S, et al. Chronic myelomonocytic leukaemia. Br J Haematol 1975;30:289–302.

[3] Miescher PA, Farguet JJ. Chronic myelomonocytic leukemia in adults. Semin Hematol 1974;11:129–39.

[4] Bennett JM, Catovsky D, Daniel MT, Flandrin G, Galton DA, Gralnick HR, et al. Proposals for the classification of the myelodysplastic syndromes. Br J Haematol 1982;51:189–99.

[5] Bennett JM, Catovsky D, Daniel MT, Flandrin G, Galton DA, Gralnick H, et al. The chronic myeloid leukaemias: guidelines for distinguishing chronic granulocytic, atypical chronic myeloid, and chronic myelomonocytic leukaemia. Proposals by the French–American–British Cooperative Leukaemia Group. Br J Haematol 1994;87:746–54.

[6] Germing U, Gattermann N, Minning H, Heyll A, Aul C. Problems in the classification of CMML—dysplastic versus proliferative type. Leuk Res 1998;22:871–8.

[7] Voglová J, Chrobák L, Neuwirtová R, Malasková V, Straka L. Myelodysplastic and myeloproliferative type of chronic myelomonocytic leukemia—distinct subgroups or two stages of the same disease? Leuk Res 2001;25:493–9.

[8] Onida F, Kantarjian HM, Smith TL, Ball G, Keating MJ, Estey EH, et al. Prognostic factors and scoring systems in chronic myelomonocytic leukemia: a retrospective analysis of 213 patients. Blood 2002;99:840–9.

[9] Vardiman JW, Harris NL, Brunning RD. The World Health Organization (WHO) classification of the myeloid neoplasms. Blood 2002;100:2292–302.

[10] Germing U, Strupp C, Knipp S, Kuendgen A, Giagounidis A, Hildebrandt B, et al. Chronic myelomonocytic leukemia in the light of the WHO proposals. Haematologica 2007;92:974–7.

[11] Schuler E, Schroeder M, Neukirchen J, Strupp C, Xicoy B, Kündgen A, et al. Refined medullary blast and white blood cell count based classification of chronic myelomonocytic leukemias. Leuk Res 2014;38:1413–9.

[12] Vardiman JW, Thiele J, Arber DA, Brunning RD, Borowitz MJ, Porwit A, et al. The 2008 revision of the World Health Organization (WHO) classification of myeloid neoplasms and acute leukemia: rationale and important changes. Blood 2009;114:937–51.

[13] Apperley JF, Gardembas M, Melo JV, Russell-Jones R, Bain BJ, Baxter EJ, et al. Response to imatinib mesylate in patients with chronic myeloproliferative diseases with rearrangements of the platelet-derived growth factor receptor beta. N Engl J Med 2002;347:481–7.

[14] Li B, Gale RP, Xiao Z. Molecular genetics of chronic neutrophilic leukemia, chronic myelomonocytic leukemia and atypical chronic myeloid leukemia. J Hematol Oncol 2014;7:93.

[15] Meggendorfer M, Haferlach T, Jeromin S, Haferlach C, Kern W, Schnittger S. Molecular analyses of MDS/MPN overlap entities according to WHO classification reveal a distinct molecular pattern for MDS/MPN, unclassifiable. Blood 2014;124:4618–8.

[16] Selimoglu-Buet D, Wagner-Ballon O, Saada V, Bardet V, Itzykson R, Bencheikh L, et al. Characteristic repartition of monocyte subsets as a diagnostic signature of chronic myelomonocytic leukemia. Blood 2015;125:3618–26.

[17] Visser O, Trama A, Maynadié M, Stiller C, Marcos-Gragera R, De Angelis R, et al. Incidence, survival and prevalence of myeloid malignancies in Europe. Eur J Cancer 2012;48:3257–66.

[18] Dinmohamed AG, van Norden Y, Visser O, Posthuma EFM, Huijgens PC, Sonneveld P, et al. The use of medical claims to assess incidence, diagnostic procedures and initial treatment of myelodysplastic syndromes and chronic myelomonocytic leukemia in the Netherlands. Leuk Res 2015;39:177–82.

[19] Takahashi K, Pemmaraju N, Strati P, Nogueras-Gonzalez G, Ning J, Bueso-Ramos C, et al. Clinical characteristics and outcomes of therapy-related chronic myelomonocytic leukemia. Blood 2013;122:2807–11.

[20] Subari S, Patnaik M, Alfakara D, Gangat N, Elliott M, Hogan W, et al. Patients with therapy-related CMML have shorter median overall survival than those with De Novo CMML: Mayo Clinic long-term follow-up experience. Clin Lymphoma Myeloma Leuk 2015;15:546–9.

[21] Onida F, Beran M. Chronic myelomonocytic leukemia: myeloproliferative variant. Curr Hematol Rep 2004;3:218–26.

[22] Mathew RA, Bennett JM, Liu JJ, Komrokji RS, Lancet JE, Naghashpour M, et al. Cutaneous manifestations in CMML: indication of disease acceleration or transformation to AML and review of the literature. Leuk Res 2012;36:72–80.

[23] Morita Y, Ohyama Y, Rai S, Kawauchi M, Yamaguchi T, Shimada T, et al. A case of chronic myelomonocytic leukemia who developed pericardial effusion during stably controlled leukocytosis. Intern Med 2011;50:1737–40.

[24] Bane AL, Enright H, Sweeney EC. Chronic myelomonocytic leukemia revealed by uncontrollable hematuria. Arch Pathol Lab Med 2001;125:657–9.

[25] Hyams ES, Gupta R, Melamed J, Taneja SS, Shah O. Renal involvement by chronic myelomonocytic leukemia requiring nephroureterectomy. Rev Urol 2009;11:33–7.

[26] Peker D, Padron E, Bennett JM, Zhang X, Horna P, Epling-Burnette PK, et al. A close association of autoimmune-mediated processes and autoimmune disorders with chronic myelomonocytic leukemia: observation from a single institution. Acta Haematol 2015;133:249–56.

[27] Hadjadj J, Michel M, Chauveheid M-P, Godeau B, Papo T, Sacre K. Immune thrombocytopenia in chronic myelomonocytic leukemia. Eur J Haematol 2014;93:521–6.

[28] Goasguen JE, Bennett JM, Bain BJ, Vallespí T, Brunning R, Mufti GJ. Morphological evaluation of monocytes and their precursors. Haematologica 2009;94:994–7.

[29] Such E, Cervera J, Costa D, Solé F, Vallespí T, Luño E, et al. Cytogenetic risk stratification in chronic myelomonocytic leukemia. Haematologica 2011;96:375–83.

[30] Wassie EA, Itzykson R, Lasho TL, Kosmider O, Finke CM, Hanson CA, et al. Molecular and prognostic correlates of cytogenetic abnormalities in chronic myelomonocytic leukemia: a Mayo Clinic-French Consortium Study. Am J Hematol 2014;89:1111–5.

[31] Meggendorfer M, Roller A, Haferlach T, Eder C, Dicker F, Grossmann V, et al. SRSF2 mutations in 275 cases with chronic myelomonocytic leukemia (CMML). Blood 2012;120:3080–8.

[32] Haferlach T, Nagata Y, Grossmann V, Okuno Y, Bacher U, Nagae G, et al. Landscape of genetic lesions in 944 patients with myelodysplastic syndromes. Leukemia 2014;28:241–7.

[33] Zoi K, Cross NCP. Molecular pathogenesis of atypical CML, CMML and MDS/MPN-unclassifiable. Int J Hematol 2015;101:229–42.

[34] Padron E, Painter JS, Kunigal S, Mailloux AW, McGraw K, McDaniel JM, et al. GM-CSF-dependent pSTAT5 sensitivity is a feature with therapeutic potential in chronic myelomonocytic leukemia. Blood 2013;121:5068–77.

[35] Smith AE, Mohamedali AM, Kulasekararaj A, Lim Z, Gäken J, Lea NC, et al. Next-generation sequencing of the TET2 gene in 355 MDS and CMML patients reveals low-abundance mutant clones with early origins, but indicates no definite prognostic value. Blood 2010;116:3923–32.

[36] Figueroa ME, Abdel-Wahab O, Lu C, Ward PS, Patel J, Shih A, et al. Leukemic IDH1 and IDH2 mutations result in a hypermethylation phenotype, disrupt TET2 function, and impair hematopoietic differentiation. Cancer Cell 2010;18:553–67.

[37] Itzykson R, Kosmider O, Renneville A, Morabito M, Preudhomme C, Berthon C, et al. Clonal architecture of chronic myelomonocytic leukemias. Blood 2013;121:2186–98.

[38] Pronier E, Almire C, Mokrani H, Vasanthakumar A, Simon A, da Costa Reis Monte Mor B, et al. Inhibition of TET2-mediated conversion of 5-methylcytosine to 5-hydroxymethylcytosine disturbs erythroid and granulomonocytic differentiation of human hematopoietic progenitors. Blood 2011;118:2551–5.

[39] Kosmider O, Gelsi-Boyer V, Ciudad M, Racoeur C, Jooste V, Vey N, et al. TET2 gene mutation is a frequent and adverse event in chronic myelomonocytic leukemia. Haematologica 2009;94:1676–81.

[40] Itzykson R, Kosmider O, Renneville A, Gelsi-Boyer V, Meggendorfer M, Morabito M, et al. Prognostic score including gene mutations in chronic myelomonocytic leukemia. J Clin Oncol 2013;31:2428–36.

[41] Patnaik MM, Itzykson R, Lasho TL, Kosmider O, Finke CM, Hanson CA, et al. ASXL1 and SETBP1 mutations and their prognostic contribution in chronic myelomonocytic leukemia: a two-center study of 466 patients. Leukemia 2014;28:2206–12.

[42] Mughal TI, Cross NCP, Padron E, Tiu RV, Savona M, Malcovati L, et al. An International MDS/MPN Working Group's perspective and recommendations on molecular pathogenesis, diagnosis and clinical characterization of myelodysplastic/myeloproliferative neoplasms. Haematologica 2015;100:1117–30.

[43] Such E, Germing U, Malcovati L, Cervera J, Kuendgen A, Porta Della MG, et al. Development and validation of a prognostic scoring system for patients with chronic myelomonocytic leukemia. Blood 2013;121:3005–15.

[44] Patnaik MM, Wassie EA, Padron E, Onida F, Itzykson R, Lasho TL, et al. Chronic myelomonocytic leukemia in younger patients: molecular and cytogenetic predictors of survival and treatment outcome. Blood Cancer J 2015;5:e270.

[45] Wattel E, Guerci A, Hecquet B, Economopoulos T, Copplestone A, Mahé B, et al. A randomized trial of hydroxyurea versus VP16 in adult chronic myelomonocytic leukemia. Groupe Français des Myélodysplasies and European CMML Group. Blood 1996;88:2480–7.

[46] Fenaux P, Mufti GJ, Hellstrom-Lindberg E, Santini V, Finelli C, Giagounidis A, et al. Efficacy of azacitidine compared with that of conventional care regimens in the treatment of higher-risk myelodysplastic syndromes: a randomised, open-label, phase III study. Lancet Oncol 2009;10:223–32.

[47] Xicoy B, Germing U, Jimenez M-J, Garcia O, Garcia R, Schemenau J, et al. Response to erythropoietic-stimulating agents in patients with chronic myelomonocytic leukemia. Eur J Haematol 2015. doi:10.1111/ejh.12679. [Epub ahead of print].

[48] Symeonidis A, van Biezen A, de Wreede L, Piciocchi A, Finke J, Beelen D, et al. Achievement of complete remission predicts outcome of allogeneic haematopoietic stem cell transplantation in patients with chronic myelomonocytic leukaemia. A study of the Chronic Malignancies Working Party of the European Group for Blood and Marrow Transplantation. Br J Haematol 2015;98:983–91.

[49] Warlick ED, Cioc A, Defor T, Dolan M, Weisdorf D. Allogeneic stem cell transplantation for adults with myelodysplastic syndromes: importance of pretransplant disease burden. Biol Blood Marrow Transplant 2009;15:30–8.

[50] Kongtim P, Popat U, Jimenez A, Gaballa S, Fakih El R, Rondon G, et al. Treatment with hypomethylating agents before allogeneic stem cell transplant improves progression-free survival for patients with chronic myelomonocytic leukemia. Biol Blood Marrow Transplant 2016;22:47–53.

[51] Beran M, Kantarjian H, O'Brien S, Koller C, Al-Bitar M, Arbuck S, et al. Topotecan, a topoisomerase I inhibitor, is active in the treatment of myelodysplastic syndrome and chronic myelomonocytic leukemia. Blood 1996;88:2473–9.

[52] Oscier DG, Worsley A, Hamblin TJ, Mufti GJ. Treatment of chronic myelomonocytic leukaemia with low dose etoposide. Br J Haematol 1989;72:468–71.

[53] Wattel E, De Botton S, Luc Laï J, Preudhomme C, Lepelley P, Bauters F, et al. Long-term follow-up of de novo myelodysplastic syndromes treated with intensive chemotherapy: incidence of long-term survivors and outcome of partial responders. Br J Haematol 1997;98:983–91.

[54] Ades L, Sekeres MA, Wolfromm A, Teichman ML, Tiu RV, Itzykson R, et al. Predictive factors of response and survival among chronic myelomonocytic leukemia patients treated with azacitidine. Leuk Res 2013;37:609–13.

[55] Fianchi L, Criscuolo M, Breccia M, Maurillo L, Salvi F, Musto P, et al. High rate of remissions in chronic myelomonocytic leukemia treated with 5-azacytidine: results of an Italian retrospective study. Leuk Lymphoma 2013;54:658–61.

[56] Pleyer L, Germing U, Sperr WR, Linkesch W, Burgstaller S, Stauder R, et al. Azacitidine in CMML: matched-pair analyses of daily-life patients reveal modest effects on clinical course and survival. Leuk Res 2014;38:475–83.

[57] Aribi A, Borthakur G, Ravandi F, Shan J, Davisson J, Cortes J, et al. Activity of decitabine, a hypomethylating agent, in chronic myelomonocytic leukemia. Cancer 2007;109:713–7.

[58] Braun T, Itzykson R, Renneville A, de Renzis B, Dreyfus F, Laribi K, et al. Molecular predictors of response to decitabine in advanced chronic myelomonocytic leukemia: a phase 2 trial. Blood 2011;118:3824–31.

[59] Wijermans PW, Ruter B, Baer MR, Slack JL, Saba HI, Lubbert M. Efficacy of decitabine in the treatment of patients with chronic myelomonocytic leukemia (CMML). Leuk Res 2008;32:587–91.

[60] Meldi K, Qin T, Buchi F, Droin N, Sotzen J, Micol J-B, et al. Specific molecular signatures predict decitabine response in chronic myelomonocytic leukemia. J Clin Investig 2015;125:1857–72.

[61] Subari S, Patnaik M, Alfakara D, Zblewski D, Hook C, Hashmi S, et al. Hypomethylating agents are effective in shrinking splenomegaly in patients with chronic myelomonocytic leukemia. Leuk Lymphoma 2015;1–7 [Epub ahead of print].

[62] Feldman EJ, Cortes J, DeAngelo DJ, Holyoake T, Simonsson B, O'Brien SG, et al. On the use of lonafarnib in myelodysplastic syndrome and chronic myelomonocytic leukemia. Leukemia 2008;22:1707–11.

[63] Kurzrock R, Kantarjian HM, Cortes JE, Singhania N, Thomas DA, Wilson EF, et al. Farnesyltransferase inhibitor R115777 in myelodysplastic syndrome: clinical and biologic activities in the phase 1 setting. Blood 2003;102:4527–34.

[64] Buresh A, Perentesis J, Rimsza L, Kurtin S, Heaton R, Sugrue M, et al. Hyperleukocytosis complicating lonafarnib treatment in patients with chronic myelomonocytic leukemia. Leukemia 2005;19:308–10.

[65] Buckstein R, Kerbel R, Cheung M, Shaked Y, Chodirker L, Lee CR, et al. Lenalidomide and metronomic melphalan for CMML and higher risk MDS: a phase 2 clinical study with biomarkers of angiogenesis. Leuk Res 2014;38:756–63.

[66] Padron E, Dezern A, Andrade-Campos M, Vaddi K, Scherle P, Zhang Q, et al. A multi-institution phase 1 trial of ruxolitinib in patients with chronic myelomonocytic leukemia (CMML). Clin Cancer Res 2016

Chapter 7

Different Mechanisms of Drug Resistance in Myelodysplastic Syndromes and Acute Myeloid Leukemia

Lucia Messingerova, Denisa Imrichova,
Martina Coculova, Marian Zelina, Lucia Pavlikova,
Helena Kavcova, Mario Seres, Viera Bohacova,
Boris Lakatos, Zdena Sulova and Albert Breier

Additional information is available at the end of the chapter

http://dx.doi.org/10.5772/63483

Abstract

Myelodysplastic syndromes (MDSs) represent clonal hematopoietic stem cell (HSC) disorders in which genetic and/or epigenetic alteration are involved in the normal function of hematopoietic stem and progenitor cells. This results in the development of blood cytopenias and bone marrow dysplasia. In recent years, therapy with hypomethylating agents (HMAs) in combination with supportive therapies is recommended as frontline treatment for patients with high-risk MDSs according to International Prognostic Scoring System (IPSS HR-MDS). Therapy with HMAs is essential namely for IPSS HR-MDS patients who do not proceed to immediate allogeneic stem cell transplantation (alloSCT). For IPSS LR-MDS (International Prognostic Scoring System, low-risk MDSs) patients, however, supportive therapies and growth factors are the mainstay of treatment. Some patients in this group are treated with immunomodulatory agents derived from thalidomide (lenalidomide) or using immunosuppressive therapy (IST). The therapeutic decisions can change during the course of the disease based on changes in risk-category and the functional status of patients, in response to prior therapies, changes in patient preferences, and other factors.

Resistance to chemotherapy is a serious obstacle to the successful treatment of overall malignancies, including AML and MDS. The failure of therapeutic treatment may be due to the development of multidrug resistance (MDR) phenotype. MDR represents the induction of large-scale defensive mechanisms from which the upregulation of membrane transporters (like P-glycoprotein – P-gp) effluxing chemotherapeutic drugs from tumor cells represents the most observed molecular causality. Other mechanisms of MDR include drug metabolism, alterations in drug-induced apoptosis, epigenetic changes, epithelial-mesenchymal transition, alteration in drug targets structures, and acceleration of DNA repair.

The present contribution represents a state-of-the-art review of available knowledge about this issue.

Keywords: myelodysplastic syndromes, acute myeloid leukemia, multidrug resistance, lenalidomide, 5-azacytidine, 5-aza-2-deoxyazacytidine

1. Introduction

Myelodysplastic syndromes (MDSs) represent the group of disorders associated with altered hematopoietic stem cells (HSCs) that lead to inefficient hematopoiesis [1]. This clinically results in dysplasia in one or more myeloid cell lineages, and variable degrees of cytopenias. The mean age of MDS patients' diagnosis ranges from 60 to 70 years. The incidence of MDS varied from 4.3 to 1.8 per 100,000 individuals per year in the US and Europe, respectively. Incidence slightly favors Caucasian males. MDS can lead to acute myeloid leukemia (AML) in 10–15% of patients.

Improvements in cytogenetic analysis techniques enable predicting the risk of MDS patients lapse into AML and the selection of optimal therapy [2]. The International Prognostic Scoring System (IPSS) described in the 1990s [3] is still commonly used. This scoring system defines how to measure the risk of patients' development from MDS to AML, and recommends dividing patients into four groups (low, intermediate 1, intermediate 2, and high risk). In lower risk patients, a combination of supportive care (includes transfusions of blood products, antibiotics) with substance improving erythropoiesis, immunosuppressive therapy, immunomodulatory therapy, and stem cell transplantation has been used. Treatment options for patients diagnosed as higher risk include demethylating agents, cytotoxic chemotherapy, bone marrow HSC transplantation, and experimental treatments in clinical trials [4].

2. Treatment options

The only curative option for patients with MDS represents hematopoietic bone marrow stem cell transplantations. However, alloSCT is not available for all patients because of the comorbidities of elderly patients [1]. Therefore some patients cannot be treated with alloSCT and other treatment options have to be used.

2.1. IPSS low-risk MDS patients' treatment option

Supportive care is an important therapy for the management of patients with low-risk MDS, as well as patients with poor disease prognosis which due to age or physical condition could not be treated with more intensive forms of therapy [5]. Several low-risk patients are dependent on blood transfusions. However, patients treated with blood transfusions may be overloaded with iron ions, so that iron chelation therapy is required [6]. Due to the partial dysfunction of immunity, antibiotics are needed for treatable infections [7].

There are three commonly used therapies for low-risk MDS patients: i. erythropoiesis-stimulating agents (ESAs); ii. immunosuppressive therapy; and iii. immunomodulatory therapy with thalidomide derivative lenalidomide (revlimid). The treatment of patients with ESAs leads to significant erythroid response in 20–70% of unselected patients with MDS [1]. A median response for treatment with erythropoietin and colony-stimulating factor (CSF) applied together was 2 years and improves life quality [8]. Several immunosuppressants such as antithymocyte globulin and cyclosporine A were studied in a randomized phase III clinical trial. This treatment seems to be associated with hematologic responses in a subset of patients, however, it was not found to reduce the 2-year transformation and overall survival [9].

Over recent years, attention has been paid to immunomodulatory-acting drugs (IMIDs). The anti-MDS activity of these drugs involves antiproliferative effects, downregulation of crucial cytokines, and costimulatory effects on T and NK cells [10]. The IMIDs are thalidomide analogs which have greater immunological and anticancer properties, but lack the toxicity associated with thalidomide [11]. Lenalidomide (LEN) was proven to be effective in the treatment of patients with low-risk MDS, particularly in cases with special molecular feature, i.e., deletions in the long arm of chromosome 5 [12, 13].

2.2. IPSS high-risk MDS patients' treatment option

Patients with high-risk MDS have poor outcomes, high probability of AML development, and without intensive treatment or alloSCT their median survival is limited to 1 year [3]. The treatment of high-risk MDS patients is based on three commonly used therapies: i. alloSCT; ii. intensive chemotherapy; and iii. drugs with epigenetic mechanism of action such as demethylation agents and histone deacetylase inhibitors (HDACi) [1]. Similarly as in low-risk patients, the application of alloSCT is limited by the patients' age and overall condition.

About 50% of patients with high-risk MDS achieve complete remission with standard anti-leukemic chemotherapy with fludarabine, idarubicin, or topotecan. This therapy could be improved by a combination of these drugs with intermediate- or high-dose cytosine arabinoside [14]. The combination of such therapy with granulocyte colony-stimulating factor (G-CSF) is well tolerated and highly effective in the remission of both high-risk MDS patients and AML patients [15].

Inhibitors of histone deacetylase block the deacetylation of histones molecules, i.e., they protect histones in acetylation forms. The acetylation of histones occurs in the replication- and transcription-active euchromatin. HDACi could protect euchromatin against formation changes to heterochromatin that is replication and transcription inactive. The effect of HDACi could be pleiotropic, leading to the induction of differentiation, growth arrest, and finally to the apoptosis of tumor cells. The mechanisms of HDACi's effectiveness are under intensive debate, and it may be p53 dependent or independent [16]. Valproic acid, entinostat, vorinostat, and other HDCAi are under intensive research with the aim of characterizing their effectiveness against MDS [16].

The cytosine analogs 4-amino-1-(β-D-ribofuranosyl)-1,3,5-triazin-2(1H)-one – azacytidine (AzaC) and 4-amino-1-(β-D-deoxyribofuranosyl)-1,3,5-triazin-2(1H)-one – deoxyazacytidine (decitabine, DAC), which were described as cancerostatic agents in the late 1960s and the early 1970s [17, 18], were found to effectively block DNA methylation [19]. Their effectiveness in inducing beneficial effects in the treatment of MDS [20] and AML [21] was already proven. The downregulation of DNA methylation induced by AzaC and DAC is related to the ability of this substance to be artificially incorporated into DNA instead of cytosine, which has to be methylated by DNA methyltransferase [22]. This could be considered as a major principle of DAC action. In contrast to DAC's effects, AzaC is more complex and also involves incorporation into mRNA, tRNA, and rRNA, which disrupts nucleic acid and protein metabolism leading to apoptosis in addition to the incorporation of substances into DNA [22, 23]. Consistently AzaC induced more pronounced cell damage effects than DAC [24].

3. Drug resistance of MDS and AML patients

3.1. Mechanisms of drug resistance of neoplastic cells

The multidrug resistance (MDR) of neoplastic cells represents a real obstacle in the effective treatment of neoplastic diseases [25]. MDR could be an inherent property of tissue from which neoplastic cells were developed – primary (intrinsic) MDR, or could be induced by prior treatment with anticancer drugs – secondary (acquired) MDR (reviewed in [26]). In both cases the neoplastic cells exert reduced sensitivity to more than one drug that differs in structure and pharmacological efficiency. In many cases, cells with resistance to a large scale of diverse drugs are present in cancer tissue. Several mechanisms are involved in the mediation of MDR, which can be divided into seven groups (**Figure 1**, reviewed in [27]):

i. Potentiating drug metabolism via the induction/activation of phase I and phase II detoxification enzymes

ii. Potentiating cell drug efflux via the induction/activation of membrane drug transporter predominantly members of the ABC family

iii. Alteration in drug target structures

iv. Acceleration of DNA-repair

v. Changes in epigenetic regulation

vi. Programmed cell death inhibition

vii. Epithelial-mesenchymal transition

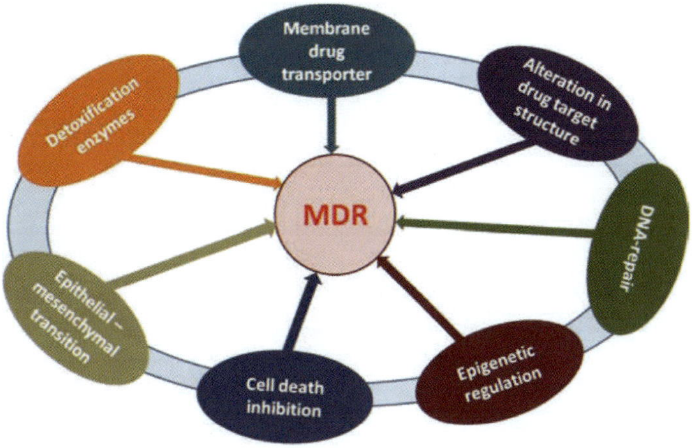

Figure 1. Mechanisms of multidrug resistance.

These mechanisms could act independently or cooperate in the development of MDR in relation to cancer cells' specific character. The expression of drug transporters represents the most observed molecular causality of MDR (reviewed in [28, 29]). At least three transporters are involved in the reduction of drug sensitivity of neoplastic cells. The best known is P-glycoprotein (P-gp) that represents an ABCB1 member of the ABC transporter family and was discovered as the first ABC transporter in 1976 [30]. P-gp could efflux a large scale of different uncharged substances from cells. Drugs such as colchicine, tacrolimus, and quinidine; chemotherapeutic agents such as etoposide, doxorubicin, and vinblastine; different lipids and steroids; xenobiotics; DNA-intercalators such as ethidium bromide; linear or circular peptides like valinomycin and gramicidin; bilirubin; cardiac glycosides like digoxin; different immunosuppressive agents; glucocorticoids like dexamethasone; HIV-type 1 antiretroviral therapy agents like protease inhibitors and nonnucleoside reverse transcriptase inhibitors; and many others are known to be P-gp substrates. When P-gp is expressed in neoplastic tissue it can depress cell sensitivity to its substrates several hundred times [31]. Besides this generally accepted role as a drug transporter, this protein may also play another role as an antiapoptotic regulatory protein and this role is independent of P-gp efflux activity [29, 32]. This additional role also enables P-gp to reduce cell sensitivity to substances that are not its substrates, such as cisplatin several times [33, 34].

Other important transporters involved in MDR are ABCC1-3 members of the ABC transporters' family, also known as multidrug-resistant associate proteins 1–3 (MRP1-MRP3) that in contrast to P-gp are specific to negatively charged organic anions (reviewed in [35]). They are also specific for drug conjugates with glucuronic acid and glutathione as a product of phase II enzyme drug detoxification.

One more transporter ABCG2 member of the ABC transporter family is often described to be involved in MDR [36]. This transporter also known as breast cancer-resistant protein (BCRP) may efflux substances such as mitoxantrone, methotrexate, topotecan, imatinib, and others. The substrate specificity of P-gp, MRP1-3, and BCRP overlaps, and each could be responsible for the efflux of common substrate.

The drug could be detoxified by phase I and phase II detoxification enzymes that secure oxidative and conjugative ways of drug modification which are mediated by cytochrome P450 (CYP) monooxygenases and conjugating enzymes (glutathione S-transferases [GSTs] and UDP-glucuronyl-transferase), respectively [37]. The CYP family, particularly the CYP3A members of the CYP family, may be involved in the reduction of cell sensitivity to several drugs. The transcriptional control of the CYP family is mediated by pregnane X nuclear receptor, i.e., the same nuclear receptor involved in P-gp expression [38].

GSTs represent a group of enzymes that are often involved in the protection of cells against toxic stress [39]. These enzymes catalyze the conjugation of several xenobiotics with reduced glutathione [40]. The actions of GSTs are often coordinated with MRPs that transport several conjugates of drugs and reduced glutathione [41]. While P-gp cannot transport glutathione conjugates, coordinated coexpression of P-gp and GST was observed in vitro using AML cell lines [42].

Alteration in drug target structures such as the mechanism of MDR represents a large group of diverse changes in regulatory pathways, which is finally responsible for the downregulation or upregulation of drug molecular target. An example of this behavior alteration of topoisomerase II, such as the molecular causality of neoplastic cell resistance to topoisomerase poisons, could be performed (reviewed in [28]).

The repair of DNA primarily damaged by drugs' direct action, or secondarily by the elevation of oxygen reactive species formation, clearly yields to the drug resistance of neoplastic cells [27]. The therapeutic effects of DNA-damaging drugs in cancer treatment are given by the equilibrium between drug-induced DNA damage and the effectiveness of DNA repair mechanisms. The inhibition of repair pathways used in conjunction with DNA damaging chemotherapy could sensitize cancer cells and therefore increase the efficacy of therapy [27].

Epithelial-mesenchymal transition is a mechanism predominantly taking part in solid tumor metastatic processes. This mechanism could play only a minor role (if any) in drug resistance development in MDS and AML patients.

The high expression levels of antiapoptotic proto-oncogene of the Bcl-2 family (such as BCL-2, Bcl-XL, Mcl-1, Bcl-w, and Bfl-1) were often reported to be associated with in vitro resistance to chemotherapeutic agents, poor clinical outcomes in cases of AML [43], and in cases of adults with acute lymphoblastic leukemia [44]. Bcl-2 was shown to be restricted in tissues characterized by apoptotic cell death [45]. Antiapoptotic proteins of the Bcl-2 family hetero-oligomerize in vivo with a conserved homolog – proapoptotic member of the Bcl-2 family (such as Bax), and this process is known to modulate apoptosis [46]. The translocation of the Bax (or other proapoptotic protein) monomer from the cytosol to the mitochondria followed by the formation of BAX homo-oligomers represents a physiological death stimulus, which may be prevented by the presence of the Bcl-2 protein (or other antiapoptotic proteins) [47]. Therefore for apoptosis progression, an equilibrium between anti- and proapoptotic proteins plays a

http://dx.doi.org/10.5772/63483

crucial role. This is molecularly regulated by the p53 known as the central regulator of apoptosis [48]. This is consistent with known data about the role of the mutated form of TP53 in cancer [49, 50].

Epigenetic regulations are involved in the development of MDR directly by the downregulation or upregulation of important genes responsible for cell death or survival. For example, tumor-suppressor genes are often silenced via hypermethylation, and oncogenes are overexpressed via hypomethylation [27]. Epigenetics could also play an indirect role in cell drug sensitivity by the following mechanism: the opening of the chromatin structure, which is prerequisite for DNA replication and transcription, and to produce uncovered DNA that is more accessible for drug-induced DNA damage. This is consistent with more pronounced DNA damage induced with drugs in more proliferating and/or transcriptionally active cells.

Hypermethylation of the MDR1 promoter was associated with transcriptional repression and chromatin structural changes [51]. The demethylation of this promoter in cancer cell lines was found to elevate the multidrug-resistant phenotype [52].

Epigenetic mechanisms can also influence DNA damage repair. For example, DNA mismatch repair processes can be lost due to the hypermethylation of the human mutL homolog 1 (hMLH1) gene promoter, which can lead to cancer development [27].

Demethylation by DAC may have a role in increasing the efficacy of chemotherapy for patients with tumors, as characterized by high hMLH1 promoter methylation and low hMLH1 expression [53].

3.2. Resistance to immunomodulatory drugs

Over recent years, attention has been paid to exploiting the immunomodulatory effects primarily obtained for thalidomide [54], which has resulted in novel IMIDs. The anti-MDS activity of these drugs (namely LEN) was proven for low-risk MDS, particularly with 5q deletion (del[5q]) [55]. This action is attributed to several mechanisms that involve antiproliferative effects, downregulation of crucial cytokines, and costimulatory effects on T and NK cells [10]. However, the exact mechanism of IMIDs' action in MDS treatment is still not fully understood. The IMIDs' immunomodulatory compounds derived from the thalidomide structure have greater immunological and anticancer properties, but lack the toxicity associated with thalidomide [11]. LEN (Revlimid) was approved for use in low- and intermediate-1-risk MDS patients who have the deletion 5q chromosome and no other chromosomal abnormalities, are dependent on red blood cell transfusions, and for whom other treatment options have been found to be insufficient or inadequate by EMA (European Medicines Agency) and the FDA (Food and Drug Administration). After LEN treatment, blood transfusion-independent rates were 56–67%, and median response duration was longer than 104 weeks [1]. Additionally, a significant proportion of these responders achieved cytogenetic responses (50–76%), indicating a direct cytotoxic effect of LEN on the neoplastic clones, although a significant proportion of patients develop resistance to this treatment. The study of cytogenetics and molecular predictors of responses in patients with myeloid malignancies without del[5q] treated with LEN indicated that treatment could be effective in patients with normal karyotype and a gain of 8 chromosome is present [55]. The LEN response was achieved by one quarter of MDS patients lacking the 5q abnormality. Ebert et al. [56] found that mononuclear cells from bone marrow aspirates of patients who respond to LEN have a decreased expression of genes, which are specific to terminal erythroid differentiation, regardless of the presence or absence of a 5q deletion. Moreover, LEN acts directly on hematopoietic progenitor cells to increase erythropoiesis relative to other lineages.

The mechanism of LEN's therapeutic effects and the mechanisms that depress its effectiveness in MDS treatment are not fully understood, but could be related to TP53 mutation (reviewed in [57]).

TP53-mutated populations seem to be associated with the early stage of low-risk MDS in patients with del[5q] [58]. However, these authors stated that TP53 mutations could not be predicted by general clinical features but were associated with p53 overexpression. Specific R72P polymorphism of TP53 results in two molecular forms of p53. Molecular variant p53-R72 with better mitochondrial localization activates apoptosis more efficiently (by direct induction of cytochrome c release) than p53-P72 variant [59]. McGraw et al. [60] underscore the distribution of R72P in MDS and highlight differences between del(5q) and non-del(5q) subtypes by gene polymorphism and the relationship to LEN response. However, to prove the potential interaction of R72P variants with germline variants in other key regulators or effectors of the p53 pathway that may modify MDS risk and LEN treatment response, further research will be necessary.

Allelic deletion of the RPS14 gene is a key effector of the hypoplastic anemia in patients with MDS and chromosome 5q deletion [61]. Disruption of ribosome integrity liberates free ribosomal proteins to bind to and trigger the degradation of E3 ubiquitin-protein ligase MDM2 (a negative regulator of p53), with consequent p53 transactivation. Consistently, p53 is overexpressed in erythroid precursors of primary bone marrow del(5q) MDS specimens accompanied by reduced cellular MDM2. LEN may act in the stabilization of MDM2 that leads to p53 degradation [61].

When LEN was used in establishing human AML cell lines SKM-1 and MOLM-13 for resistance, only SKM-1 but not MOLM-13 cells developed MDR phenotype with massive expression of P-gp [62]. Both these cell lines were derived from AML patients, whose disease developed from MDS. In contrast to MOLM-13 with wild type of p53 [63, 64], SKM-1 represents cells expressing a mutated p53 form [65]. Thus cells with mutated TP53 could express P-gp under long-term LEN treatment, which leads to typical P-gp mediated MDR.

3.3. Resistance to hypomethylating agents

In pathogenesis of MDS, both genetics and epigenetics alterations are cooperated. Disruption of genetic pathways regulating the processes of self-renewal, differentiation, quiescence, and stem cell-niche signaling contributes to AML transformation. The hypermethylation of different genes was discussed to be partially responsible for the poor prognosis of MDS patients [66]. Demethylating agents, such as AzaC and DAC, were shown to induce clinical responses in 40–70% of MDS patients [67, 68]. Although hypomethylation is considered the dominant mode of therapeutic action of these drugs, it may also induce DNA damage and consequent apoptosis [69]. Interestingly, clinically significant responses to decitabine without significant toxicity can be seen in patients after nonsuccessful azacitidine therapy [70].

Changes in the expression profile of genes like CD9, GPNMB, FUCA1, ANGPT1, PLA2G7, TPM1, and ARHGEF3 were observed when CD34+ cells isolated from the bone marrow of high-risk MDS patients treated in vitro with DAC were compared with CD34+ cells isolated from patients with untreated early stage Hodgkin's lymphoma taken as a control [66].

AzaC resistance represents a real obstacle for the effective treatment of MDS patients, which focused the attention of scientists on alternative therapeutic strategies for nonresponsive patients. For this reason, AzaC-resistant MDS/AML cell lines are established. AzaC-resistant SKM-1 cells exhibited increased expression of the BCL2L10 member of the antiapoptotic Bcl-2 family that altered apoptosis progression [71]. Interestingly we described the downregulation and changed molecular form of the Bcl-2 protein identified by polyclonal antibody (sc-492, Santa Cruz Biotechnology, USA) in our variant of SKM-1 AzaC-resistant cells [42]. Moreover, other AzaC-resistant AML cells derived from the MOLM-13 cell line exerted similar changes in the Bcl-2 protein. Significant correlation of AzaC resistance with a percentage of MDS or AML cells expressing BCL2L10 was established on a group of 77 patients [71].

AzaC resistance could include impaired mitochondrial membrane permeabilization and caspase activation when AzaC resistant and sensitive SKM-1 myeloid were compared [72]. In our experiments, when the same cell model was used resistance to AzaC was associated with strong over expression of P-gp that secured additional resistance to P-gp substrates [42]. This is a rather interesting finding because AzaC is not a P-gp substrate, and P-gp was not responsible for AzaC resistance. We obtained similar results using MOLM-13 cells. The activity of GST was found to be elevated 8 times when AzaC resistant and sensitive SKM-1 and MOLM-13 cells were compared [42].

AzaC induced the upregulation of LC3-II and elevation of cathepsin B activity (both autophagy markers). Increased basal autophagy was observed in SKM-1 AzaC-resistant cells, but these cells were resistant to AzaC-mediated autophagy [72]. Autophagy depression using a LC3 silencer revealed the protective function of autophagy in AzaC-sensitive and AzaC-resistant cells in basal condition [72]. Taking all the facts about apoptosis and autophagy progression in AML cell models together, it could be concluded that resistance to AzaC is associated with alterations of both processes via impaired homeostasis of its key regulators such as Bcl-2 family proteins and LC3. However, the exact mechanism of this feature is not fully understood and future research will be necessary.

Enzymes involved in cytidine metabolism such as cytidine deaminase (CDA) and deoxycytidine kinase (DCK) seem to be responsible for the primary (intrinsic) AzaC resistance, because nonresponders of AzaC have a 3-fold higher CDA/CDK ratio. There were no significant differences at relapse in DAC metabolism genes, and no CDK mutations were detected [73].

MDSs are characterized by mutations in genes encoding epigenetic modifiers and aberrant DNA methylation. Clonal mutation of TP53 and non-receptor type 11 protein tyrosine phosphatase were associated with shorter overall survival, but not the drug response of patients. Clonal tet methylcytosine dioxygenase 2 (TET2) mutations predicted a response when subclones were treated as wild type. The highest response rate was observed in patients with a mutation in the TET2 gene without a clonal mutation of the trancriptional regulator encoded by ASXL1 gene. [74].

While somatic mutations did not differentiate responders from nonresponders for DAC treatment, differentially methylated regions of DNA at baseline distinguished responders from nonresponders. In responders, the upregulated genes included those that are associated with the cell cycle, potentially contributing to effective DAC incorporation [75].

While DAC is generally accepted as a hypomethylating agent, it may exert a therapeutic effect also in another way. The acceleration of reactive oxygen species induced with DAC could take place in the overall DAC effect. However, reactive oxygen species accumulation was not always present in the sample of AML patients after DAC treatment. Therefore, the relevance of reactive oxygen species generation in the mechanism of DAC pharmacological effectiveness should be studied more intensively in the future [76].

3.4. Resistance to intensive chemotherapy

MDS intermediate- or high-risk patients may be treated with an intensive chemotherapy regimen that is similar as used for AML treatment. A combination of drugs such as cytosine arabinoside, fludarabine, idarubicin, and topotecan, etc. could be used [14]. This chemotherapy is oriented on destroying abnormal blood cells or preventing their growth. For patients who are eligible, bone marrow transplantation is recommended after this therapy.

The development of MDR resistance during the application of this protocol is similar as for other types of neoplastic diseases, and may involve each of the mechanisms described in Chapter 3. The combination of drug-resistant mechanisms that are included in MDR phenotype development during high intensive treatment depends on the specific patient molecular feature, previous therapeutic history, and drugs applied during previous treatment.

3.5. Resistance to CD33-targeted therapy

Progressive methods of MDS treatment represent antibody targeting therapy with cytotoxic agents linked to humanized antibodies against antigens specific to neoplastic cells. Both MDS and AML are characterized by the presence of undifferentiated CD33-positive myeloblast in peripheral blood and bone marrow, compared with healthy control [77]. CD33 is a 67 kDa glycoprotein present on the surface of myeloid cells, and is a member of the sialic acid binding immunoglobulin-like lectin family of proteins [78]. After binding to an appropriate antibody, CD33 is rapidly internalized into leukemia cells [79, 80]. This action enables the use of a humanized CD33 antibody, conjugated to cytotoxic agents for targeted immunotherapy [78, 79]. Gemtuzumab ozogamicin represents antibody drug (from a class of calicheamicins) conjugates [7, 78–81]. This therapy has proven to be effective, but resistance to treatment could be developed. Another immune-targeting preparation is AVE9633 (immunoconjugate of humanized monoclonal CD33 antibody, linked through a disulfide bond to the maytansine derivative DM4) that was used in the treatment of several leukemia cell lines [82]. The activity of P-gp was attributed as a critical factor in depressing the success of this therapy. P-gp mediated the efflux of drug liberated from linkage with antibody due to intracellular enzymes was attributed as being responsible for this resistance [82]. However, a significant inverse correlation was determined for the expression of P-gp and CD33 in the AML blast obtained from patients [81]. We described the strong downregulation of CD33 on mRNA and the protein level in P-gp positive SKM-1 cells selected for resistance by LEN, vincristine, mitoxantrone, or in P-gp positive MOLM-13 cells selected for resistance by vincristine or mitoxantrone [62]. Upregulation of CD33 expression level was also observed in P-gp silenced cell lines. Therefore, the failure of CD33-targeted therapy of patients with AML blast overexpressing P-gp could be caused by a lack of CD33 as an antibody target structure on the cell surface.

3.6. Detection of drug-resistant markers in neoplastic cells

Cellular expression of drug-resistant markers could be monitored on mRNA level (RT-PCR methods) or protein level (Western blot and immunofluorescence flow cytometry) [83]. Proteins active in MDR development like ABC transporters, drug metabolizing enzymes, antiapoptotic proteins, and many others could be detected by these methods. Transport activity of drug transporters could be measured using depressed intracellular retention of their fluorescent substrates by flow cytometry. Retentions of calcein/AM, rhodamine 123, or doxorubicin were often used for P-gp efflux activity detection directly in cells isolated from patients [84]. Activities of detoxification enzymes could be monitored by appropriate substrates, which enzymatic modifications induce changes in either fluorescence or light absorbance properties. Conjugation of 1-chloro-2,4-dinitrobenzene with reduced glutathione as a result of GST activity could be taken as example [42]. Specific mutations of genes active in MDR development (like *TP53*) could be detected using mutation analysis including specifically designed PCR reaction, denaturing high-performance liquid chromatography, or DNA-sequencing techniques. Alteration in drug-induced apoptosis could be monitored as difference in drug-induced DNA-fragmentation by electrophoresis or using comet assay [85]. Application of oligonucleotide microarray for human genome represents available methods to obtain complex information about expression profiles of MDR-associated genes in patients [86]. Moreover, when nonresponders and responders will be compared using oligonucleotide microarrays, new information about involving different genes' expression in MDR development could be obtained. Cytotoxic effects of several drugs could be monitored directly in cells isolated from patient samples using assays based on reduction of formazan (like MTT assay) by intracellular dehydrogenases, or liberation of fluorescent label from its esters (like fluorescein diacetate) by intracellular esterases.

4. Perspectives

MDSs represent a very diverse group of hematological malignancies. Treatment of this disease involves several drugs such as LEN, AzaC, and DAC. Unfortunately, the exact mechanism of action is still not fully understood. Therefore, prediction of the response to this treatment is still very complicated. For this reason, a detailed knowledge of the molecular causality of MDS and AML progression will be necessary. Moreover, unclear questions about the molecular mechanisms of these drugs should be answered. Resistance to treatment use for AML and MDS still represents serious problems with causality not fully understood. Research oriented on these topics will bring new knowledge and new predictive molecular markers that will enable the better selection of effective therapy for each patient.

Acknowledgements

This research was supported by grants from the Slovak APVV grant agency (No. APVV-14-0334) and the VEGA grant agency (Vega 2/0182/13, 2/0028/15, 2/0156/16) and the project: "Diagnostics of socially important disorders in Slovakia, based on modern biotechnologies" ITMS 26240220058, supported by the Research & Developmental Operational Programme funded by the ERDF.

Author details

Lucia Messingerova[1,2], Denisa Imrichova[2], Martina Coculova[1], Marian Zelina[2], Lucia Pavlikova[2], Helena Kavcova[2], Mario Seres[2], Viera Bohacova[2], Boris Lakatos[1], Zdena Sulova[2] and Albert Breier[1,2*]

*Address all correspondence to: albert.breier@stuba.sk

1 Institute of Biochemistry and Microbiology, Faculty of Chemical and Food Technology, Slovak University of Technology, Bratislava, Slovakia

2 Institute of Molecular Physiology and Genetics, Slovak Academy of Sciences, Bratislava, Slovakia

References

[1] Zeidan A.M., Linhares Y., Gore S.D., Current therapy of myelodysplastic syndromes, Blood Rev 2013;27: 243–259. DOI: 10.1016/j.blre.2013.07.003.

[2] Garcia-Manero G., Myelodysplastic syndromes: 2015 update on diagnosis, risk-stratification and management, Am J Hematol 2015;90: 831–841. DOI: 10.1002/ajh.24102.

[3] Greenberg P., Cox C., LeBeau M.M., Fenaux P., Morel P., Sanz G., Sanz M., Vallespi T., Hamblin T., Oscier D., Ohyashiki K., Toyama K., Aul C., Mufti G., Bennett J., Interna-

tional scoring system for evaluating prognosis in myelodysplastic syndromes, Blood 1997;89: 2079–2088.

[4] Barzi A., Sekeres M.A., Myelodysplastic syndromes: a practical approach to diagnosis and treatment, Cleve Clin J Med 2010;77: 37–44. DOI: 10.3949/ccjm.77a.09069.

[5] Bowen D., Culligan D., Jowitt S., Kelsey S., Mufti G., Oscier D., Parker J., Guidelines for the diagnosis and therapy of adult myelodysplastic syndromes, Br J Haematol 2003;120: 187–200.

[6] Gattermann N., Overview of guidelines on iron chelation therapy in patients with myelodysplastic syndromes and transfusional iron overload, Int J Hematol 2008;88: 24–29. DOI: 10.1007/s12185-008-0118-z.

[7] Shipley J.L., Butera J.N., Acute myelogenous leukemia, Exp Hematol 2009;37: 649–658. DOI: 10.1016/j.exphem.2009.04.002.

[8] Jadersten M., Montgomery S.M., Dybedal I., Porwit-MacDonald A., Hellstrom-Lindberg E., Long-term outcome of treatment of anemia in MDS with erythropoietin and G-CSF, Blood 2005;106: 803–811. DOI: 10.1182/blood-2004-10-3872.

[9] Passweg J.R., Giagounidis A.A., Simcock M., Aul C., Dobbelstein C., Stadler M., Ossenkoppele G., Hofmann W.K., Schilling K., Tichelli A., Ganser A., Immunosuppressive therapy for patients with myelodysplastic syndrome: a prospective randomized multicenter phase III trial comparing antithymocyte globulin plus cyclosporine with best supportive care--SAKK 33/99, J Clin Oncol 2011;29: 303–309. DOI: 10.1200/JCO.2010.31.2686.

[10] Quach H., Ritchie D., Stewart A.K., Neeson P., Harrison S., Smyth M.J., Prince H.M., Mechanism of action of immunomodulatory drugs (IMiDS) in multiple myeloma, Leukemia 2010;24: 22–32. DOI: 10.1038/leu.2009.236.

[11] Bartlett J.B., Dredge K., Dalgleish A.G., The evolution of thalidomide and its IMiD derivatives as anticancer agents, Nat Rev Cancer 2004;4: 314–322. DOI: 10.1038/nrc1323.

[12] List A., Dewald G., Bennett J., Giagounidis A., Raza A., Feldman E., Powell B., Greenberg P., Thomas D., Stone R., Reeder C., Wride K., Patin J., Schmidt M., Zeldis J., Knight R., Lenalidomide in the myelodysplastic syndrome with chromosome 5q deletion, N Engl J Med 2006;355: 1456–1465. DOI: 10.1056/NEJMoa061292.

[13] List A., Kurtin S., Roe D.J., Buresh A., Mahadevan D., Fuchs D., Rimsza L., Heaton R., Knight R., Zeldis J.B., Efficacy of lenalidomide in myelodysplastic syndromes, N Engl J Med 2005;352: 549–557. DOI: 10.1056/NEJMoa041668.

[14] Beran M., Intensive chemotherapy for patients with high-risk myelodysplastic syndrome, Int J Hematol 2000;72: 139–150.

[15] Hofmann W.K., Heil G., Zander C., Wiebe S., Ottmann O.G., Bergmann L., Hoeffken K., Fischer J.T., Knuth A., Kolbe K., Schmoll H.J., Langer W., Westerhausen M., Koelbel C.B., Hoelzer D., Ganser A., Intensive chemotherapy with idarubicin, cytarabine,

etoposide, and G-CSF priming in patients with advanced myelodysplastic syndrome and high-risk acute myeloid leukemia, Ann Hematol 2004;83: 498–503. DOI: 10.1007/s00277-004-0889-0.

[16] Stintzing S., Kemmerling R., Kiesslich T., Alinger B., Ocker M., Neureiter D., Myelodysplastic syndrome and histone deacetylase inhibitors: "to be or not to be acetylated"?, J Biomed Biotechnol 2011;2011: 214143. DOI: 10.1155/2011/214143.

[17] Doskocil J., Sorm F., The mode of action of 5-aza-2'-deoxycytidine in Escherichia coli, Eur J Biochem 1970;13: 180–187.

[18] Sorm F., Piskala A., Cihak A., Vesely J., 5-Azacytidine, a new, highly effective cancerostatic, Experientia 1964;20: 202–203.

[19] Jones P.A., Taylor S.M., Cellular differentiation, cytidine analogs and DNA methylation, Cell 1980;20: 85–93.

[20] Buckstein R., Yee K., Wells R.A., 5-Azacytidine in myelodysplastic syndromes: a clinical practice guideline, Cancer Treat Rev 2011;37: 160–167. DOI: 10.1016/j.ctrv.2010.05.006.

[21] Ivanoff S., Gruson B., Chantepie S.P., Lemasle E., Merlusca L., Harrivel V., Charbonnier A., Votte P., Royer B., Marolleau J.P., 5-Azacytidine treatment for relapsed or refractory acute myeloid leukemia after intensive chemotherapy, Am J Hematol 2013;88: 601–605. DOI: 10.1002/ajh.23464.

[22] Christman J.K., 5-Azacytidine and 5-aza-2'-deoxycytidine as inhibitors of DNA methylation: mechanistic studies and their implications for cancer therapy, Oncogene 2002;21: 5483–5495. DOI: 10.1038/sj.onc.1205699.

[23] Stresemann C., Lyko F., Modes of action of the DNA methyltransferase inhibitors azacytidine and decitabine, Int J Cancer 2008;123: 8–13. DOI: 10.1002/ijc.23607.

[24] Hollenbach P.W., Nguyen A.N., Brady H., Williams M., Ning Y., Richard N., Krushel L., Aukerman S.L., Heise C., MacBeth K.J., A comparison of azacitidine and decitabine activities in acute myeloid leukemia cell lines, PLoS One 2010;5: e9001. DOI: 10.1371/journal.pone.0009001.

[25] Patane S., Cancer multidrug resistance-targeted therapy in both cancer and cardiovascular system with cardiovascular drugs, Int J Cardiol 2014;176: 10.1016/j.ijcard.2014.07.158.

[26] Kvackajova-Kisucka J., Barancik M., Breier A., Drug transporters and their role in multidrug resistance of neoplastic cells, Gen Physiol Biophys 2001;20: 215–237.

[27] Housman G., Byler S., Heerboth S., Lapinska K., Longacre M., Snyder N., Sarkar S., Drug resistance in cancer: an overview, Cancers (Basel) 2014;6: 1769–1792. DOI: 10.3390/cancers6031769.

[28] Breier A., Barancik M., Sulova Z., Uhrik B., P-glycoprotein – implications of metabolism of neoplastic cells and cancer therapy, Curr Cancer Drug Targets 2005;5: 457–468. DOI: 10.2174/1568009054863636.

[29] Breier A., Gibalova L., Seres M., Barancik M., Sulova Z., New insight into p-glycoprotein as a drug target, Anticancer Agents Med Chem 2013;13: 159–170. DOI: 10.2174/1871520611307010159.

[30] Juliano R.L., Ling V., A surface glycoprotein modulating drug permeability in Chinese hamster ovary cell mutants, Biochim Biophys Acta 1976;455: 152–162. DOI: 10.1016/0005-2736(76)90160-7.

[31] Breier A., Drobna Z., Docolomansky P., Barancik M., Cytotoxic activity of several unrelated drugs on L1210 mouse leukemic cell sublines with P-glycoprotein (PGP) mediated multidrug resistance (MDR) phenotype, A QSAR study, Neoplasma 2000;47: 100–106.

[32] Tainton K.M., Smyth M.J., Jackson J.T., Tanner J.E., Cerruti L., Jane S.M., Darcy P.K., Johnstone R.W., Mutational analysis of P-glycoprotein: suppression of caspase activation in the absence of ATP-dependent drug efflux, Cell Death Differ 2004;11: 1028–1037. DOI: 10.1038/sj.cdd.4401440.

[33] Gibalova L., Sedlak J., Labudova M., Barancik M., Rehakova A., Breier A., Sulova Z., Multidrug resistant P-glycoprotein positive L1210/VCR cells are also cross-resistant to cisplatin via a mechanism distinct from P-glycoprotein-mediated drug efflux activity, Gen Physiol Biophys 2009;28: 391–403.

[34] Gibalova L., Seres M., Rusnak A., Ditte P., Labudova M., Uhrik B., Pastorek J., Sedlak J., Breier A., Sulova Z., P-glycoprotein depresses cisplatin sensitivity in L1210 cells by inhibiting cisplatin-induced caspase-3 activation, Toxicol In Vitro 2012;26: 435–444. DOI: 10.1016/j.tiv.2012.01.014.

[35] Borst P., Evers R., Kool M., Wijnholds J., A family of drug transporters: the multidrug resistance-associated proteins, J Natl Cancer Inst 2000;92: 1295–1302.

[36] Doyle L., Ross D.D., Multidrug resistance mediated by the breast cancer resistance protein BCRP (ABCG2), Oncogene 2003;22: 7340–7358. DOI: 10.1038/sj.onc.1206938.

[37] Li J., Bluth M.H., Pharmacogenomics of drug metabolizing enzymes and transporters: implications for cancer therapy, Pharmgenomics Pers Med 2011;4: 11–33. DOI: 10.2147/PGPM.S18861.

[38] Christians U., Schmitz V., Haschke M., Functional interactions between P-glycoprotein and CYP3A in drug metabolism, Expert Opin Drug Metab Toxicol 2005;1: 641–654. DOI: 10.1517/17425255.1.4.641.

[39] Di Pietro G., Magno L.A., Rios-Santos F., Glutathione S-transferases: an overview in cancer research, Expert Opin Drug Metab Toxicol 2010;6: 153–170. DOI: 10.1517/17425250903427980.

[40] Armstrong R.N., Glutathione S-transferases: reaction mechanism, structure, and function, Chem Res Toxicol 1991;4: 131–140.

[41] Morrow C.S., Smitherman P.K., Diah S.K., Schneider E., Townsend A.J., Coordinated action of glutathione S-transferases (GSTs) and multidrug resistance protein 1 (MRP1) in antineoplastic drug detoxification. Mechanism of GST A1-1- and MRP1-associated resistance to chlorambucil in MCF7 breast carcinoma cells, J Biol Chem 1998;273: 20114–20120.

[42] Messingerova L., Imrichova D., Kavcova H., Turakova K., Breier A., Sulova Z., Acute myeloid leukemia cells MOLM-13 and SKM-1 established for resistance by azacytidine are crossresistant to P-glycoprotein substrates, Toxicol In Vitro 2015;29: 1405–1415. DOI: 10.1016/j.tiv.2015.05.011.

[43] Campos L., Oriol P., Sabido O., Guyotat D., Simultaneous expression of P-glycoprotein and BCL-2 in acute myeloid leukemia blast cells, Leuk. Lymphoma 1997;27: 119–125. DOI: 10.3109/10428199709068278.

[44] Del Principe M.I., Del Poeta G., Maurillo L., Buccisano F., Venditti A., Tamburini A., Bruno A., Cox M.C., Suppo G., Tendas A., Gianni L., Postorino M., Masi M., Del Principe D., Amadori S., P-glycoprotein and BCL-2 levels predict outcome in adult acute lymphoblastic leukaemia, Br J Haematol 2003;121: 730–738.

[45] Hockenbery D.M., Zutter M., Hickey W., Nahm M., Korsmeyer S.J., BCL2 protein is topographically restricted in tissues characterized by apoptotic cell death, Proc Natl Acad Sci U S A 1991;88: 6961–6965.

[46] Oltvai Z.N., Milliman C.L., Korsmeyer S.J., Bcl-2 heterodimerizes in vivo with a conserved homolog, Bax, that accelerates programmed cell death, Cell 1993;74: 609–619. DOI: 10.1016/0092-8674(93)90509-O.

[47] Brunelle J.K., Letai A., Control of mitochondrial apoptosis by the Bcl-2 family, J Cell Sci 2009;122: 437–441. DOI: 10.1242/jcs.031682.

[48] Meek D.W., Regulation of the p53 response and its relationship to cancer, Biochem J 2015;469: 325–346. DOI: 10.1042/BJ20150517.

[49] Muller P., Nenutil R., Vojtesek B., Relevance of p53 protein and its mutations for novel strategies in cancer therapy, Cas Lek Cesk 2004;143: 313–317.

[50] Muller P.A., Vousden K.H., p53 mutations in cancer, Nat Cell Biol 2013;15: 2–8. DOI: 10.1038/ncb2641.

[51] Baker E.K., El-Osta A., The rise of DNA methylation and the importance of chromatin on multidrug resistance in cancer, Exp Cell Res 2003;290: 177–194. DOI: S0014482703003422 [pii].

[52] Kantharidis P., El-Osta A., deSilva M., Wall D.M., Hu X.F., Slater A., Nadalin G., Parkin J.D., Zalcberg J.R., Altered methylation of the human MDR1 promoter is associated with acquired multidrug resistance, Clin Cancer Res 1997;3: 2025–2032.

[53] Arnold C.N., Goel A., Boland C.R., Role of hMLH1 promoter hypermethylation in drug resistance to 5-fluorouracil in colorectal cancer cell lines, Int J Cancer 2003;106: 66–73. DOI: 10.1002/ijc.11176.

[54] Corral L.G., Kaplan G., Immunomodulation by thalidomide and thalidomide analogues, Ann Rheum Dis 1999;58 Suppl 1: 107–113.

[55] Sugimoto Y., Sekeres M.A., Makishima H., Traina F., Visconte V., Jankowska A., Jerez A., Szpurka H., O'Keefe C.L., Guinta K., Afable M., Tiu R., McGraw K.L., List A.F., Maciejewski J., Cytogenetic and molecular predictors of response in patients with myeloid malignancies without del[5q] treated with lenalidomide, J Hematol Oncol 2012;5: 4. DOI: 0.1186/1756-8722-5-4.

[56] Ebert B.L., Galili N., Tamayo P., Bosco J., Mak R., Pretz J., Tanguturi S., Ladd-Acosta C., Stone R., Golub T.R., Raza A., An erythroid differentiation signature predicts response to lenalidomide in myelodysplastic syndrome, PLoS Med 2008;5: e35. DOI: 0.1371/journal.pmed.0050035.

[57] Fuchs O., Important genes in the pathogenesis of 5q- syndrome and their connection with ribosomal stress and the innate immune system pathway, Leuk Res Treatment 2012;2012: 179402. DOI: 10.1155/2012/179402.

[58] Jadersten M., Saft L., Smith A., Kulasekararaj A., Pomplun S., Gohring G., Hedlund A., Hast R., Schlegelberger B., Porwit A., Hellstrom-Lindberg E., Mufti G.J., TP53 mutations in low-risk myelodysplastic syndromes with del(5q) predict disease progression, J Clin Oncol 2011;29: 1971–1979. DOI: 10.1200/JCO.2010.31.8576.

[59] Murphy M.E., Leu J.I., George D.L., p53 moves to mitochondria: a turn on the path to apoptosis, Cell Cycle 2004;3: 836–839.

[60] McGraw K.L., Zhang L.M., Rollison D.E., Basiorka A.A., Fulp W., Rawal B., Jerez A., Billingsley D.L., Lin H.Y., Kurtin S.E., Yoder S., Zhang Y., Guinta K., Mallo M., Sole F., Calasanz M.J., Cervera J., Such E., Gonzalez T., Nevill T.J., Haferlach T., Smith A.E., Kulasekararaj A., Mufti G., Karsan A., Maciejewski J.P., Sokol L., Epling-Burnette P.K., Wei S., List A.F., The relationship of TP53 R72P polymorphism to disease outcome and TP53 mutation in myelodysplastic syndromes, Blood Cancer J 2015;5: e291. DOI: 10.1038/bcj.2015.11.

[61] Wei S., Chen X., McGraw K., Zhang L., Komrokji R., Clark J., Caceres G., Billingsley D., Sokol L., Lancet J., Fortenbery N., Zhou J., Eksioglu E.A., Sallman D., Wang H., Epling-Burnette P.K., Djeu J., Sekeres M., Maciejewski J.P., List A., Lenalidomide promotes p53 degradation by inhibiting MDM2 auto-ubiquitination in myelodysplastic syndrome with chromosome 5q deletion, Oncogene 2013;32: 1110–1120. DOI: 10.1038/onc. 2012.139.

[62] Imrichova D., Messingerova L., Seres M., Kavcova H., Pavlikova L., Coculova M., Breier A., Sulova Z., Selection of resistant acute myeloid leukemia SKM-1 and MOLM-13 cells by vincristine-, mitoxantrone- and lenalidomide-induced upregulation of P-glycoprotein activity and downregulation of CD33 cell surface exposure, Eur J Pharm Sci 2015;77: 29–39. DOI: 10.1016/j.ejps.2015.05.022.

[63] Kojima K., Konopleva M., Samudio I.J., Shikami M., Cabreira-Hansen M., McQueen T., Ruvolo V., Tsao T., Zeng Z., Vassilev L.T., Andreeff M., MDM2 antagonists induce p53-dependent apoptosis in AML: implications for leukemia therapy, Blood 2005;106: 3150–3159. DOI: 10.1182/blood-2005-02-0553.

[64] Thompson T., Andreeff M., Studzinski G.P., Vassilev L.T., 1,25-dihydroxyvitamin D3 enhances the apoptotic activity of MDM2 antagonist nutlin-3a in acute myeloid leukemia cells expressing wild-type p53, Mol Cancer Ther 2010;9: 1158–1168. DOI: 10.1158/1535-7163.MCT-09-1036.

[65] Nakagawa T., Matozaki S., Murayama T., Nishimura R., Tsutsumi M., Kawaguchi R., Yokoyama Y., Hikiji K., Isobe T., Chihara K., Establishment of a leukaemic cell line from a patient with acquisition of chromosomal abnormalities during disease progression in myelodysplastic syndrome, Br J Haematol 1993;85: 469–476.

[66] Giachelia M., D'Alo F., Fabiani E., Saulnier N., Di Ruscio A., Guidi F., Hohaus S., Voso M.T., Leone G., Gene expression profiling of myelodysplastic CD34+ hematopoietic stem cells treated in vitro with decitabine, Leuk Res 2011;35: 465–471. DOI: 10.1016/j.leukres.2010.07.022.

[67] Fenaux P., Mufti G.J., Hellstrom-Lindberg E., Santini V., Finelli C., Giagounidis A., Schoch R., Gattermann N., Sanz G., List A., Gore S.D., Seymour J.F., Bennett J.M., Byrd J., Backstrom J., Zimmerman L., McKenzie D., Beach C., Silverman L.R., Efficacy of azacitidine compared with that of conventional care regimens in the treatment of higher-risk myelodysplastic syndromes: a randomised, open-label, phase III study, Lancet Oncol 2009;10: 223–232. DOI: 10.1016/S1470-2045(09)70003-8.

[68] Kantarjian H., Oki Y., Garcia-Manero G., Huang X., O'Brien S., Cortes J., Faderl S., Bueso-Ramos C., Ravandi F., Estrov Z., Ferrajoli A., Wierda W., Shan J., Davis J., Giles F., Saba H.I., Issa J.P., Results of a randomized study of 3 schedules of low-dose decitabine in higher-risk myelodysplastic syndrome and chronic myelomonocytic leukemia, Blood 2007;109: 52–57. DOI: blood-10.1182/blood-2006-05-021162.

[69] Stresemann C., Bokelmann I., Mahlknecht U., Lyko F., Azacytidine causes complex DNA methylation responses in myeloid leukemia, Mol Cancer Ther. DOI: 10.1158/1535-7163.MCT-08-0411.

[70] Borthakur G., Ahdab S.E., Ravandi F., Faderl S., Ferrajoli A., Newman B., Issa J.P., Kantarjian H., Activity of decitabine in patients with myelodysplastic syndrome previously treated with azacitidine, Leuk Lymphoma 2008;49: 690–695. DOI: 10.1080/10428190701882146.

[71] Cluzeau T., Robert G., Mounier N., Karsenti J.M., Dufies M., Puissant A., Jacquel A., Renneville A., Preudhomme C., Cassuto J.P., Raynaud S., Luciano F., Auberger P., BCL2L10 is a predictive factor for resistance to azacitidine in MDS and AML patients, Oncotarget 2012;3: 490–501. DOI: 10.18632/oncotarget.481.

[72] Cluzeau T., Robert G., Puissant A., Jean-Michel K., Cassuto J.P., Raynaud S., Auberger P., Azacitidine-resistant SKM1 myeloid cells are defective for AZA-induced mitochondrial apoptosis and autophagy, Cell Cycle 2011;10: 2339–2343. DOI: 10.4161/cc. 10.14.16308.

[73] Qin T., Castoro R., El Ahdab S., Jelinek J., Wang X., Si J., Shu J., He R., Zhang N., Chung W., Kantarjian H.M., Issa J.P., Mechanisms of resistance to decitabine in the myelodysplastic syndrome, PLoS One 2011;6: e23372. DOI: 10.1371/journal.pone.0023372.

[74] Bejar R., Lord A., Stevenson K., Bar-Natan M., Perez-Ladaga A., Zaneveld J., Wang H., Caughey B., Stojanov P., Getz G., Garcia-Manero G., Kantarjian H., Chen R., Stone R.M., Neuberg D., Steensma D.P., Ebert B.L., TET2 mutations predict response to hypomethylating agents in myelodysplastic syndrome patients, Blood 2014;124: 2705–2712. DOI: 10.1182/blood-2014-06-582809.

[75] Meldi K., Qin T., Buchi F., Droin N., Sotzen J., Micol J.B., Selimoglu-Buet D., Masala E., Allione B., Gioia D., Poloni A., Lunghi M., Solary E., Abdel-Wahab O., Santini V., Figueroa M.E., Specific molecular signatures predict decitabine response in chronic myelomonocytic leukemia, J Clin Invest 2015;125: 1857–1872. DOI: 10.1172/JCI78752.

[76] Fandy T.E., Jiemjit A., Thakar M., Rhoden P., Suarez L., Gore S.D., Decitabine induces delayed reactive oxygen species (ROS) accumulation in leukemia cells and induces the expression of ROS generating enzymes, Clin Cancer Res 2014;20: 1249–1258. DOI: 10.1158/1078-0432.CCR-13-1453.

[77] Jilani I., Estey E., Huh Y., Joe Y., Manshouri T., Yared M., Giles F., Kantarjian H., Cortes J., Thomas D., Keating M., Freireich E., Albitar M., Differences in CD33 intensity between various myeloid neoplasms, Am J Clin Pathol 2002;118: 560–566. DOI: 10.1309/1WMW-CMXX-4WN4-T55U.

[78] Jurcic J.G., What happened to anti-CD33 therapy for acute myeloid leukemia? Curr Hematol Malig Rep 2012;7: 65–73. DOI: 10.1007/s11899-011-0103-0.

[79] Cianfriglia M., The biology of MDR1-P-glycoprotein (MDR1-Pgp) in designing functional antibody drug conjugates (ADCs): the experience of gemtuzumab ozogamicin, Ann Ist Super Sanita 2013;49: 150–168. DOI: DOI: 10.4415/ANN_13_02_07.

[80] Naito K., Takeshita A., Shigeno K., Nakamura S., Fujisawa S., Shinjo K., Yoshida H., Ohnishi K., Mori M., Terakawa S., Ohno R., Calicheamicin-conjugated humanized anti-CD33 monoclonal antibody (gemtuzumab zogamicin, CMA-676) shows cytocidal effect on CD33-positive leukemia cell lines, but is inactive on P-glycoprotein-expressing sublines, Leukemia 2000;14: 1436–1443.

[81] Walter R.B., Appelbaum F.R., Estey E.H., Bernstein I.D., Acute myeloid leukemia stem cells and CD33-targeted immunotherapy, Blood 2012;119: 6198–6208. DOI: 10.1182/blood-2011-11-325050.

[82] Tang R., Cohen S., Perrot J.Y., Faussat A.M., Zuany-Amorim C., Marjanovic Z., Morjani H., Fava F., Corre E., Legrand O., Marie J.P., P-gp activity is a critical resistance factor against AVE9633 and DM4 cytotoxicity in leukaemia cell lines, but not a major mechanism of chemoresistance in cells from acute myeloid leukaemia patients, BMC Cancer 2009;9: 199. DOI: 10.1186/1471-2407-9-199.

[83] Beck W.T., Grogan T.M., Methods to detect P-glycoprotein and implications for other drug resistance-associated proteins, Leukemia 1997;11: 1107–1109.

[84] Jovelet C., Benard J., Forestier F., Farinotti R., Bidart J.M., Gil S., Inhibition of P-glycoprotein functionality by vandetanib may reverse cancer cell resistance to doxorubicin, Eur J Pharm Sci 2012;46: 484–491. DOI: 10.1016/j.ejps.2012.03.012.

[85] Kundu T., Bhattacharya R.K., Siddiqi M., Roy M., Correlation of apoptosis with comet formation induced by tea polyphenols in human leukemia cells, J Environ Pathol Toxicol Oncol 2005;24: 115–128. DOI: 10.1615/JEnvPathToxOncol.v24.i2.50.

[86] Zhao Y.P., Chen G., Feng B., Zhang T.P., Ma E.L., Wu Y.D., Microarray analysis of gene expression profile of multidrug resistance in pancreatic cancer, Chin Med J (Engl) 2007;120: 1743–1752.

22509356R00123

Printed in Poland
by Amazon Fulfillment
Poland Sp. z o.o., Wrocław